Digital Mammography:
A Practical Approach

Digital Mammography: A Practical Approach

Edited by

Gary J. Whitman, MD
Professor, Departments of Diagnostic Radiology and Radiation Oncology,
The University of Texas MD Anderson Cancer Center, Houston, TX, USA

Tamara Miner Haygood, PhD, MD
Associate Professor, Department of Diagnostic Radiology,
The University of Texas MD Anderson Cancer Center, Houston, TX, USA

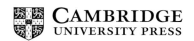
CAMBRIDGE
UNIVERSITY PRESS

CAMBRIDGE UNIVERSITY PRESS
Cambridge, New York, Melbourne, Madrid, Cape Town,
Singapore, São Paulo, Delhi, Mexico City

Cambridge University Press
The Edinburgh Building, Cambridge CB2 8RU, UK

Published in the United States of America
by Cambridge University Press, New York

www.cambridge.org
Information on this title: www.cambridge.org/9780521763721

© Cambridge University Press 2013

First published 2013

Printed and bound in the United Kingdom by the MPG Books Group

*A catalogue record for this publication is available from the
British Library*

Library of Congress Cataloguing in Publication data

Digital mammography : a practical approach / edited by Gary
J. Whitman, Tamara Miner Haygood.
    p. cm.
  Includes index.
  ISBN 978-0-521-76372-1 (Hardback)
  1. Breast–Radiography. 2. Breast–Imaging. 3. Breast–Cancer–
Diagnosis. I. Whitman, Gary J. II. Haygood, Tamara Miner,
1956–
  RG493.5.R33D539 2012
  618.1'907572–dc23
                               2012020420

ISBN 978-0-521-76372-1 Hardback

To my wife, Susan, and my children, Sam and Kayla, who help me every step of the way

GJW

To my children, Anya and Costa, who make the journey more interesting

TMH

Contents

Contributors

Valerie Andolina, RT (R) (M)
Elizabeth Wende Breast Care, LLC, Rochester, NY, USA

Callie Cheatham
Texas A & M University, College Station, TX, USA

Shannon DeMay, CIIP
Elizabeth Wende Breast Care, LLC, Rochester, NY, USA

Stamatia Destounis MD, FACR
Elizabeth Wende Breast Care, LLC; Clinical Associate Professor, School of Medicine and Dentistry, University of Rochester, Rochester, NY, USA

Basak E. Dogan, MD
Assistant Professor, Department of Diagnostic Radiology, The University of Texas MD Anderson Cancer Center, Houston, TX, USA

William R. Geiser, MS
Senior Medical Physicist, Department of Imaging Physics, The University of Texas MD Anderson Cancer Center, Houston, TX, USA

Tamara Miner Haygood, PhD, MD
Associate Professor, Department of Diagnostic Radiology, The University of Texas MD Anderson Cancer Center, Houston, TX, USA

Lindsay Hwang, BS
Case Western Reserve University School of Medicine, Cleveland, OH, USA

Malak Itani, MD
Department of Diagnostic Radiology, American University of Beirut Medical Center, Beirut, Lebanon

Andrew Karellas, PhD, FACR
Professor of Radiology and Director of Radiological Physics, University of Massachusetts Medical School, Worcester, MA, USA

Raunak Khisty, MBBS, MPH
Resident, Department of Psychiatry, Wake Forest School of Medicine, Winston-Salem, NC, USA

Diana Kissel, MS, CIIP
Elizabeth Wende Breast Care, LLC, Rochester, NY, USA

Chao-Jen Lai, PhD
Department of Imaging Physics, The University of Texas MD Anderson Cancer Center, Houston, TX, USA

Michael N. Linver, MD, FACR
Director of Mammography, Breast Imaging Center of X-Ray Associates of New Mexico; Clinical Professor of Radiology, University of New Mexico School of Medicine, Albuquerque, NM, USA

Xinming Liu, PhD
Department of Imaging Physics, The University of Texas MD Anderson Cancer Center, Houston, TX, USA

Alexis V. Nees, MD
Clinical Associate Professor, Department of Diagnostic Imaging, University of Michigan Health System, Ann Arbor, MI, USA

Robert D. Rosenberg, MD, FACR
Radiology Associates of Albuquerque; Professor Emeritus, Department of Radiology, University of New Mexico Albuquerque, NM, USA

Michael Ryan, MD
Saint Alphonsus Regional Medical Center, Boise, ID, USA

Karla A. Sepulveda, MD
Assistant Professor of Radiology, Smith Breast Center, Baylor Clinic, Houston, TX, USA

Chris C. Shaw, PhD
Professor, Department of Imaging Physics, The University of Texas MD Anderson Cancer Center, Houston, TX, USA

Tanya W. Stephens, MD
Associate Professor, Department of Diagnostic Radiology, The University of Texas MD Anderson Cancer Center, Houston, TX, USA

Stephen Switzer
Switzer Business Solutions, LLC, Rochester, NY, USA

Philip M. Tchou, PhD
Wilford Hall Medical Center, Lackland Air Force Base, San Antonio, TX, USA

Srinivasan Vedantham, PhD
Associate Professor of Radiology, University of Massachusetts Medical School, Worcester, MA, USA

Jihong Wang, PhD
Associate Professor, Department of Imaging Physics, Division of Diagnostic Imaging, The University of Texas MD Anderson Cancer Center, Houston, TX, USA

Nancy Wayne, MS
Elizabeth Wende Breast Care, LLC, Rochester, NY, USA

Gary J. Whitman, MD, FACR
Professor, Departments of Diagnostic Radiology and Radiation Oncology, The University of Texas MD Anderson Cancer Center, Houston, TX, USA

Preface

This book represents the culmination of a decade of conversations and queries regarding digital mammography. When digital mammography was introduced, my colleague Dr. Tamara Haygood and I wondered how digital systems would change mammographic image acquisition and interpretation. Some observers thought that transitioning to digital mammography was similar to converting to a new film-screen combination. We quickly realized that the new digital units had no screens, and thereafter we stopped printing films.

Dr. Haygood and I talked and questioned more. Why did it take longer to read a digital mammogram compared to a film-screen mammogram? What percentage of mammography units were digital? Could digital mammography be successfully implemented on a mobile van? What is the effect of enterprise-wide distribution of mammographic images? What type of a network is needed to support digital mammography? What monitors are required for digital mammography interpretation?

The list of questions keeps going. Currently, we question if tomosynthesis will replace standard planar digital mammography. Is there a role for breast CT? Is digital breast imaging improved with the addition of intravenous contrast material?

The aim of the book is to provide information to practicing radiologists and physicists about all facets of digital mammography. We hope that this book will help you solidify your understanding of digital mammography, from detectors to display to interpretation. Our aim is that this book will provide a core of knowledge, enabling practitioners to understand digital mammography and its derivatives, pose new questions, and find new answers.

This book contains information that we hope will be relevant to radiologists and physicists in many different geographic locations. Nonetheless, it does have an American slant. The book is written in "United States" English. For example, we use etiology rather than aetiology, hematoma rather than haematoma, and color rather than colour. In addition, discussions of legal and regulatory aspects of mammographic practice usually emphasize American law. Even within the United States relevant law can vary among the states. Therefore all readers should take such discussions in this book as generalizations that need to be verified with respect to specific jurisdictions.

Gary J. Whitman

Acknowledgments

Writing a book takes a lot of time and a great deal of hard work. We thank our authors, who got their writing done on time, covered the topics requested, and were invariably gracious whenever we had changes to suggest. Most of the authors have heavy clinical loads with very little "free" time for writing. We could not have written this book by ourselves, so we are very grateful to our chapter authors, without whom there would be no book at all.

The difference between a good manuscript and a good book is a good editor, and we were blessed with dedicated professionals at Cambridge University Press. We would like to thank Joanna Chamberlin, Hugh Brazier, and Lucy Edwards for diligent and talented attention to our manuscript. We hope that working with us was not too very similar to herding cats.

We also could not have done this without the able and cheerful help of our administrative assistants. We would like to thank Bobbie Blaylock for assistance with correspondence, in editing and in preparation of several tables, as well as proofreading of chapters assigned to Tamara. We extend a big Texas-style thank you to Barbara Almarez Mahinda, who worked with Gary on all facets of this project. We thank Joyce Bradley, Patty Castro, and Tamika Martin for secretarial support. In addition, we thank Camilla Ramagli and Kelly Duggan for assistance in image preparation.

We have worked with some incredible colleagues who have taught us and helped guide us. We thank Beatriz Adrada, Elsa Arribas, Geetha Ayyar, Deepak Bedi, Rosalind Candelaria, Selin Carkaci, Paul Davis, Peter Dempsey, Basak Dogan, Mark Dryden, Beth Edeiken, Bruno Fornage, Irwin Freudlich, Revathy Iyer, Marc Jacobson, Anne Kushwaha, Deanna Lane, Carisa Le-Petross, John Martin, Victoria Nguyen, David Paulus, Bhaskara Rao, Gaiane Rauch, Barry Samuels, Lumarie Santiago, Marion Scoggins, Veronica Selinko, Carol Stelling, Tanya Stephens, and Wei Yang, all of whom are or have recently been associated with MD Anderson's breast imaging section for helping to create an environment of thinking and questioning that led to this book. We must further thank Behrang Amini, Colleen Costelloe, Rajendra Kumar, John Madewell, Kevin McEnery, and Bill Murphy of MD Anderson's musculoskeletal radiology section, who have not merely tolerated but actively encouraged Tamara's interest in breast imaging and have provided support and opportunities essential to her role in editing this book. Also, we have been privileged to work with great residents, fellows, technologists, sonographers, physicists, nurses, and aides. To all of you— muchas gracias!

A "big" project like this takes time away from family and friends. We would especially like to thank our families for patiently supporting our efforts from start to finish.

Gary J. Whitman, MD
Tamara Miner Haygood, PhD, MD

Detectors for digital mammography

Andrew Karellas and Srinivasan Vedantham

Introduction

Mammography is the most technically demanding radiographic modality, requiring high spatial resolution, excellent low contrast discrimination, and wide dynamic range. The development of dedicated mammography systems [1] in the mid-1960s and the refinements in film-screen technology over its long evolution [2,3] were of critical importance in establishing the benefits of mammography in reducing breast cancer mortality [4–10]. The use of film-screen technology over 30 years ensured excellent spatial resolution under optimal conditions. The high spatial resolution requirement was thought to be essential for imaging small and subtle calcifications as small as 100–200 µm, in particular for visualizing its morphology. In spite of the excellent imaging characteristics of film-screen technology under optimal exposure and film development conditions, intrinsically images are more susceptible to artifacts. Small deviations from optimal exposure and processing conditions can have profound effects on mammographic image quality, such as its ability to provide a balanced image over regions of the breast that vary in radiographic density. The well-documented weaknesses of film-screen technology [11–13] include limited dynamic range, limited tolerance to exposure conditions, complexity and instabilities due to the chemical processing of film, and the lack of ability to digitally communicate, store, and enhance the images.

Digital mammography, a term coined for electronic image capture of x-rays transmitted through the breast, is a concept that was formed about 30 years ago as a means of circumventing some of the major limitations of film-screen technology. An electronic imaging detector that replaces film-screen for image capture would minimize the possibility of suboptimally exposed mammograms, which can potentially conceal subtle soft tissue lesions and microcalcifications. Digital mammography can provide wide dynamic range, wide exposure latitude, and the ability to communicate, store, and digitally manipulate images. The concept of computer-aided detection and diagnosis (CADe and CADx) [14,15] was envisioned even before digital mammography became a reality, and the idea of obtaining mammograms using electronic image capture was

certainly very attractive as an enabling technology for further development and proliferation of computer-aided techniques. Convenient digital storage and communication of mammographic images was another potential advantage that fueled the early development of digital mammography. The ensemble of all these positive attributes served as the overall motivation for seeking replacement of film-screen with digital mammography, in the belief that the benefits provided by digital mammography would improve detection, diagnosis, and management of breast cancer.

In the early days of investigations into the potential of digital mammography, particularly those pertaining to digital communication, image enhancement, and computer-aided techniques, digitization of film mammograms was used as a proxy because of the unavailability of digital mammography detectors. Digitization was accomplished by flying spot scanners, video cameras, and eventually high-resolution digital scanners. This early experience with digitized mammograms was important, because it provided an early experience of digital enhancement techniques, understanding the need for digital communication and storage, and most importantly it acted as a platform for the development and evaluation of CADe/CADx. Creation of databases with digitized mammograms for teaching and research that were readily accessible through the internet [16] was also particularly important in improving our understanding of image display (monitor) requirements and the tools needed by the user for digital image manipulation. Several studies demonstrated techniques for enhancing digitized mammograms, and others reported on the "equivalence" of digitized mammograms to the original film mammograms. Digitized mammograms added another dimension to film-screen mammography, and considering some of the initial challenges in the development of digital mammography detectors, it appeared that replacing film-screen mammography was a nearly impossible task.

One of the beliefs during the developmental stages of digital mammography was that the detectors designed for digital mammography should replicate many of the desirable characteristics of film-screen technology while circumventing

Digital Mammography: A Practical Approach, ed. Gary J. Whitman and Tamara Miner Haygood. Published by Cambridge University Press.
© Cambridge University Press 2013.

all of its limitations. This assumption made it particularly challenging during the development of digital mammography detectors, considering that film-screen technology had undergone many improvements such as development of screens and film with increased sensitivity and refinements in chemical processing. The development of digital detectors to cover the entire breast, and with spatial resolution comparable to film-screen technology, required digital detectors with an effective pixel size of 20 μm or less. Attaining this spatial resolution seemed impossible then, and it is still unrealistic even with current technology. The theoretical basis of the complex interplay between resolution, image noise, and radiation dose was well known [17–19]. The construction and characterization of early prototypes of digital mammography detectors allowed comparison of their physical imaging properties with film-screen technology, in particular understanding the trade-off between spatial resolution and image noise that was essential in mitigating some of the concerns about the pixel size used by digital mammography detectors.

The term digital mammography is generally used for any technology that performs electronic image capture of x-rays transmitted through the breast. However, the technological implementations of digital mammography utilize various principles for image formation that also affect the resultant image quality. This necessitates a discussion of the image quality metrics used to describe the performance of digital mammography systems.

Image quality metrics

Mammography systems must possess certain desired characteristics in terms of spatial resolution, image noise transfer, dynamic range, fixed pattern noise, artifacts, and dose efficiency. Several universally accepted metrics have been developed that can be used for the evaluation of the performance of digital mammography systems. These metrics can be either observer-independent or observer-dependent. The observer-independent metrics may be based on analysis in the spatial or image domain or in the spatial frequency domain. These metrics are summarized in Table 1.1. If one considers a continuous spatial distribution of x-rays on the detector surface, then the resultant signal is sampled by the pixels which are spatially separated by the pixel pitch, represented as Δ. Then, the cut-off spatial frequency (ω_c) is defined as $\omega_c = 1/\Delta$, and the spatial frequency above which aliasing (degradation due to undersampling) occurs is defined by the Nyquist frequency $\omega_N = 1/2\Delta$. In terms of spatial resolution, three of the metrics are related: resolution in the spatial domain, typically represented by the point spread function (PSF) or the related spread functions such as the line spread function (LSF) and the edge spread function (ESF); the observer-dependent limiting resolution, which is the smallest spacing between "line-pairs" or the highest line-pairs/mm the observer is able to visualize; and the modulation transfer function (MTF) in the spatial frequency domain. The

Table 1.1 Observer-dependent and observer-independent image quality metrics that are used to assess digital mammography system performance.

Image quality metrics	
Objective (observer-independent)	**Perceptual (observer-dependent)**
Spatial domain metrics	Limiting resolution
Resolution (PSF)	Threshold contrast-detail
Noise (standard deviation, variance)	Alternative forced choice (AFC)
Contrast (signal difference to noise ratio)	Receiver operating characteristics (ROC)
Spatial frequency domain metrics	
Modulaton transfer function	
Noise power spectrum	
Noise equivalent quanta	
Detective quantum efficiency	

modulation transfer function is a measure of the signal transfer property of the imaging system and provides the factor by which the output signal amplitude is reduced compared to the sinusoidal input at different spatial frequencies. The spatial domain objective metric LSF is related to the spatial frequency domain MTF by the modulus of its Fourier transform normalized to a peak of unity at zero spatial frequency. MTF is a dimensionless quantity. Figure 1.1 shows an example, where system A has a narrower point spread function (reduced blur) than system B. The corresponding MTF shown on the right indicates that system A has improved MTF compared to system B. The concept of presampling MTF is used with digital imaging systems so as to minimize the phase/sampling effects that can affect the measurements [20–22].

The observer-dependent limiting resolution is typically the spatial frequency at which the MTF is approximately in the range of 0.05–0.1, provided the detector sampling (pixel pitch) does not result in aliasing. As an example, let us assume systems A and B shown in Figure 1.1 have pixel pitch of 100 μm and the x-ray source focal spot is too small to have an effect. The Nyquist spatial frequency for both systems is 5 cycles/mm [$=1/(2\times0.1$-mm)] and the cut-off frequency is 10 cycles/mm [$=1/(0.1$-mm)]. The spatial frequency at which the MTF is 0.1 is approximately 3 and 6 cycles/mm for systems B and A, respectively. Let us assume that a high-contrast line-pair test object, such as that shown in Figure 1.2, is imaged after positioning on the detector surface so that there is negligible magnification and it is aligned with the pixel orientation. For system B, an observer would be able to perceive approximately 3 line-pairs/mm, corresponding to the spatial frequency at which the MTF is 0.1, as it is lower than the Nyquist frequency. For system A, the limiting resolution that the observer perceives without aliasing effects would be approximately 5 line-pairs/mm, corresponding to the Nyquist frequency, even though the spatial frequency at which MTF is 0.1 is 6 cycles/mm. However, if the test object is moved closer to

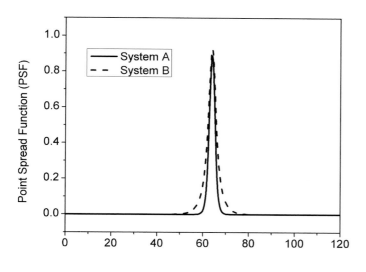 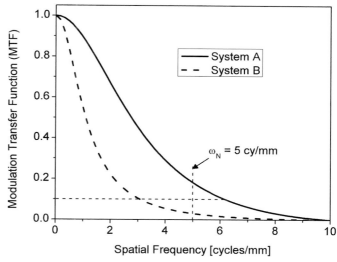

Figure 1.1 Relationship between point spread function (PSF) and modulation transfer function (MTF). System A has a narrower PSF, resulting in a higher MTF, compared to system B.

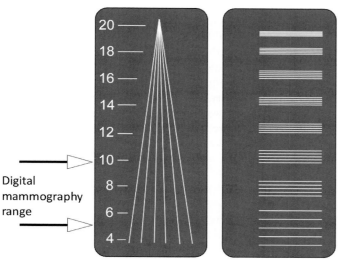

Figure 1.2 Examples of resolution test patterns used for assessing perceived limiting resolution (not to scale).

the source, resulting in magnification (for example 1.8 times, as typically used in magnification mammography), and assuming the x-ray focal spot size does not contribute to blur, then it would be possible to perceive a limiting resolution of 6 line-pairs/mm with system A. Thus under conditions of negligible magnification, the limiting resolution that is perceived using a line-pair test object without aliasing effects is the minimum of the Nyquist spatial frequency or the spatial frequency at which the modulation transfer function has a value of approximately 0.1. Perceived limiting resolution with a test pattern is often used for monitoring system image quality, and is performed as part of annual quality control procedures for mammography systems.

The noise power spectrum (NPS) provides the spatial frequency domain representation of the image noise, and the integral of the NPS is identical to the second-order spatial domain noise metric, the variance. This implies that for Poisson-distributed incident x-ray quanta at a given exposure or air kerma, measurement of the NPS can provide the noise transfer properties of the system at that exposure. NPS is determined by ensemble average of the squares of the magnitude of Fourier-transformed images or regions of interest acquired with uniform exposure to the detector. If the acquired images are represented in digital units (DU), then the NPS has units of $DU^2 \cdot mm^2$. Alternatively, if the images are transformed from DU to electrons, exposure (mR), or air kerma (mGy), then the units for NPS are correspondingly altered. It is important to note that the measured NPS includes aliasing effects and hence the NPS is only defined up to the Nyquist sampling limit. Often the term "normalized NPS" is also used to represent the image noise at a given exposure, which represents the measured NPS divided by the square of the mean large-area signal at that exposure. If one considers an x-ray spectrum with x-ray photon fluence per unit (mR) exposure of q_0/X photons/$(mm^2 \cdot mR)$ and exposure incident on the detector of X_i mR, then the photon fluence is $(q_0/X)X_i$ photons/mm^2. The large-area mean signal at uniform exposure to the detector, X_i, can be represented as S_i. Then the normalized NPS is represented as $\hat{W}(u, v) = W(u, v)/S_i^2$, where $W(u, v)$ is the NPS measured at the exposure X_i. Typically, the signal S_i increases with increase in exposure X_i either in a linear fashion or in a predefined manner such as logarithmic or square-root response, depending on the detector readout technology. The NPS, $W(u, v)$ will also exhibit a similar response with increasing exposure provided the additive system noise is not dominant. Hence, the normalized NPS, $\hat{W}(u, v)$ will exhibit decreased amplitude when exposure X_i is increased. Thus, the exposure dependency will be reversed between the NPS and the normalized NPS. In addition, normalization by S_i, which is represented in DU, would also result in change of units for the normalized NPS to mm^2.

Noise equivalent quanta (NEQ) is an important metric derived from the large-area mean signal, MTF, and NPS and represents the square of the signal-to-noise ratio at a given exposure to the detector. It is computed as $NEQ(u, v) = S_i^2 MTF^2(u, v)/W(u, v)$, or equivalently as $NEQ(u, v) = MTF^2(u, v)/\hat{W}(u, v)$. From the above mathematical description, it is apparent that NEQ has units of mm^{-2}, as MTF is dimensionless and the normalized NPS has units of mm^2. NEQ facilitates task-specific system optimization [23] such as selecting the appropriate applied tube voltage (kVp) and x-ray beam filtration so as to maximize the signal-to-noise ratio. It also facilitates comparison across multiple detector technologies. Another important derived metric is the detective quantum efficiency (DQE), which provides the signal-to-noise ratio transfer characteristics of the system and is a measure of dose efficiency. It is computed as,

$$DQE(u, v) = \frac{S_i^2 MTF^2(u, v)}{[(q_0/X)X_i]W(u, v)} = \frac{NEQ(u, v)}{[(q_0/X)X_i]}.$$

Since, NEQ has units of mm^{-2} and the photon fluence (q_0/X) X_i also has units of mm^{-2}, DQE is a dimensionless quantity. For Poisson-distributed x-ray quanta, where the mean is equal to its variance, the term $(q_0/X)X_i$ represents the variance of the x-ray beam incident on the detector at the exposure X_i. Thus, DQE represents the ratio of the square of the signal-to-noise ratio at image output to that at detector input, providing the signal-to-noise ratio transfer characteristics of the system. Also, for a defined x-ray beam quality (kVp, filtration), the term $(q_0/X)X_i$ is proportional to the radiation dose, and hence DQE can also provide a measure of dose efficiency.

The spatial domain metric contrast provides the difference in signal values between two locations that differ in x-ray attenuation properties. However, with digital imaging systems that allow easy manipulation of image data values, contrast is usually computed as the signal difference to noise ratio (SDNR). It is computed as $SDNR = |S_b - S_o|/\sigma_b$, where S_b and S_o represent the mean signal values of the background and the signal object, and σ_b represents the standard deviation of the background. Alternative descriptions for the standard deviation such as $\sqrt{\sigma_b^2 + \sigma_o^2}$, which takes into account the standard deviation of the signal intensities within the object, may also be used in SDNR computation. Contrast measurements with test phantoms, such as the American College of Radiology (ACR)-recommended accreditation phantom, are often used for monitoring system image quality and are performed as part of annual quality control procedures for mammography systems [24].

All of the image quality metrics described above, with the exception of the perceived limiting resolution, do not involve the observer. Threshold contrast-detail measurements provide a powerful tool that takes into account the signal object size, its contrast, and the image noise as perceived by the observer. A typical contrast-detail phantom contains a homogeneous background with circular disk-shaped signal objects that are arranged in a square matrix and vary in diameter along one direction that provides changes in object size, and in disk thickness along the orthogonal direction that provides changes in image contrast. The observer or group of observers determines for each row and column the signal objects that are visualized. For each disk diameter (detail size), the disk thickness (contrast) that is just visualized by the observer or group of observers is plotted to generate the contrast-detail diagram, which provides the threshold contrast-detail characteristics of the system. One major limitation of this approach is that the ordered matrix of signal objects allows observers to predict the location of objects that may be difficult to visualize without this prior knowledge.

Alternative forced choice (AFC) methodology can overcome this limitation. In this approach the signal object may be located in one of multiple locations, and the observer has to indicate its location even if the signal object is difficult to visualize because of its size, contrast, or the noise present in the images. Since the observer is "forced" to choose the location of the signal from multiple locations (alternative choice), the term "alternative forced choice" is used. Additionally, the methodology allows estimating contrast-detail characteristics at different threshold levels. Figure 1.3 shows an example of a phantom that is designed for conducting AFC studies in mammography [25]. This phantom has a homogeneous background with a matrix of cells that contain circular disk-shaped signal objects, which vary in diameter along one direction and in thickness along the orthogonal direction. Each cell has two signal objects, one at its center and the other at one of its four corners. For the AFC study, the signal object located at the center of a cell is ignored and the observer has to select one of the four corners, i.e., four alternative choices, in which the signal object is perceived. The probability that an observer may randomly pick the correct corner is 1/4 (0.25). Thus the fraction of correct responses, often referred to as percent correct detection, will range from 0.25 to 1.0. Figure 1.4 shows an example of percent correct detection for three disk diameters based on image interpretation by one observer of hard-copy digital images of the phantom [25]. The 50% threshold level is shown by the horizontal line and its intercept with the curves for the three disk diameters projected to the x-axis (disk depth that provides a measure of contrast) is used to generate the contrast-detail diagram. Figure 1.5 shows an example of contrast-detail characteristics obtained at 62.5% threshold for a film-screen mammography system and hard-copy images from a digital mammography clinical prototype system [25]. It is important to note that these are *threshold* contrast-detail characteristics, and thus a system exhibiting improved contrast-detail characteristics would be represented by a curve lower than the other. An ideal system would exhibit threshold contrast-detail characteristics that follow the axes, i.e., even a small signal object (detail size) is visualized with high contrast. While the specific phantom described above has a homogeneous background, AFC methodology can also be used for studies with heterogeneous backgrounds such as

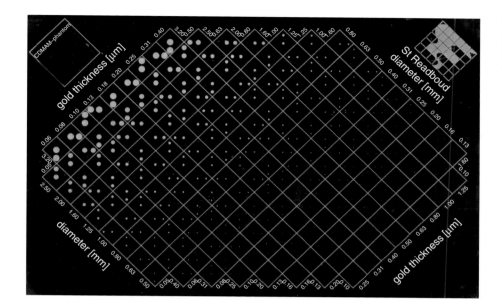

Figure 1.3 CDMAM phantom that can be used for AFC studies of mammography systems. Reproduced with permission from Suryanarayanan *et al., Radiology* 2002; **225**: 801–7 [25]. © Radiological Society of North America.

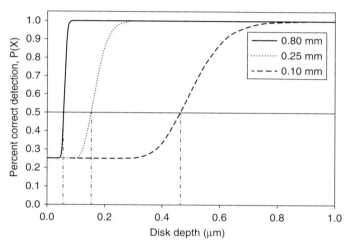

Figure 1.4 Percent correct detection for three disk diameters used for computing threshold contrast-detail characteristics using AFC methodology. Reproduced with permission from Suryanarayanan *et al., Radiology* 2002; **225**: 801–7 [25]. © Radiological Society of North America.

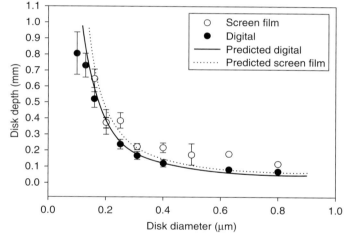

Figure 1.5 Contrast-detail characteristics obtained at 62.5% threshold using AFC methodology. Reproduced with permission from Suryanarayanan *et al., Radiology* 2002; **225**: 801–7 [25]. © Radiological Society of North America.

the anatomical background due to overlapping tissue structures encountered in mammography [26].

The standard and best-established perceptual image quality metric that is of direct clinical relevance is the receiver operating characteristic (ROC), which provides sensitivity/specificity characteristics. Considering the extensive use of ROC methodology in medical imaging, and the availability of excellent texts on this topic [27,28], only a brief description is provided. ROC methodology not only allows comparison across different technologies within the same modality, e.g., film-screen versus digital mammography, it also allows comparison across different modalities, e.g., mammography versus breast ultrasound. The methodology is suitable not only for detection tasks based

on observer's confidence in the presence of a lesion in an image, but also characterization tasks based on observer's confidence that the lesion present is malignant. In a typical ROC study, an observer provides a rating based on a predefined scale for the intended task and this rating is analyzed with knowledge of "truth." Software programs to fit observer ratings to an ROC curve and calculate the statistical significance of differences between ROC index estimates and parameters are available [29].

Description of the image quality metrics and understanding their importance is necessary to contrast the different digital mammography detector technologies that are currently used in practice. Broadly, it is convenient to classify the detector technologies into indirect and direct conversion, based on the physical principle used for image formation.

Indirect conversion with prompt readout

The indirect-conversion approach with prompt readout of the signal is similar to the basic principle used in film-screen technology. This process uses a scintillator, typically a thin layer of thallium-doped cesium iodide or gadolinium oxysulfide. X-rays transmitted though the breast pass though the breast support plate and the antiscatter grid, and interact with the scintillator primarily by the photoelectric effect. In response to the x-ray interaction the scintillator emits light predominantly in the green region of the electromagnetic spectrum and proportional to the energy of the interacting x-ray photon that is detected by an optically sensitive detector (photodetector). This seemingly simple approach had been technologically difficult to accomplish until the last decade. Technological implementation of the indirect conversion with prompt readout varies based on the scintillator and the photodetector used.

Scintillator

The physical characteristics of the scintillator are critical for attaining good spatial resolution and contrast at a low radiation dose. Gadolinium oxysulfide polycrystalline granular scintillators, which have been used widely as intensifying screens in film cassettes, were initially used with small-field-of-view digital mammography systems [30] and early full-field digital mammography system designs [31], largely because of the unavailability of alternatives. However, they were not well suited as scintillators in digital mammography. A major reason is the difference in the geometry of x-ray projection between film-screen and digital mammography. As depicted in Figure 1.6 (right), x-rays must first pass though the film to reach the screen, and this is done by design in order to minimize light diffusion in the screen and thereby preserve spatial resolution. This geometry ensures that scintillations generated from each x-ray photon interaction within the screen predominantly occur close to the film surface because of exponential x-ray attenuation. In digital mammography, this geometry is not replicated (Figure 1.6, left) and it is challenging to implement because x-rays must first penetrate the detector substrate and

photodetector before the scintillator. The detector substrate, depending on the optically sensitive detector and the readout technology, is typically a glass plate with a thickness of about 1 mm, which could cause partial x-ray attenuation. Therefore, with available detectors, the scintillators must be placed such that the x-ray beam interacts with the scintillator before the photodetector. In this configuration a higher fraction of x-ray interactions in the scintillator occur further from the photodetector, and the larger path length of the scintillations before reaching the photodetector contributes to increased light diffusion, which degrades spatial resolution. While reducing the scintillator layer thickness could reduce the path length and consequently improve spatial resolution, this results in reduced x-ray stopping power or quantum efficiency. Therefore, scintillators for digital mammography must possess certain characteristics that ensure high quantum efficiency with minimal degradation of the resolution.

Out of hundreds of known scintillators, currently only one, thallium-doped cesium iodide (CsI:Tl) has been deemed suitable for digital mammography. This scintillator can be vapor-deposited on a number of substrates or directly on the optically sensitive detector. Direct deposition of the scintillator on the detector is desirable for efficient light transmission that will deliver adequate signal to the silicon photodetector. The vapor deposition is important, as it forms a needle-like structure that reduces lateral diffusion of the scintillations caused by x-ray interaction by predominantly channeling the light through the process of internal reflection, in essence acting like pseudo-fiberoptics. This structure is shown in the scanning electron microscope image in Figure 1.7. The pseudo-fiberoptic structure allows the use of a thicker scintillator layer to improve quantum efficiency, with minimal degradation in spatial resolution. On average, each interacting 1 keV x-ray photon generates approximately 50–55 optical photons. This scintillator has good transparency to the scintillations generated, i.e., reduced self-attenuation of optical photons, that transports most of the scintillations to the photodetector. In addition, the wavelength of emission is well matched to the absorption characteristics of silicon-based photodetectors, resulting in good efficiency. Typically, digital mammography systems use a layer of CsI:Tl 100–150 μm thick, and the quantum efficiency as a function of incident x-ray photon energy is shown for the energy range of 5–40 keV in Figure 1.8. A nominal value for packing fraction, which defines the volume occupied by the phosphor

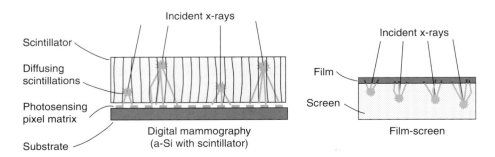

Figure 1.6 Comparison of imaging geometry used with film-screen mammography and digital mammography based on indirect conversion with prompt readout.

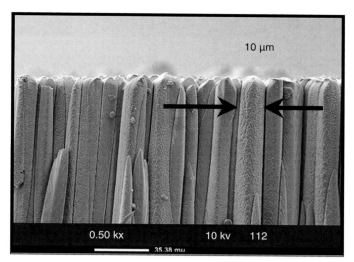

Figure 1.7 Scanning electron microscope image of a CsI:Tl scintillator, showing the needle-like structures. Courtesy of Vivek Nagarkar, PhD, RMD Inc., Watertown, MA.

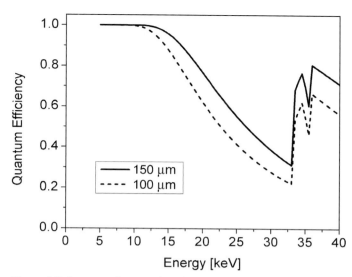

Figure 1.8 Quantum efficiency of CsI:Tl 100 and 150 μm thick, with 80% packing fraction in the energy range 5–40 keV.

grains within this layer, of 80% was assumed for these calculations. The integration of CsI:Tl with the photodetector presented several challenges in manufacturing, particularly in the direct deposition onto the photodetector array and protection from humidity, because of the hygroscopic nature of CsI:Tl. These early challenges have been overcome, and integrated digital mammographic detector assemblies of this type are now produced routinely by at least one major manufacturer.

Photodetector

Currently, the most commonly used photodetector technology is the flat-panel amorphous silicon photodiode array with thin-film transistor readout. Although scintillator development for mammography presented some challenges for the industry in terms of optimizing CsI:Tl thickness, optimizing thallium dopant concentration, which can affect light output, and refining direct deposition techniques, the properties of CsI have been known for many years. However, pixilated amorphous silicon detectors are a relatively new technology, and the first commercially intended devices were manufactured only in the mid-1990s. The detector consists of a thin layer of amorphous silicon (a-Si) with a thickness of a few μm that is deposited on a glass substrate with a thickness of about 1 mm (Figure 1.6, left). The photodetector consists of an array of approximately 2400 × 3000 photosensitive elements (pixels) for a 24 × 30 cm detector. The detector consists of the hydrogenated amorphous silicon (a-Si:H) photodiode, the photosensitive part of the detector that responds to the optical signal from the scintillator, the a-Si:H thin-film transistor, and the bias, gate, and data channels. The a-Si layer is the light-sensitive part of the flat-panel plate with a quantum efficiency of about 50–65% for the light emitted by a CsI:Tl scintillator. The bias channels supply the voltage, and the gate channels control the signal readout of the panel. It is important to note that the signal-detecting a-Si

photodiode occupies only a fraction of the pixel area on the a-Si flat-panel detector with the remainder taken up by other structures such as the bias, gate, and data lines and the thin-film transistor. The size of each a-Si detector element is about 100 μm. Geometrical fill factor, defined as the ratio of the area occupied by the optically sensitive region (a-Si photodiode) to the pixel area, can vary with different flat-panel detector designs, but with current technology achieving approximately 75% fill factor is considered high. Higher fill factors approaching unity are desirable so as to maximize the capture of the optical signal from the scintillator. It is relevant to note that the CsI:Tl scintillator layer is deposited as a continuous layer covering the entire detector, and only the a-Si photodiode array with thin-film transistor readout is a discrete array.

The a-Si with scintillator (indirect-conversion) approach was the first large-scale attempt for full-breast digital mammography, also known as full-field digital mammography (FFDM). Initially, a-Si flat-panel detectors did not appear suitable for digital mammography. Early results with a-Si with a scintillator for x-ray imaging applications seemed promising, but their adaptation to mammography seemed a distant goal because of the electronic noise levels and the relatively large 100 μm detector elements. The resulting limiting resolution of 5 line-pairs/mm, compared to about 18 line-pairs/mm for film-screen mammography, was also perceived as a severe limitation. Despite these concerns, clinical performance [32,33], physical [34,35], and perceptual [25] evaluations have demonstrated important advantages over film-screen mammography. Figure 1.9 shows the objective physical performance metric, DQE, measured for a clinical FFDM system at 28 kVp with a molybdenum anode, rhodium-filtered (Mo/Rh) x-ray spectrum after transmitting through 45 mm of polymethyl methacrylate (PMMA) [34]. Continuing evolution of this detector technology [36], in part to address the needs of breast imaging techniques such as digital breast tomosynthesis and contrast-enhanced digital mammography, can be observed with

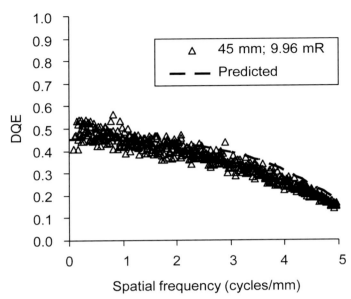

Figure 1.9 DQE measurements performed on an amorphous silicon (a-Si)-based full-field digital mammography (FFDM) system at 28 kVp Mo/Rh x-ray spectrum filtered with 45 mm of PMMA. Reproduced with permission from Suryanarayanan *et al.*, *Nucl Instrum Methods Phys Res A*, 2004; **533**: 560–70 [34]. © Elsevier B.V.

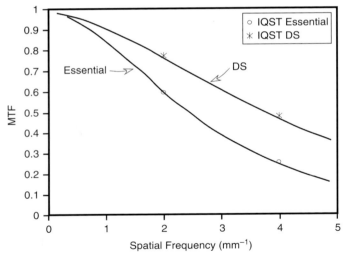

Figure 1.10 MTF measurements performed on two versions of amorphous silicon (a-Si)-based FFDM systems. Adapted with permission from Ghetti *et al.*, *Med Phys* 2008; **35**: 456–63 [36]. © American Association of Physicists in Medicine.

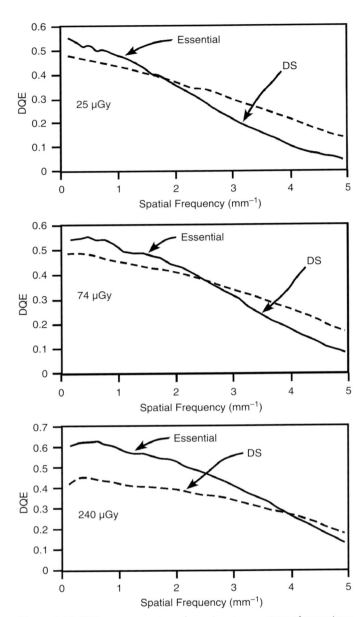

Figure 1.11 DQE measurements performed on two versions of amorphous silicon (a-Si)-based FFDM systems. Adapted with permission from Ghetti *et al.*, *Med Phys* 2008; **35**: 456–63 [36]. © American Association of Physicists in Medicine.

changes in MTF and DQE shown in Figures 1.10 and 1.11, respectively. Thus, current versions of CsI:Tl coupled a-Si-based indirect-conversion detectors provide a low-frequency DQE, in the range of 0.5–0.6 for exposure levels relevant to mammography.

Alternative photodetector technologies such as charge-coupled devices (CCDs) and complementary metal-oxide semiconductors (CMOS) are also of interest in the indirect-conversion approach with prompt readout. Small-field-of-view digital mammography systems [30] used for spot compression views and stereotactic locations, as well as early generations of

FFDM systems [31,37], used charge-coupled devices for readout. CMOS technology, in particular systems employing on-pixel amplification to increase signal intensity relative to noise, is being actively researched as a possible candidate for digital mammography [38,39].

Direct conversion

The direct-conversion approach eliminates the scintillator, and a photoconductive amorphous selenium (a-Se) layer with a thickness of about 200–250 µm is used as the primary detector

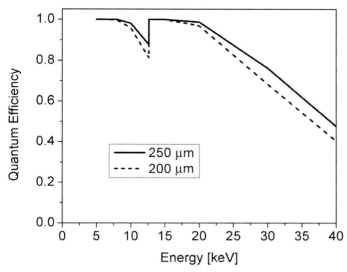

Figure 1.12 Quantum efficiency of a-Se layers 200 and 250 µm thick with 80% packing fraction.

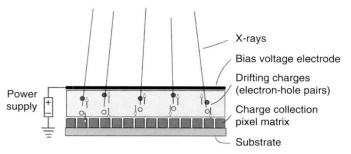

Figure 1.13 Schematic of an amorphous selenium (a-Se)-based direct-conversion detector.

of x-rays. Figure 1.12 shows the computed quantum efficiency for a-Se layers 200 and 250 µm thick as a function of incident x-ray photon energy in the range of 5–40 keV. X-rays are transmitted past the breast, traverse through a thin continuous electrode layer, and interact in the a-Se layer. This interaction generates electron-hole pairs primarily through photoelectric effect. An electric field is applied across the a-Se layer, typically 10–15 V per µm thickness of a-Se layer, and approximately 15–20 electron-hole pairs are generated for each interacting 1 keV x-ray photon [40]. The generated charges produce a signal at the readout electrode. Figure 1.13 shows a schematic representation of the detector.

Until recently, amorphous selenium-based direct-conversion detectors utilized flat-panel amorphous silicon thin-film transistor (TFT) arrays for charge readout. Figure 1.14 shows a schematic of such a thin-film transistor readout. Similar to the readout used in amorphous silicon-based indirect-conversion detectors, the presence of bias, gate, and data lines and the thin-film transistor results in a fill factor that is approximately 70%. Currently, a-Se detectors with TFT readout are available either with 70 µm pixels or with 85 µm pixels. One important characteristic that direct-conversion amorphous selenium exhibits is excellent spatial resolution. This high spatial resolution can be observed through their MTF characteristics [41], shown in Figure 1.15 for an a-Se detector with 70 µm pixel pitch. The MTF approaches the theoretical expectation of an ideal pixel response with small degradation due to charge trapping [42]. Measured DQE characteristics [41] using a 28 kVp Mo/Mo spectrum with 2 mm of Al added to the x-ray tube port for an a-Se detector with 70 µm pixel pitch are shown in Figure 1.16. Low-frequency DQE of approximately 60% is observed at exposure levels relevant to mammography. Similar results have also been reported for a system using 85 µm pixel pitch [42].

There has been considerable research interest in developing optical readout technology in an effort to minimize the electronic noise that arises from TFT readout [43–46]. Recently, an a-Se-based system that utilizes an additional photoconductive layer with a 50 µm pixel pitch has been developed, and this has shown desirable physical characteristics [46].

Digital cassette mammography

Digital mammography with flat-panel detectors using direct and indirect-conversion methods represents a top-tier technology in terms of radiation dose efficiency, contrast, and spatial resolution. These devices are completely integrated with the x-ray system and cannot be used to upgrade film-screen systems to digital mammography. Therefore, with the rapid conversion from film-screen to digital mammography, even relatively recent film-screen mammography units will have to be discarded if a facility decides to upgrade to digital mammography. The conversion to digital by using a digital cassette is a concept that has been discussed for many years. Photo-stimulable phosphor plates (also called CR, for computed radiography) incorporated in a portable cassette have been widely used in general radiography for many years and they are now the most widely used digital technology for general radiography. CR-based digital cassette mammography provides a cost-efficient approach for upgrading a facility with multiple film-screen systems to digital mammography, but is yet to demonstrate objective image quality metrics that are similar to dedicated flat-panel detector-based digital mammography systems.

In computed radiography, a photostimulable phosphor plate, also called an image plate (IP), is used as the primary detector of x-rays similar to film-screen mammography or scintillator-based indirect-conversion detectors. This IP is incorporated in a cassette that is identical in dimensions and form to a film-screen mammography cassette, and it is intended to be used in place of a film-screen cassette in mammography units. During mammographic exposure, x-rays transmit past the breast, breast support plate, antiscatter grid, and the digital cassette cover, prior to absorption in the photostimulable phosphor primarily by the photoelectric effect. This generates electron-hole pairs and a fraction of the generated charge is trapped in the crystal structure, creating a latent image proportional to the energy of the

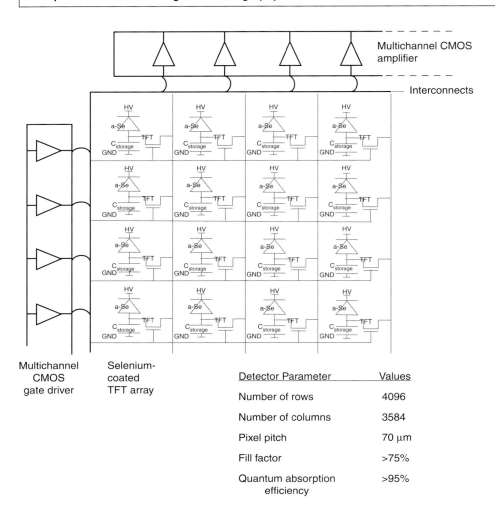

Figure 1.14 Schematic of a thin-film transistor (TFT) array used for charge readout in a-Se detectors. Courtesy of Hologic, Inc., Bedford, MA.

Detector Parameter	Values
Number of rows	4096
Number of columns	3584
Pixel pitch	70 μm
Fill factor	>75%
Quantum absorption efficiency	>95%

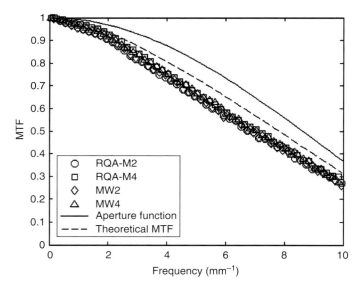

Figure 1.15 MTF characteristics of a prototype a-Se-based digital mammography system with 70 μm pixel pitch. Reproduced with permission from Saunders *et al.*, *Med Phys* 2005; **32**: 588–99 [41]. © American Association of Physicists in Medicine.

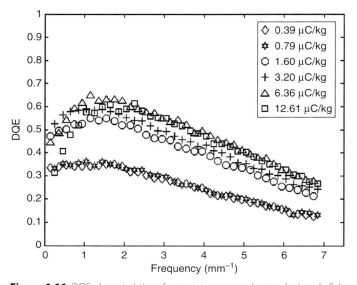

Figure 1.16 DQE characteristics of a prototype amorphous selenium (a-Se)-based digital mammography system with 70 μm pixel pitch. Reproduced with permission from Saunders *et al.*, *Med Phys* 2005; **32**: 588–99 [41]. © American Association of Physicists in Medicine.

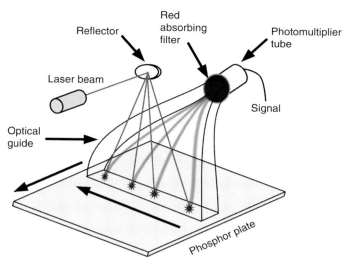

Figure 1.17 Schematic of computed radiography (CR) readout process.

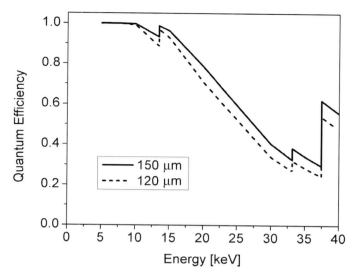

Figure 1.18 Quantum efficiency of $BaFBr_{0.85}I_{0.15}$ photostimulable phosphor 120 and 150 μm thick (60% packing fraction).

interacting x-rays. The CR cassette is then transported to a reader, which uses optical stimulation, typically from a laser source that emits in the 630–680 nm wavelength (red), and the trapped electrons are released in a process that radiates energy in the form of light, typically in the ultraviolet-blue region (400–450 nm). This process is referred to as photostimulated luminescence, and it is shown schematically in Figure 1.17. In this readout process a raster scan of the laser beam is performed by moving the plate in the longitudinal direction while the laser beam is scanned in the transverse direction. Alternatively, the plate may remain stationary and the laser beam may be scanned in two directions for a complete point-by-point readout. The emitted light intensity from any point of the imaging plate is approximately proportional to the radiation absorbed at that point. Therefore, detection of the spatial distribution of photostimulated luminescence provides a mammographic image that is proportional to x-ray energy absorbed in the imaging plate.

One key component of the CR technology is the photostimulable phosphor. Most digital cassette mammography systems utilize barium fluorohalide grains as the phosphor. While early generations of CR technology used europium-doped barium fluorobromide (BaFBr:Eu) as the phosphor, current generations incorporate iodine (typically, $BaFBr_{0.85}I_{0.15}$:Eu) and strontium (BaSrFBrI:Eu). Incorporation of iodine allowed the use of a semiconductor laser source that emits at 680 nm, whereas a 633 nm He-Ne laser source was needed for optimal stimulation of BaFBr:Eu phosphors. The addition of iodine and strontium improves the x-ray attenuation characteristics. The phosphor layer in the imaging plate is typically 120–150 μm thick, and the packing fraction is approximately 60%. Figure 1.18 shows the quantum efficiency computation for various barium fluorohalide photostimulable phosphors of 150 μm thickness and with a packing fraction of 60%. In addition to these granular phosphors, needle-like cesium bromide phosphors (CsBr:Eu) similar to the CsI:Tl scintillator have been developed and can provide improvements in spatial resolution. In addition to the phosphor layer, the imaging plate also contains the substrate that provides mechanical rigidity, an electroconductive layer for electrostatic discharge, an anti-halation layer that limits the lateral spread of the laser light, and a protective layer to prevent dust adhesion and abrasion.

Another key component of this technology is the CR reader. One key distinction that needs to be made with CR technology is that the laser beam is incident on the same surface of the imaging plate that was irradiated with x-rays, replicating an imaging geometry similar to that used in film-screen systems (Figure 1.6, right). This is necessary for preserving spatial resolution. The general approach for image readout was shown in Figure 1.17. In principle, the readout process appears to be simple, but there were many challenges that had to be overcome to generate the high spatial resolution required for mammography and to maximize the stimulated signal from the plate. The readout requires a well-defined laser beam with a smaller cross-section than that used for general radiography, and a finer sampling pitch defined by the spacing between consecutive readout points during the laser scan. This sampling pitch is referred to as "pixel size" in such systems. However, even with "pixel sizes" that are typically 50 μm for mammography, scattering of laser light within the phosphor layer that stimulates adjacent regions results in photostimulated emission from these regions and contributes to degradation of the spatial resolution. This scattering effect is more dominant in barium fluorohalide granular phosphors than in needle-like CsBr phosphors. Therefore, depending on the phosphor employed, a "pixel size" of 50 μm may not yield a limiting resolution of 10 line-pairs/mm. Image plates may also incorporate additive colorants (dyes) to minimize scattering of laser light within the imaging plate. An additional challenge in CR mammography has been efficient capture of the photostimulated emissions. Careful design of the light guide or a reflecting cavity is necessary to maximize collection of these

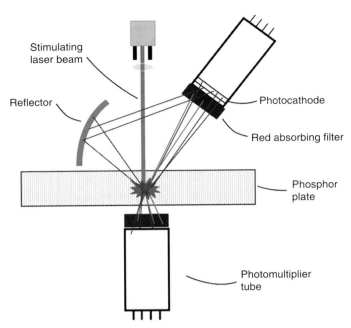

Figure 1.19 Readout of photostimulated emissions from both sides of a storage phosphor, referred to as "dual-side" read.

emissions. The stimulating laser light incident on the imaging plate has an intensity that is several orders of magnitude greater than the photostimulated emissions. Therefore, even a small fraction of the laser light, if collected by the photodetector, could have detrimental effects on dynamic range and contrast. An optical band-pass filter is used to transmit most of the photostimulated emissions (blue light), while absorbing any scattered laser stimulation light. The photostimulated emissions are detected by a photodetector, typically a photomultiplier tube (PMT). Another approach that has been used in digital cassette mammography to improve efficiency is to read the photostimulated luminescence from both sides of the imaging plate, as shown in Figure 1.19: this is referred to as "dual-side" read CR mammography. This necessitated changes to the imaging plate by making it optically transparent in both directions. Currently single-side and dual-side read versions of CR mammography are used.

After readout, the imaging plates must be erased, and this is accomplished in an automated manner within the CR reader. Complete erasure is essential to ensure that subsequent image acquisitions are not degraded by residual image from prior image acquisition with the same imaging plate. Performance characterization of dual-side read CR mammography systems [47–49] with 50 μm "pixel size" has shown limiting resolution (10% MTF) of approximately 7 line-pairs/mm and a low-frequency DQE of approximately 40–50% for conditions relevant to mammography.

Photon-counting mammography

In all of the aforementioned digital mammography detectors, the signal generated in each pixel is proportional to the energy of the interacting x-ray. This implies that a higher-energy x-ray photon that interacts with the detector would generate a stronger signal than a lower-energy x-ray photon. Hence, the resulting images typically contain an increased fraction of higher-energy x-ray photons, provided the quantum efficiency is similar throughout the energy range of the x-ray spectrum. It is known that x-ray attenuation differences in breast tissues decrease with increasing energy. Thus, energy-integrating detectors result in some contrast degradation. Additionally, in scintillator-coupled amorphous silicon or direct-conversion amorphous selenium flat-panel digital mammography detectors, the generated electronic signal (charge) in each pixel is integrated over the duration of image acquisition. Individual x-ray interactions are not recorded. Since charges are integrated, electronic noise generated in the detector panel is also included in the resultant image, which results in performance degradation and is readily observed at DQE measurements performed at low x-ray exposure levels incident on these flat-panel detectors.

In comparison, in photon-counting detectors, where the generated signal is proportional to the number of x-ray photons interacting with the detector, the resulting image gives equal weight to the interacting x-rays irrespective of their energy. Thus, photon-counting detectors inherently provide improved contrast. In addition, inclusion of a threshold to discriminate electronic noise allows for rejection of electronic noise in the acquired images. Therefore, counting each individual x-ray photon can alleviate some of the problems with image noise. Historically this has been very difficult to implement because of the relatively large x-ray photon fluence (approximately 5×10^5 x-ray photons/mm^2) for the image region attenuated by the breast in a typical mammogram. The x-ray photon fluence can increase substantially, as much as three orders of magnitude higher at the skin line of a typical mammogram. Further, the duration of image acquisition for a typical mammogram with non-scanning area detectors such as film-screen mammography and digital mammography with flat-panel detectors and CR technology is approximately 1–2 seconds. At this high incident x-ray photon fluence rate, effective discrimination and counting of electronic signal from each x-ray interaction within the detector is extremely difficult. However, recent progress on detectors and electronics has enabled mammography with photon counting using specially designed multi-strip silicon detectors in a slot-scanning acquisition approach. One advantage of the slot-scanning approach is the ability to reject a large fraction of the scattered x-ray photons by virtue of the restrictive collimation provided by the slot without the need for an antiscatter grid that partially attenuates a fraction of the primary x-ray beam. Figure 1.20 shows a schematic of this approach. In one implementation, a detector pixel size of about 50 μm is used in the direction perpendicular to the chest wall but the effective pixel in the lateral direction is determined by the object sampling by the scanning mechanism. Performance characterization of such slot-scan photon-counting detectors has shown asymmetric MTF characteristics [50].

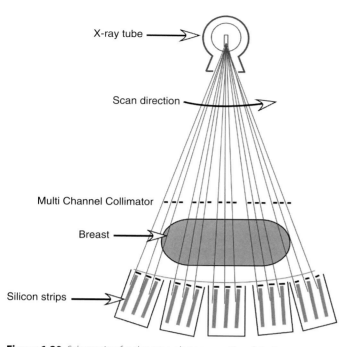

Figure 1.20 Schematic of a slot-scan photon-counting detector.

(labels: X-ray tube, Scan direction, Multi Channel Collimator, Breast, Silicon strips)

Current status and future trends

Digital mammography is now considered equivalent to film-screen in terms of clinical performance and is becoming the new "gold standard." In developed countries the majority of mammographic units are now digital; for example, it is estimated that approximately 90% (or perhaps more) of all units in the USA will be digital by the end of the year 2012. Therefore, film-screen mammography will be completely replaced by digital, and in facilities where the entire mammographic unit cannot be replaced for economic reasons they are likely to

be upgraded with digital cassette-type CR or even with solid-state detectors in a cassette format.

As described previously, digital mammography is represented by a number of different types of detector technologies and acquisition approaches. Image correction techniques aimed at reducing artifacts are necessary with digital mammography detectors to account for pixel inhomogeneities. Image processing techniques can be used to enhance resolution and for improving image uniformity such as visualizing regions of the breast close to the skin. Images of test objects with homogeneous background such as the accreditation phantom recommended by the American College of Radiology can reveal certain differences in perceived image noise and contrast characteristics between the detectors. These differences may be less apparent in clinical images because of the anatomical structure. However, high image noise levels in "flat-field" images are likely to affect the quality of clinical images.

In general, the limiting spatial resolution (10% MTF) achieved by these digital mammography systems is lower than that of film-screen mammography and is highly variable depending on the detector technology [51], as shown in Figure 1.21. Pixel sizes currently implemented with digital mammography systems vary between 50 and 100 μm; however, pixel size is one of the physical characteristics that affect spatial resolution. Additional factors, depending on the detector technology, such as scattering of light within scintillator or photostimulable phosphor to a large extent and charge trapping to a small extent, contribute to degradation of spatial resolution. While the reduced spatial resolution observed with digital mammography systems does not seem to have a substantial impact on their clinical performance, certain clinical situations, such as visualizing the morphology of subtle microcalcifications, can test their resolution and contrast capabilities. In such cases, the usefulness of an artifact-free high-resolution detector cannot be overstated. Digital mammography with greatly increased spatial resolution is not considered

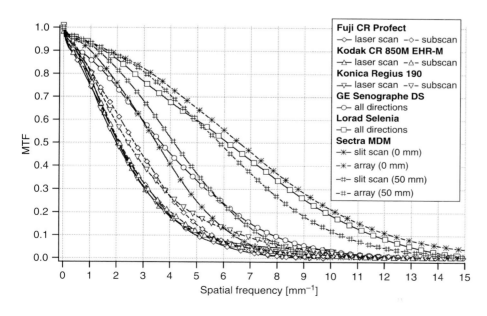

Fuji CR Profect
–◇– laser scan –◇– subscan
Kodak CR 850M EHR-M
–△– laser scan –△– subscan
Konica Regius 190
–▽– laser scan –▽– subscan
GE Senographe DS
–○– all directions
Lorad Selenia
–□– all directions
Sectra MDM
–✳– slit scan (0 mm)
-✳- array (0 mm)
-╫- slit scan (50 mm)
-╫- array (50 mm)

Figure 1.21 MTF characteristics of various digital mammography systems. Reproduced with permission from Monnin *et al., Med Phys* 2007; **34**: 906–14 [51]. © American Association of Physicists in Medicine.

a critically needed improvement, but modest improvements in resolution without negatively affecting the DQE and dose efficiency could be useful in characterizing the morphology of microcalcifications. Given this consideration and the technological and economical barriers, increases in the spatial resolution of digital mammography are likely to be gradual over the next few years.

All digital mammography detection technologies represent an improvement over film-screen mammography in dynamic range, penetration through dense tissue, and reduced repeat rate. In terms of dose efficiency, all digital mammography detectors exhibit good DQE characteristics that exceed film-screen mammography. In general, a-Si, a-Se, and photon-counting detectors exhibit improved DQE characteristics at mammographic exposure levels compared to CR technology [51], as shown in Figures 1.22 and 1.23. CR technology performs at dose levels that are comparable to film-screen mammography. Therefore, it is a suitable replacement for film-screen mammography, but substantial dose reduction with CR mammography is yet to be demonstrated. Digital mammography detectors exhibit low-frequency DQE that does not typically exceed 65–70%. Depending on the detector, as much as 30% of all available x-rays are not effectively utilized for image formation. Additional reduction in dose can potentially be achieved by using detectors with improved DQE characteristics.

One approach to increase low-frequency DQE is to increase the quantum efficiency of these detectors, but this may result in further degradation of spatial resolution. In scintillator-based detectors, increasing the thickness of the scintillator for better quantum efficiency will degrade spatial resolution because of increased light diffusion. In a-Se detectors, increasing the thickness of the photoconductor may

increase charge trapping, which could affect overall image quality. Overall, DQE characteristics of digital mammography systems will gradually continue to improve, driven primarily by advancements in readout technology and low-noise electronics, and substantial improvements will likely require new developments in material science pertaining to scintillators, photoconductors, and related materials used in x-ray detection. Figure 1.24 shows on example on how both DQE and spatial resolution may be improved by changing the geometry of mammographic image acquisition in scintillator-based detectors. In this approach, the amorphous silicon layer of the detector is deposited in a very thin substrate that exhibits very low absorption to x-rays. Currently, approximately 1 mm thick glass substrate is used, and this is prohibitively thick for mammographic x-ray energies. It is now technically feasible to use thinner and lower-density substrates for a-Si detectors, and this substrate material may be a polymer or other low x-ray attenuating material. X-rays that are transmitted through the breast pass though the substrate and the thin layer (typically about 1 μm thickness) of a-Si matrix and reach the scintillator. This geometry replicates the geometry with film-screen mammography by minimizing the path length between locations at which x-ray interaction occurs and the a-Si matrix layer. The reduced path length would limit lateral light diffusion, which will better preserve spatial resolution. The approach would also facilitate the use of thicker scintillator layers to improve quantum efficiency, and potentially the DQE.

The advent of digital breast tomosynthesis has meant that detector technology that was originally designed for mammography must also now perform digital breast tomosynthesis. This adaptation presents several challenges in terms of temporal

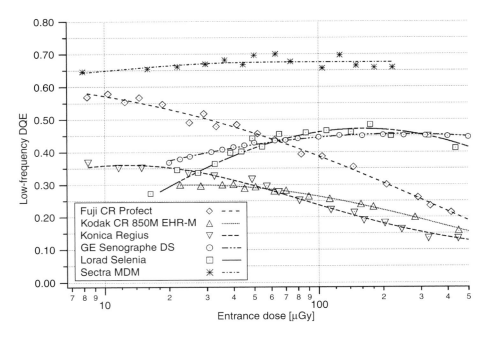

Figure 1.22 Low-frequency DQE characteristics of various digital mammography systems. Reproduced with permission from Monnin *et al.*, *Med Phys* 2007; **34**: 906–14 [51]. © American Association of Physicists in Medicine.

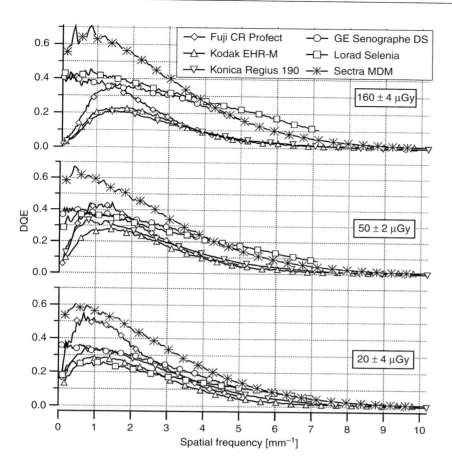

Figure 1.23 Frequency-dependent DQE characteristics of various digital mammography systems. Reproduced with permission from Monnin *et al.*, *Med Phys* 2007; **34**: 906–14 [51]. © American Association of Physicists in Medicine.

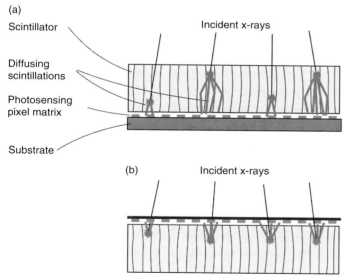

Figure 1.24 Improving digital mammography system performance by changing the geometry of mammographic image acquisition: (a) current approach, where x-rays interact on the surface furthest from the a-Si matrix; (b) reversing the geometry can improve spatial resolution.

response and fast readout characteristics, and low-dose perform-ance. Breast tomosynthesis requires the acquisition of multiple projection images (approximately 11–21 images) in as short a time as possible to minimize patient motion. Also, each x-ray projection is acquired with a dose that is approximately the dose of a single mammogram divided by the number of projection images. This creates a condition where for each projection image the detector receives very small x-ray fluence, and under these conditions the contribution of noise from the detector electronics becomes substantial, resulting in degradation of DQE and dose efficiency. This effect may be remediated by using a larger pixel size (pixel binning) for the tomosynthesis acquisition, a tech-nique that has been used in a-Se detectors, or by using a more efficient scintillator, a technique that has been used with scintil-lator-coupled a-Si detectors. In the pixel-binning approach, two or more neighboring pixels are combined during signal readout, thus providing for improved signal-to-noise ratio in the com-bined (binned) pixel. In the a-Si detectors, a thicker scintillator can provide improvement in quantum efficiency and hence higher signal per pixel. In both techniques, the trade-off is in the spatial resolution compared to conventional digital mam-mography acquisition. In the case of a-Se, pixel binning may be asymmetric (1×2 pixels) or symmetric (2×2 pixels) and is performed only during tomosynthesis. In a-Si detectors, the same pixel size and scintillator are used for mammography and tomo-synthesis acquisition. This reduced resolution in the plane of the breast parallel to the detector is tolerated, because of the limited depth information that is provided by tomosynthesis. The spatial resolution in the depth direction is poor (~1 mm slice with substantial out-of-slice artifacts), and is limited by the projection geometry and reconstruction and not by the detector pixel. The current trend is to develop hybrid systems that perform digital mammography and tomosynthesis, and the challenge is to develop detectors that can perform in a dual-use mode that can be optimized for both types of image acquisitions.

and the National Institute of Biomedical Imaging and Bioengineering. The contents are solely the responsibility of the authors and do not necessarily represent the official views of the NIH, NCI, or NIBIB.

Acknowledgments

This work reflects in part the experience and insight obtained while working under the support from grants R01 EB004015 (to Andrew Karellas), R21 CA134128 (to Andrew Karellas), and R01 CA128906 (to Srinivasan Vedantham) from the National Institutes of Health, the National Cancer Institute,

Disclosures

The authors have collaborated in the past with GE Global Research Center and they have a current collaboration with Hologic, Inc. There is an institutional research agreement between the University of Massachusetts Medical School and Koninklijke Philips Electronics N.V.

References

1. Egan RL. Experience with mammography in a tumor institution: evaluation of 1,000 studies. *Radiology* 1960; **75**: 894–900.

2. Bassett LW, Gold RH. The evolution of mammography. *AJR Am J Roentgenol* 1988; **150**: 493–8.

3. Price JL, Bler PD. The reduction of radiation and exposure time in mammography. *Br J Radiol* 1970; **43**: 251–5.

4. Shapiro S, Strax P, Venet L. Periodic breast cancer screening in reducing mortality from breast cancer. *JAMA* 1971; **215**: 1777–85.

5. Thurfjell EJ, Lindgren JA. Breast cancer survival rates with mammographic screening: similar favorable survival rates for women younger and those older than 50 years. *Radiology* 1996; **201**: 421–6.

6. Duffy SW, Tabar L, Chen HH, *et al.* The impact of organized mammography service screening on breast carcinoma mortality in seven Swedish counties. *Cancer* 2002; **95**: 458–69.

7. Tabar L, Vitak B, Chen HH, *et al.* Beyond randomized controlled trials: organized mammographic screening substantially reduces breast carcinoma mortality. *Cancer* 2001; **91**: 1724–31.

8. Swedish Organized Service Screening Evaluation Group. Reduction in breast cancer mortality from organized service screening with mammography: 1. Further confirmation with extended data. *Cancer Epidemiol Biomarkers Prev* 2006; **15**: 45–51.

9. Swedish Organized Service Screening Evaluation Group. Reduction in breast cancer mortality from the organised service screening with mammography: 2. Validation with alternative analytic methods. *Cancer Epidemiol Biomarkers Prev* 2006; **15**: 52–6.

10. Berry DA, Cronin KA, Plevritis SK, *et al.* Effect of screening and adjuvant therapy on mortality from breast cancer. *N Engl J Med* 2005; **353**: 1784–92.

11. Nishikawa RM, Mawdsley GE, Fenster A, Yaffe MJ. Scanned-projection digital mammography. *Med Phys* 1987; **14**: 717–27.

12. Maidment AD, Fahrig R, Yaffe MJ. Dynamic range requirements in digital mammography. *Med Phys* 1993; **20**: 1621–33.

13. Oestmann JW, Kopans D, Hall DA, *et al.* A comparison of digitized storage phosphors and conventional mammography in the detection of malignant microcalcifications. *Invest Radiol* 1988; **23**: 725–8.

14. Chan HP, Doi K, Vyborny CJ, *et al.* Improvement in radiologists' detection of clustered microcalcifications on mammograms: the potential of computer-aided diagnosis. *Invest Radiol* 1990; **25**: 1102–10.

15. Nishikawa RM, Giger ML, Doi K, Vyborny CJ, Schmidt RA. Computer-aided detection of clustered microcalcifications: an improved method for grouping detected signals. *Med Phys* 1993; **20**: 1661–6.

16. Kallergi M, Clark RA, Clarke LP. Medical image databases for CAD applications in digital mammography: design issues. *Stud Health Technol Inform* 1997; **43**: 601–5.

17. Kundel HL. Images, image quality and observer performance. *Radiology* 1979; **132**: 265–71.

18. Barrett HH, Swindell W. *Radiological Imaging: the Theory of Image Formation, Detection and Processing*, revised edn. New York, NY: Academic Press, 1981.

19. Dainty JC, Shaw R. *Image Science*. San Diego, CA: Academic Press, 1974.

20. Fujita H, Tsai DY, Itoh T, *et al.* A simple method for determining the modulation transfer-function in digital radiography. *IEEE Trans Med Imaging* 1992; **11**: 34–9.

21. Dobbins JT. Effects of undersampling on the proper interpretation of modulation transfer function, noise power spectra, and noise equivalent quanta of digital imaging systems. *Med Phys* 1995; **22**: 171–81.

22. Dobbins JT, Ergun DL, Rutz L, *et al.* DQE(f) of four generations of computed radiography acquisition devices. *Med Phys* 1995; **22**: 1581–93.

23. International Commission on Radiation Units and Measurements. *Medical Imaging: the Assessment of Image Quality*. Bethesda, MD: ICRU, 1996.

24. American College of Radiology. *Mammography Quality Control Manual*. Reston, VA: ACR, 1999.

25. Suryanarayanan S, Karellas A, Vedantham S, *et al.* Flat-panel digital mammography system: contrast-detail comparison between screen-film radiographs and hard-copy images. *Radiology* 2002; **225**: 801–7.

26. Burgess AE, Jacobson FL, Judy PF. Human observer detection experiments with mammograms and power-low noise. *Med Phys* 2001; **28**: 419–37.

27. Egan JP. *Signal Detection Theory and ROC Analysis*. New York, NY: Academic Press, 1975.

28. Pepe MS. *The Statistical Evaluation of Medical Tests for Classification and Prediction*. Oxford: Oxford University Press, 2003.

29. ROCKIT. Kurt Rossmann Laboratories for Radiologic Image Research, Department of Radiology, University of Chicago.

30. Vedantham S, Karellas A, Suryanarayanan S, *et al.* Mammographic imaging with a small format CCD-based digital cassette: physical characteristics of a clinical system. *Med Phys* 2000; **27**: 1832–40.

31. Williams MB, Simoni PU, Smilowitz L, *et al.* Analysis of the detective quantum efficiency of a developmental detector for digital mammography. *Med Phys* 1999; **26**: 2273–85.

32. Lewin JM, Hendrick RE, D'Orsi CJ, *et al.* Comparison of full-field digital mammography with screen-film mammography for cancer detection: results of 4,945 paired examinations. *Radiology*, 2001; **218**: 873–80.

33. Lewin JM, D'Orsi CJ, Hendrick RE, *et al.* Clinical comparison of full-field digital mammography and screen-film mammography for detection of breast cancer. *AJR Am J Roentgenol* 2002; **179**: 671–7.

34. Suryanarayanan S, Karellas A, Vedantham S. Physical characteristics of a full-field digital mammography system. *Nucl Instrum Methods Phys Res A* 2004; **533**: 560–70.

35. Vedantham S, Karellas A, Suryanarayanan S, *et al.* Full breast digital mammography with an amorphous silicon-based flat panel detector: physical characteristics of a clinical prototype. *Med Phys* 2000; **27**: 558–67.

36. Ghetti C, Borrini A, Ortenzia O, Rossi R, Ordonez PL. Physical characteristics of GE Senographe Essential and DS digital mammography detectors. *Med Phys* 2008; **35**: 456–63.

37. Tesic MM, Piccaro MF, Munier B. Full field digital mammography scanner. *Eur J Radiol* 1999; **31**: 2–17.

38. Arvanitis CD, Bohndiek SE, Blakesley J, Olivo A, Speller RD. Signal and noise transfer properties of CMOS based active pixel flat panel imager coupled to structured CsI:Tl. *Med Phys* 2009; **36**: 116–26.

39. Arvanitis CD, Bohndiek SE, Royle G, *et al.* Empirical electro-optical and x-ray performance evaluation of CMOS active pixels sensor for low dose, high resolution x-ray medical imaging. *Med Phys* 2007; **34**: 4612–25.

40. Stone MF, Zhao W, Jacak BV, *et al.* The x-ray sensitivity of amorphous selenium for mammography. *Med Phys* 2002; **29**: 319–24.

41. Saunders RS, Samei E, Jesneck JL, Lo JY. Physical characterization of a prototype selenium-based full field digital mammography detector. *Med Phys* 2005; **32**: 588–99.

42. Zhao W, Ji WG, Debrie A, Rowlands JA. Imaging performance of amorphous selenium based flat-panel detectors for digital mammography: characterization of a small area prototype detector. *Med Phys* 2003; **30**: 254–63.

43. Rowlands JA, Hunter DM, Araj N. X-ray imaging using amorphous selenium: a photoinduced discharge readout method for digital mammography. *Med Phys* 1991; **18**: 421–31.

44. MacDougall RD, Koprinarov I, Rowlands JA. The x-ray light valve: a low-cost, digital radiographic imaging system – spatial resolution. *Med Phys* 2008; **35**: 4216–27.

45. Reznik N, Komljenovic PT, Germann S, Rowlands JA. Digital radiography using amorphous selenium: photoconductively activated switch (PAS) readout system. *Med Phys* 2008; **35**: 1039–50.

46. Rivetti S, Lanconelli N, Bertolini M, *et al.* Physical and psychophysical characterization of a novel clinical system for digital mammography. *Med Phys* 2009; **36**: 5139–48.

47. Fetterly KA, Schueler BA. Performance evaluation of a "dual-side read" dedicated mammography computed radiography system. *Med Phys* 2003; **30**: 1843–54.

48. Seibert JA, Boone JM, Cooper VN, Lindfors KK. Cassette-based digital mammography. *Technol Cancer Res Treat* 2004; **3**: 413–27.

49. Rivetti S, Canossi B, Battista R, *et al.* Physical and clinical comparison between a screen-film system and a dual-side reading mammography-dedicated computed radiography system. *Acta Radiol* 2009; **50**: 1109–18.

50. Aslund M, Cederstrom B, Lundqvist M, Danielsson M. Physical characterization of a scanning photon counting digital mammography system based on Si-strip detectors. *Med Phys* 2007; **34**: 1918–25.

51. Monnin P, Gutierrez D, Bulling S, Guntern D, Verdun FR. A comparison of the performance of digital mammography systems. *Med Phys* 2007; **34**: 906–14.

Chapter 2

Image acquisition

Tanya W. Stephens and Jihong Wang

Introduction

One of the most recent advances in mammography is digital mammography. When first approved by the US Food and Drug Administration (FDA) in 2000, digital mammography systems were categorized as class III devices, because they were then considered novel systems for screening and diagnosing breast cancer [1]. The class III device category usually includes new technologies that have not been widely used and require proof of safety and effectiveness before the product can be approved for marketing. Other examples of class III devices include heart valves and orthopedic implants. As of January 2012, 22 digital mammography systems have been approved by the FDA (Table 2.1). From the time the first digital mammography system, the GE Senographe 2000D, was approved in 2000 until today, digital mammography has been validated by multiple scientific studies [2–4]. The benefits and risks of digital versus film-screen mammography have been well documented and well described. In November 2010 the FDA reclassified digital mammography systems as class II devices. Class I and class II devices pose lower risks and include adhesive bandages, wheelchairs, and many medical imaging technologies, such as magnetic resonance imaging (MRI) scanners and film-screen mammography. The class II device category usually requires submission of a premarket notification or a 510(k) to establish that the product is substantially equivalent to a device already on the market [1].

Physics of digital mammography

A simple, basic understanding of physics is useful in understanding digital mammography. Digital information is described by using the terms pixels, bits, and bytes. A pixel is a picture element. Digital images can be described as a two-dimensional grid of square picture elements or pixels. The size of a digital image is determined by the number of horizontal pixels and the number of vertical pixels (Figure 2.1). An image that is 200 pixels by 300 pixels is 200 pixels wide and 300 pixels high. Each pixel displays a fixed maximal number of gray shades. A bit or binary digit describes the shades of gray and has two possible values,

0 and 1. The number of shades of gray is equal to 2^x, where x is the number of bits. A 12-bit image (2^{12}) has 4096 shades of gray. A byte is a unit of digital information consisting of eight bits and is a power of two with the values 0 through 255. So eight bits or one byte has 256 shades of gray. The total size of an image is the total number of pixels multiplied by the number of bits per pixel. In an image 200 pixels by 300 pixels with a gray scale of 8 bits, the total number of bits would be 200 × 300 × 8, or 480 000 bits, or 60 000 bytes. An understanding of pixels, bits, and bytes is important because this terminology is used to express the amount of information within a digital mammogram, to describe the resolution of a workstation monitor, and to measure the amount of digital space needed for long-term storage in picture archiving and communication systems (PACS) [6,7].

Image acquistion

There are similarities and differences in image acquisition between film-screen and digital mammography. Externally, the film-screen and digital mammography units are similar in appearance. Both film-screen and digital mammograms are obtained with the use of a compression paddle, an x-ray tube, and x-rays, but image acquisition with digital mammography is achieved with a fixed or removable digital detector and a computer, rather than a film-screen cassette.

The image produced by film-screen mammography can be described by the characteristic film curve or HD curve (Figure 2.2), after Hurter and Driffield [8], where optical density is on the vertical axis and the log (exposure) is on the horizontal axis. To produce a film-screen mammogram with a wide dynamic range of tissue densities, exposures that align with the steep part of the characteristic curve are used. This set of densities is the latitude of the film. Film-screen mammography has a narrow latitude. Digital detectors allow for a wider latitude because in digital mammography there is a linear relationship between density and relative exposure. The latitude of film-screen mammography is 40 : 1; in digital mammography, the latitude is 1000 : 1 [10]. The wider latitude of digital mammography results in a broader range of exposures that will produce an acceptable image [6,10,11].

Digital Mammography: A Practical Approach, ed. Gary J. Whitman and Tamara Miner Haygood. Published by Cambridge University Press.
© Cambridge University Press 2013.

Table 2.1 FDA-approved digital mammography units [5].

System	Date
GE Senographe Care Full-Field Digital Mammography (FFDM) System	10/7/11
Planmed Nuance Excel Full-Field Digital Mammography (FFDM) System	9/23/11
Planmed Nuance Full-Field Digital Mammography (FFDM) System	9/23/11
Fuji Aspire HD Full-Field Digital Mammography (FFDM) System	9/1/11
Siemens Mammomat Inspiration Pure Full-Field Digital Mammography (FFDM) System	8/16/11
Hologic Selenia Encore Full-Field Digital Mammography (FFDM) System	6/15/11
Philips (Sectra) MicroDose L30 Full-Field Digital Mammography (FFDM) System	4/28/11
Hologic Selenia Dimensions Digital Breast Tomosynthesis (DBT) System	2/11/11
Siemens Mammomat Inspiration Full Field Digital Mammography (FFDM) System	2/11/11
Carestream Directview Computed Radiography (CR) Mammography System	11/3/10
Hologic Selenia Dimensions 2D Full Field Digital Mammography (FFDM) System	2/11/09
Hologic Selenia S Full Field Digital Mammography (FFDM) System	2/11/09
Siemens Mammomat Novation S Full Field Digital Mammography (FFDM) System	2/11/09
Hologic Selenia Full Field Digital Mammography (FFDM) System with a Tungsten target	11/2007
Fuji Computed Radiography Mammography Suite (FCRMS)	7/10/06
GE Senographe Essential Full Field Digital Mammography (FFDM) System	4/11/06
Siemens Mammomat Novation DR Full Field Digital Mammography (FFDM) System	8/20/04
GE Senographe DS Full Field Digital Mammography (FFDM) System	2/19/04
Lorad/Hologic Selenia Full Field Digital Mammography (FFDM) System	10/2/02
Lorad Digital Breast Imager Full Field Digital Mammography (FFDM) System	3/15/02
Fischer Imaging SenoScan Full Field Digital Mammography (FFDM) System	9/25/01
GE Senographe 2000D Full Field Digital Mammography (FFDM) System	1/28/00

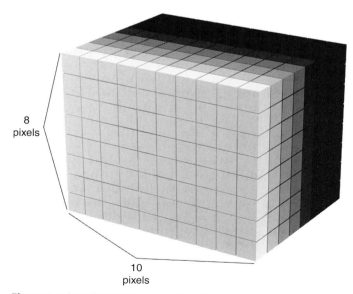

Figure 2.1 Size of a digital image. A digital image is composed of horizontal pixels and vertical pixels. This image is 10 pixels × 8 pixels.

The latitude of digital mammography is related to the dynamic range or depth of the recorded signal intensity. Dynamic range is recorded as a series of gray-scale shades. The numerical value of the dynamic range is expressed as bits or 2^x steps of digitalization. The dynamic range required for digital mammographic imaging is related to the number of gray-scale shades that will adequately display the most and least attenuating structures in the breast [6].

Spatial resolution is the ability of an imaging system to allow two adjacent structures to be visualized as being separate. Alternatively, spatial resolution can be thought of as a measure of the distinctness of an edge of a mass [12]. Digital mammography has lower spatial resolution than film-screen mammography. Film-screen mammography has a line-pair resolution of 20 line-pairs/mm; digital mammography's resolution is 5–10 line-pairs/mm. This resolution is equivalent to pixels that are 25 μm apart.

The lower spatial resolution of digital mammography is compensated for by its higher contrast resolution. The resolution of the final digital image is described by the modulation

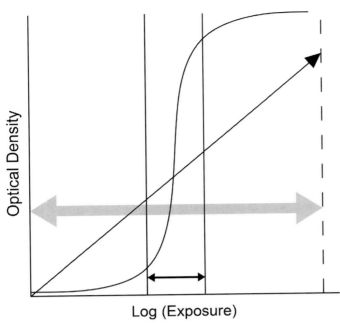

Figure 2.2 Characteristic film curve or HD curve. The relationship between optical density (vertical axis) and log (exposure) (horizontal axis) is shown by the S-shaped curve for film and the diagonal arrow for digital detectors. Film has a narrow latitude (small black arrow) versus the wide latitude (large gray arrow) of digital detectors.

transfer function (MTF). The MTF is a method to measure the spatial frequency response of an imaging component or a system. The MTF is the contrast at a given spatial frequency relative to lower frequencies.

In film-screen mammography, the focal spot and the screen both contribute to the MTF [13]. With digital mammography, the MTF is affected by the focal spot size, the detector element size, the active region of the detector, the spread of the signal in the detector, and the laser of the plate reader [13,14].

Digital images have lower noise than film-screen mammograms because of a reduction in quantum mottle and because of the elimination of granular artifacts from film emulsion [9,15,16]. In radiology, noise can be defined as any fluctuations in an image that do not correspond to variations in the x-ray attenuation of the object being imaged [12].

Digital detectors

One important difference between digital detectors and film is that digital detectors collect x-ray photons in discrete increments and image signal intensity. Film collects x-ray photons in a more continuous fashion [15]. Digital detectors offer improved detection and conspicuity of lesions compared with film-screen systems because of improved efficiency of absorption of x-ray photons, a linear response over a wide range of incident radiation intensities, and the low noise of the system [11,15]. The resolution of the digital detector is determined by the size of the DEL. The DEL is the smallest detector element. Digital detectors are usually composed of several DELs. As the

digital detector element size decreases, better spatial resolution should result.

Digital detectors may be indirect or direct. There are two subtypes of indirect detectors, those based on storage phosphor technology and those with a scintillator plus a photodetector such as amorphous silicon thin-film-transitor (TFT) array technology. Fluorescent screens such as cesium iodide (CsI) may be used to convert absorbed x-rays to visible light photons. Light-sensitive detector arrays, composed of amorphous silicon diodes or charge-coupled devices, are placed behind the screen. These arrays measure the converted light photons produced pixel by pixel.

Amorphous selenium plates can be used to acquire digital images. Amorphous selenium is an excellent absorber of x-rays and an excellent capacitor that stores the charge created by ionization at sites where x-rays are absorbed. The charge distribution from the plate is recorded by an electronic read-out. The readout is obtained by scanning the selenium plate with a laser beam or by placing a silicon diode array in contact with one side of the selenium plate.

Direct detectors capture and measure the x-rays directly. After the digital detector captures the x-ray photons, the image is processed by a computer. The image can be displayed on film or on a computer monitor.

Computed radiography (CR) and digital radiography (DR) are commonly used terms for digital radiographic detectors [12]. Computed radiography uses photostimulable phosphors (BaFBr:Eu). The plate absorbs x-rays just like film-screen cassettes; however, x-ray absorption with photostimulable phosphors causes electrons to be promoted to higher energy levels. Electrons are released when the laser scans the phosphor plate. Digital radiography is an imaging system that reads the transmitted x-ray signal immediately after exposure with the detector in place [12]. The historical nomenclature of "computed radiography" and "digital radiography" becomes less accurate as technology advances and distinct classification into these two broad categories is no longer possible. Perhaps more appropriate is a distinction based on cassette (CR) versus cassetteless (DR) operation [12].

Film-screen versus digital mammography

In film-screen mammography, the image acquisition begins with exposure of the breast to x-rays. The x-rays pass through the breast and are absorbed and scattered within the tissues. The attenuated x-rays pass through the grid, interact with image receptors, and form a latent image on the film. The exposed film is processed by reducing the silver ions to metallic silver. Fixer removes excess silver [6,17]. In screen mammography the film serves as the medium of image acquisition, display, and storage [13]. Because the processes of image acquisition, display, and storage are coupled, any problem with any one of the functions will affect the entire process. Film-screen mammograms are viewed on a viewbox and then stored in the radiology film archives.

With digital mammography, the mammogram may be viewed on a viewbox if hard copies of the images are printed on film, or viewed on a computer monitor (soft copy) and the digital images are then stored in picture archiving and communication systems (PACS). It takes several minutes to develop mammograms with film-screen mammography technology, whereas digital mammograms take less than a minute to appear on a computer monitor after image acquisition. The speed of the digital image acquisition leads to shorter examination times. With film-screen mammography, post-processing is not possible. With digital mammography, each component may be optimized independently of the other processes. The digital images may be manipulated at the workstation. The orientation, contrast, and brightness can be adjusted, images can be inverted, and digital magnification can be applied to

selected regions of the mammogram or the entire mammogram after the examination has been completed [18]. This leads to fewer repeat mammograms and optimization of the images so that lesions are more apparent to the radiologist.

Final thoughts

Over 80% of the mammographic systems in the United States are digital, and nearly all newly sold mammographic systems are digital. This phenomenon is occurring for several reasons, including the general trend of complete digital conversion of diagnostic imaging in hospital systems and the conversion to electronic medical records and PACS.

References

1. US Food and Drug Administration. FDA reclassifies certain digital mammography devices, 2010. http://www.fda.gov/ NewsEvents/Newsroom/ PressAnnouncements/ucm232505.htm (accessed January 2012).

2. Lewin JM, D'Orsi CJ, Hendrick RE, et al. Clinical comparison of full-field digital mammography and screen-film mammography for detection of breast cancer. AJR Am J Roentgenol 2002; 179: 671–7.

3. Skaane P, Skjennald A. Screen-film mammography versus full-field digital mammography with soft-copy reading: randomized trial in a population-based screening program: the Oslo II Study. Radiology 2004; 232: 197–204.

4. Skaane P, Hofvind S, Skjennald A. Randomized trial of screen-film versus full-field digital mammography with soft-copy reading in population-based screening program: follow-up and final results of Oslo II study. Radiology 2007; 244: 708–17.

5. US Food and Drug Administration. FFDM and DBT Systems, 2012. www.fda. gov/Radiation-EmittingProducts/ MammographyQualityStandardsActand Program/FacilityCertificationand

Inspection/ucm114148.htm (accessed January 2012).

6. Hashimoto BE. Physics of digital mammography. In Hashimoto BE, ed., Practical Digital Mammography. New York, NY: Thieme, 2008; pp. 4–8.

7. James JJ. The current status of digital mammography. Clin Radiol 2004; 59: 1–10.

8. Hurter F, Driffield VC. Photo-chemical investigations and a new method of the sensitivities of photographic plates. J Soc Chem Indust 1890; 9: 455–69.

9. Feig S, Yaffe MJ. Current status of digital mammography. Semin Ultrasound CT MR 1996; 17: 424–43.

10. Mahesh M. AAPM/RSNA Physics tutorial for residents: digital mammography: an overview. Radiographics 2004; 24: 1747–60.

11. Feig SA, Yaffe MJ. Digital mammography. Radiographics 1998; 18: 893–901.

12. Williams MB, Krupinshki EA, Strauss KJ, et al. Digital radiography image quality: image acquisition. J Am Coll Radiol 2007; 4: 371–88.

13. Kuzmiak CM, Pisano ED, Cole EB, et al. Comparison of full-field digital mammography to screen-film mammography with respect to contrast and spatial resolution in tissue equivalent breast phantoms. Med Phys 2005; 32: 3144–50.

14. Yaffe MJ, Mainprize JG. Detectors for digital mammography. In Pisano ED, Yaffe MJ, Kuzmiak CM, eds., Digital Mammography. Philadelphia, PA: Lippincott Williams and Wilkins, 2004; pp. 15–26.

15. Pisano E, Yaffe M. Digital mammography. Breast Dis 1998; 10: 127–36.

16. Nees A. Digital mammography: are there advantages in screening for breast cancer? Acad Radiol 2006; 15: 401–7.

17. Ikeda DM. Mammographic acquisition: screen-film and digital mammography, computer-aided detection, and the mammographic quality standards act. In Ikeda DM, ed., Breast Imaging: the Requisites. Philadelphia, PA: Mosby, 2004; pp. 1–23.

18. Smith AP, Hall PA, Marcello DM. Emerging technologies in breast cancer detection. Radiol Manage 2004; 26: 16–24.

Preparing digital mammography images for interpretation

Basak E. Dogan

Introduction

The basic advantages and disadvantages of digital mammography and the relevant technology are discussed in other chapters of this book. Results of the Digital Mammographic Imaging Screening Trial (DMIST), released in September 2005, show that digital mammography may be more accurate at detecting breast cancer in some women than standard film-screen mammography [1,2]. In that study, digital and standard film-screen mammography had similar accuracy for many women. However, digital mammography was significantly better at screening women younger than 50 years, regardless of their breast tissue density, and women of any age with very dense or extremely dense breasts. In this context, the significant advantages of digital mammography for image interpretation include the following:

- physician manipulation of breast images for more accurate detection of breast cancer
- ability to correct underexposure or overexposure of images without having to repeat the mammogram
- transmittal of images over a network for remote consultation with other physicians

The primary focus of this chapter is post-processing of raw digital mammography images for interpretation, including digital mammography display, and comparison with prior mammography studies, including analog (film-screen or digitized) mammography studies.

Image processing in digital mammography

Film-screen mammography has limited detection capability for low-contrast lesions in dense breasts. This limitation poses a problem for the estimated 40% of mammography subjects who have dense breasts [3]. The goal of image processing in digital mammography is to improve for the human observer the visibility of the signs of breast cancer and to decrease the visibility of structures and noise that may either mimic or mask the signs of cancer. All radiographic images of the breast include normal structures, among them glandular tissue, fibrous tissue, vessels, and skin pores, which under certain circumstances can mimic the signs of cancer or hide the signs of cancer. Furthermore, all breast radiographs include system-induced noise of several types, and this noise can both resemble the signs of breast cancer and obscure them. Breasts can be fatty, heterogeneously dense, or homogeneously dense. The optimum image processing will differ for these different patterns of breast composition and for individual variation within these patterns.

Digital mammography systems, unlike film-screen mammography systems, allow manipulation of fine differences in image contrast by means of image processing algorithms. As a result, very subtle differences between abnormal and normal but dense tissue can be made more obvious. Different display algorithms have advantages and disadvantages for the specific tasks required in breast imaging – diagnosis and screening. Some algorithms utilized frequently for post-processing of digital mammography are the following:

- intensity windowing (IW)
  - manual (MIW)
  - histogram-based (HIW)
  - mixture-model (MMIW)
- unsharp masking and Trex processing
- peripheral equalization
- contrast-limited adaptive histogram equalization (CLAHE)

Most manufacturers use a combination of different algorithms that include intensity windowing, unsharp masking, and peripheral equalization to optimize the digital image. This chapter discusses only clinically relevant aspects of these processing techniques, with attention to special uses of CLAHE in digitized film-screen mammography images within the context of soft-copy mammography interpretation.

Intensity windowing

Intensity windowing algorithms act on individual pixels within an image. A small portion of the full intensity range of an image is selected and then remapped to the full intensity range of the display device. This process allows selection of specific intensity values of interest. For example, intensity values that represent

Digital Mammography: A Practical Approach, ed. Gary J. Whitman and Tamara Miner Haygood. Published by Cambridge University Press.
© Cambridge University Press 2013.

(a)

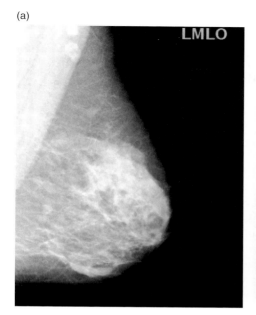

(b)

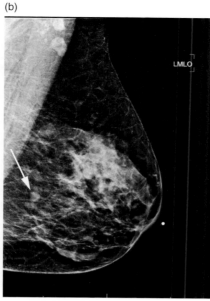

Figure 3.1 (a) Raw digital left mediolateral oblique mammogram acquired with compression thickness 58 mm, kVp 30, mAs =106. (b) After Trex processing, enhanced visibility of the breast edge and breast mass (arrow) borders is observed.

abnormal tissue or dense but normal tissue are selected to allow exaggeration of small differences in intensity values between the two objects, thus potentially increasing the conspicuity of any abnormal regions.

Unsharp masking

In order to enhance lesion edge sharpness, most digital mammography post-processing algorithms utilize unsharp masking. Unsharp masking refers to a linear or nonlinear low-pass filter that amplifies the image's high-frequency components, creating a filtered blurred, or "unsharp," positive which serves as a "mask" of the original image. The image values that result are then combined with the original image [4]. The final image preserves much of the detail of the original image, but large structures are presented with less contrast, thereby reducing the dynamic range required to display the image. The image can then be processed with an intensity windowing algorithm (manual or automated) to achieve the desired contrast levels. The intended effect of unsharp masking is to enhance the edge visibility of the borders of mass lesions. Digital unsharp masking is a flexible and powerful way to increase the sharpness of lesion borders. The pitfall of this method is that even an indistinct mass can appear more circumscribed when this algorithm is applied.

Trex processing (developed by Trex Medical Corporation) uses a histogram-based form of unsharp masking, the details of which are held confidential by the company (Figure 3.1).

Peripheral equalization

The thickness of breast tissue under compression varies. The outer edges of the breast, which are thinner than the interior,

are typically overpenetrated by x-rays at image acquisition. If the central parenchyma is presented with high contrast, then the peripheral tissue will appear very black on the film and may be difficult to distinguish visually from the black film background.

Peripheral equalization enhances visualization of tissue located near the periphery of the breast [5,6]. In peripheral equalization, a low-pass spatial filter is applied to the image to create a blurred "mask" that represents primarily the coarsest variations in signal, which are related to variations in breast thickness. The algorithm is constrained to act only on pixels that lie within the breast and where the breast thickness is changing. There are also constraints placed on the total amount of enhancement to avoid disturbing artifacts at the skin line. The result is that the digital values of pixels located near the periphery are changed so that the absolute intensities of the image become "flatter" across the mammogram. The local contrasts between pixels located near each other, which represent compositional variations in tissue, are not suppressed. In fact, because the part of the dynamic range of the film required to represent thickness changes is no longer required, it is possible to increase the contrast of the breast tissue if desired.

Abrupt changes in breast thickness or tissue density separating the central and peripheral regions of a thick breast may cause the algorithm-processing software to create a falsely exaggerated boundary (Figure 3.2). This artifact does not, however, interfere with diagnostic interpretation of images [7].

Contrast-limited adaptive histogram equalization

In mammographic imaging, use of high-contrast film-screen combinations results in underexposure of the dense mammary gland and overexposure of the breast periphery, which degrades image contrast. CLAHE is a special class of adaptive histogram equalization that maximizes contrast throughout an

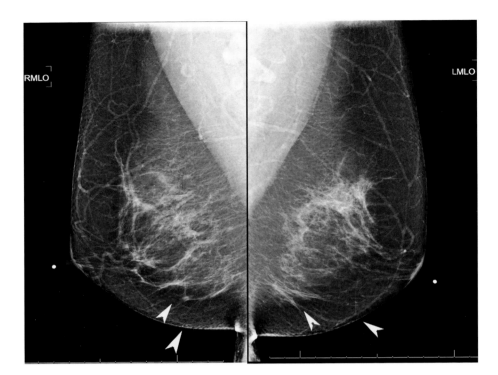

Figure 3.2 False breast "edge" created by differences in tissue thickness in the center and periphery of the breast, compared to the skin line (arrowheads). Note peripheral equalization function that helps visualize the inferior skin.

image by adaptively enhancing the contrast of each pixel relative to its local neighborhood [8,9]. This process improves contrast for all levels of contrast (small and large) in the original image. For adaptive histogram equalization to enhance local contrast, histograms are calculated for small regional areas of pixels, producing local histograms. These local histograms are then equalized or remapped from the often narrow range of intensity values indicative of a central pixel and its closest neighbors to the full range of intensity values available in the display (Figure 3.3).

CLAHE limits the maximum contrast adjustment that can be made to any local histogram. This limitation is useful in that the resulting image does not become too noisy. The size of the neighbor region is controlled by means of the region size parameter. Smaller regions allow better enhancement of the contrast of smaller spatial scale structures. In digital mammograms processed with CLAHE, lesions appear obvious relative to the background and the image detail is very good. The images do, however, have an obvious graininess, which is due to the enhanced visibility of both image signal and image noise with this algorithm. Again, this algorithm might be helpful in allowing radiologists to see subtle edge information, such as spiculation [8]. It might, however, degrade performance in the screening setting by enhancing the visibility of noise information that could simulate calcifications; therefore, it is not used routinely for image processing.

CLAHE may also have a role in improving image contrast of digitized analog mammograms by overcoming unequal areas of overexposure and underexposure, although available data regarding its feasibility for this application are limited [8].

Digital mammography soft-copy and hard-copy display

The method used for digital mammography display further defines the performance of the system and the information available to the reader. Monitors can display images at the exact same size as the original acquisition, or at smaller or larger sizes. Cathode ray tube (CRT) monitors available for soft-copy interpretation of digital mammograms provide 2048 × 2560 pixels displayed over monitor sizes of 30 × 40 cm. Over the past few years, liquid crystal display (LCD) screens have mostly replaced CRTs in clinical practice. The mechanism of image formation in LCD screens is practically the same as those used in standard computer monitors and commercial LCD televisions. The difference is only quantitative, in that medical LCDs may have a resolution of up to 3840 matrix pixels, and they lack a color mechanism. Monitor size is 18.5″ height × 15.2″ width × 4.1″ depth (470 × 387 × 103 mm). The radiologist needs to see the overview of images compared to the opposite breast, as well as old films for comparison to evaluate asymmetry, gross change, and masses; therefore, most soft-copy systems first bring up the image at less than full spatial resolution, and then allow the reader to systematically navigate through the whole image at full spatial resolution. The monitor also has the flexibility to set the gray level across the entire gray scale.

The luminance performance of a display has a significant effect on image quality. Although there are no specific threshold values for these quantities, their values need to ensure an appropriate range of luminance. The American College of Radiology (ACR) recommends that mammography monitor

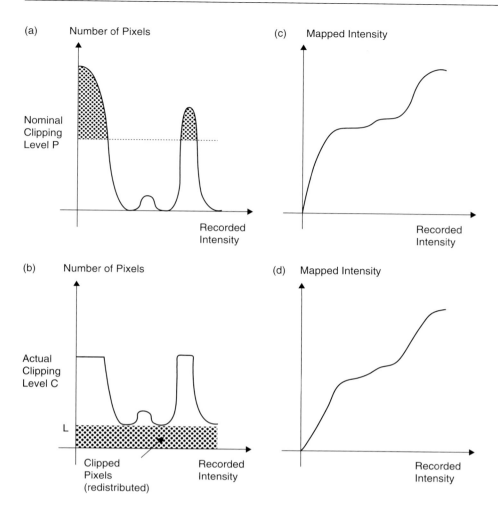

(a) Number of Pixels

Nominal Clipping Level P

Recorded Intensity

(b) Number of Pixels

Actual Clipping Level C

L

Clipped Pixels (redistributed) Recorded Intensity

(c) Mapped Intensity

Recorded Intensity

(d) Mapped Intensity

Recorded Intensity

Figure 3.3 Clipping with CLAHE. Graphs show how CLAHE redistributes the mapped intensities of the pixels in an image: (a, b) histograms; (c, d) mapping function. Adapted from Pisano *et al.*, *Radiographics* 2000; **20**: 1479–91 [9].

brightness be measured in nits (i.e. light in candelas per square meter [cd/m^2]) and maintained at a minimum of 514 nits or 150 footlambert (fL) (1 fL = 3.426 cd/m^2) [10]. Dome E5 monitors utilized in our institution have a brightness of 750 nits or 219 fL.

The existing recommendations for hard-copy film-screen printing are utilized uniformly when printing digital images. The spatial sampling of a laser printer should at least match the size of the detector element, so that the printing device is not the limiting factor. Images should be printed so that they match the real size of the imaged anatomy. When printing the digital mammogram on film, use of standard 18 × 24 cm or 24 × 30 cm films results in some loss of image size. Printing the images on smaller films shrinks the image so that the pixels occupy less absolute space than they did on the monitor, but objects appear smaller than they are on the digital image (making them more difficult for the reader to identify) or even imperceptible. If the digital mammography image is printed on a larger film than the utilized detector size, on the other hand, each pixel occupies more space on the film than the original, resulting in a magnified image. This serves only to

make the small objects more evident and may obviate the use of a magnifying glass to see these lesions, as the information available for interpretation would not change. ACR recommends that viewbox luminescence levels for mammography be maintained at 3000 nits (878 fL) or higher [10].

Soft-copy hanging protocols and image annotation

The quality of the information perceived from an image is affected not only by the inherent quality of the mammogram displayed on the soft-copy display device, but also on the manner in which the image is displayed. High-quality displays need an effective interface to enable full utilization of their capability.

In a typical mammography case interpretation, as many as 8 or 16 mammograms may need to be reviewed, corresponding to current or prior craniocaudal (CC) or mediolateral oblique (MLO) mammographic views of the left and right breasts. The interpretation usually begins with review of global views of at least four of these images. In terms of presentation ergonomics, there is no universally accepted format to display so many mammograms, and users have different display preferences. The four

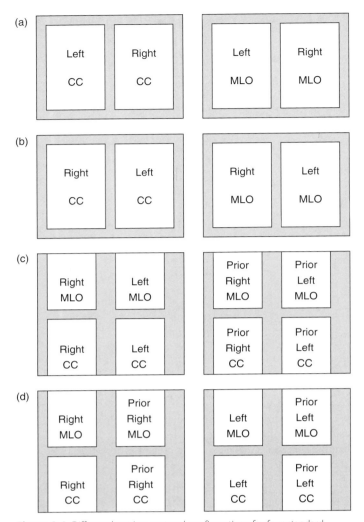

Figure 3.4 Different hanging protocol configurations for four standard screening mammography views in two monitors: (a, b) current mammography views; (c, d) comparison with prior mammograms.

images may be configured in four differing ways (Figure 3.4). Given this large potential for variability, a mammography workstation should be highly configurable, enabling the user to set up the default presentation according to his or her preferences.

Two monitors per workstation is usually optimal. Although many images may need to be viewed in a single interpretation session, multi-image comparisons rely mostly on gross differences in the images, and usually no more than two images need to be compared at high resolution at a given time. As the temporal channels of the human visual system are more sensitive than the spatial ones, there are advantages to comparing images temporally by toggling between images, as opposed to viewing images side by side. More than four monitors would interfere with the efficiency of interpretation.

The user interface must provide full visualization of the image data through the following functions:

- magnification and zoom function for full display of the spatial domain
- window and leveling
- image processing
- advanced processing and computer-aided techniques

The interface should be intuitive and ideally imitate the radiologist's established reading protocol.

Maintaining and monitoring the quality of the display device is of prime importance in maintaining a high-quality mammography operation. At the outset, a mammographic display device should be acceptance tested by a qualified medical physicist. An annual inspection and quarterly or monthly evaluation should follow. The display must also be examined on a daily basis by the user to ensure proper performance. Within this spectrum of testing, the tests range from objective quantitative tests at acceptance testing to fast visual tests performed daily.

References

1. Pisano ED, Gatsonis C, Hendrick E, *et al.* Digital Mammographic Imaging Screening Trial (DMIST) Investigators Group. Diagnostic performance of digital versus film mammography for breast-cancer screening. *N Engl J Med* 2005; **353**: 1773–83.

2. Pisano ED, Gatsonis CA, Yaffe MJ, *et al.* American College of Radiology Imaging Network digital mammographic imaging screening trial: objectives and methodology. *Radiology* 2005; **236**: 404–12.

3. Shtern F. Digital mammography and related technologies: a perspective from the National Cancer Institute. *Radiology* 1992; **183**: 629–30.

4. Chan HP, Vyborny CJ, MacMahon H, *et al.* Digital mammography ROC studies of the effects of pixel size and unsharp-mask filtering on the detection of subtle microcalcifications. *Invest Radiol* 1987; **22**: 581–9.

5. Byng JW, Critten JP, Yaffe MJ. Thickness equalization processing for mammographic images. *Radiology* 1997; **203**: 564–8.

6. Bick U, Giger ML, Schmidt RA, Nishikawa RM, Doi K. Density correction of peripheral breast tissue on digital mammograms. *Radiographics* 1996; **16**: 403–11.

7. Ayyala RS, Chorlton M, Behrman RH, Kornguth PJ, Slanetz PJ. Digital mammographic artifacts on full field

systems: what are they and how do I fix them? *Radiographics* 2008; **28**: 1999–2008.

8. Pisano ED, Zong S, Hemminger BM, *et al.* Contrast limited adaptive histogram equalization image processing to improve the detection of simulated spiculations in dense mammograms. *J Digit Imaging* 1998; **11**: 193–200.

9. Pisano ED, Cole EB, Hemminger BM, *et al.* Image processing algorithms for digital mammography: a pictorial essay. *Radiographics* 2000; **20**: 1479–91.

10. Siegel E., Krupinsky E, Samei E, *et al.* Digital mammography image quality: image display. *J Am Coll Radiol* 2006; **3**: 615–27.

Image display and visualization in digital mammography

Jihong Wang and William R. Geiser

Introduction

Image display and visualization is the final but a critical step in the entire process of digital mammography. Using picture archiving and communication systems (PACS) workstations, radiologists can review digital mammographic images on computer monitors instead of on film to make their diagnoses. The computer monitors that are used for display and visualization of digital mammographic images are extremely important parts of digital mammography systems. Since the quality and characteristics of the monitors will directly affect the image quality and thus the radiologist's diagnostic accuracy and efficiency, these monitors need to be optimized and checked for quality on a regular basis.

In traditional film-screen mammography, mammographic images are captured directly on film and the films are displayed and viewed on light boxes for interpretation. The film's inherent characteristics directly determine the final quality of the mammographic images. One of the major changes brought about by digital mammography and the implementation of PACS/electronic medical record (EMR) systems is the separation of image acquisition and image display, enabling simultaneous access to the same images at multiple locations. This arrangement has overcome some of the inefficiencies in the workflow for traditional film-based mammography operation and introduced some challenges in quality control (QC) and quality assurance (QA) in digital mammography in order to ensure consistent and optimal image quality.

It is important to realize that unlike film-screen mammography, digital mammography images displayed on PACS workstations can be adjusted for contrast and brightness after the image data have been acquired. In digital mammography patient images are captured by a digital receptor and converted into digital image data consisting of bits and bytes. Unlike film-based mammography, these digital images can be immediately accessed from any connected PACS workstations by different individuals at the same time, tremendously improving workflow efficiency and information access, and thus patient care. On the other hand, it is also important for images displayed on these workstations to have consistent and optimal

quality to ensure high-quality mammographic interpretations. Ironically, in the early days of digital mammography, because of the lack of adequate digital image display devices (i.e., computer display monitors with adequate spatial and contrast resolution for mammography), mammographic images acquired digitally were printed on film using laser printers for image interpretation.

Since the late 1990s, advancement in liquid crystal display (LCD) flat-panel monitor technology has made high-resolution flat-panel monitors readily available for medical use. Flat-panel LCD monitors used for today's medical image display have higher resolution, less power consumption, much lighter weight, and less size than their cathode ray tube (CRT) predecessors, making LCDs the dominant image display devices used in medicine. Other new image display technologies, such as organic light-emitting diodes (OLEDs), which promise brighter images and less power consumption, are also under development and may become commercially available in the near future.

Image display workstations for digital mammography

Today's digital image display workstations for digital mammography interpretation usually consist of two or more high-resolution medical-grade monitors and one or two color monitors (Figure 4.1). The high-resolution medical-grade monitors are usually monochromatic and with high brightness. Connected to these high-resolution monitors are specialized graphics cards, which are an integral part of the digital image display system. Such cards are typically located inside the computer box. The function of a graphics card is to convert the digital image data matrix to a video signal output to a display device (e.g., LCD monitor), on which the image is formed. Some newer computer motherboards have graphics cards integrated into their chipsets. However, most medical-grade monitors still use separate graphics cards because of the special requirements of medical image display devices.

Digital Mammography: A Practical Approach, ed. Gary J. Whitman and Tamara Miner Haygood. Published by Cambridge University Press.
© Cambridge University Press 2013.

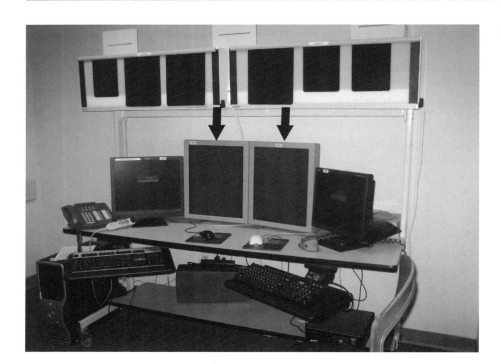

Figure 4.1 A digital mammography workstation with two high-resolution 5 MP monitors centrally (arrows) and two color monitors (one on each side).

For digital mammography, there are several steps in the process of converting the bits and bytes of the digital image data matrix into the final image visible by a human observer on the computer monitor. From image acquisition to image display, several conversions are performed on the digital image data; the conversion functions are contained in and are therefore sometimes referred to as look-up tables (LUTs). The LUTs are applied to the digital image data before the data are finally presented on computer display monitors as a gray-scale or a color image that can be viewed by human viewers.

The first conversion (via LUT) applied to the digital image data usually occurs on the graphics card, whereby pixel values of the digital mammography image data are converted to digital driving levels; these in turn are converted to video signal voltages. The video signal voltages are then sent from the graphics card through a standard interface (e.g., video graphics array [VGA] or digital visual interface [DVI]) to the monitor. Within the monitor, the input video signal voltage from the graphics card is converted to a specific luminance level for each image pixel. These pixels form a dot matrix image, which can be seen by human viewers. Usually, after these conversions, the relationship between the input pixel value of the mammography image data and the luminance level of the corresponding pixel on the monitor surface is nonlinear.

Monitors used in digital mammography

The diagnostic quality and accuracy in digital mammography is partially dependent on whether the information contained in the digital mammographic image data can be displayed with high fidelity. In the end, radiologists or other human observers cannot "see" the bits and bytes in a digital image, and the quality of an image display system (consisting of both the monitor and the graphics card) will affect the ability to present high-quality images. Computer monitors used for medical image displays (or medical-grade monitors) usually have higher spatial and contrast resolution, especially for those used for digital mammography. Matching graphics cards and driver software are also required. Because of the limited market size, medical-grade display monitors are usually much more expensive than computer monitors designed for general consumer use.

Since the introduction of medical-grade flat-panel LCD monitors in the late 1990s, these monitors have became dominant in the medical image display arena due to their low energy consumption (~30–50% less than their predecessors, equivalently sized CRT monitors), high luminance output, light weight, smaller footprint, and virtually no glare. Earlier flat-panel LCD monitors had been limited to spatial resolution of less than 3 megapixels (MP) and were monochromatic. Today 5 MP monitors, some with even higher resolution and in color, are readily available and have become more common in digital mammography. Almost 100% of all medical-grade monitors sold today are the flat-panel LCD type. The most common configuration of digital mammography image review workstations is two high-resolution medical-grade monitors (5 MP) and one color consumer-grade monitor.

The flat-panel LCD monitor is based on active matrix liquid crystal display (AMLCD) technology, which started in the late 1980s, driven mainly by the demand of the general consumer computer market. These monitors then came into the medical display marketplace, benefiting from the consumer market demand for flat-panel monitors, which drove manufacturing costs down dramatically. LCD display devices rely on the electro-optical characteristics of liquid crystals (LCs). The polarization properties of LC molecules can be altered by applying an external electrical field. Consequently, the optical characteristics of the LC material can be controlled electronically. More specifically, the polarization orientation of a light beam passing through the LC material layer can be modified by varying the applied voltage of this electrical field. This modification is called the "electro-optical effect," and it is used in LCD monitors to modulate light transmission. An LCD-based image display device utilizes a large number of such LC cells, with each representing a pixel on the monitor.

One of the unique aspects of LCD devices is that the light emitted from the monitor surface is non-Lambertian. As a consequence, the intensity of the light emitted from the LCD monitor surface is not symmetrical. In other words, the intensity of the light measured at different angles from the central axis of the monitor surface may differ markedly due to the specific designs of the LCD flat-panel monitors, resulting in a potentially severe angular dependence of the output luminance level or light intensity. The angular dependence of LCD monitors can be quite severe and may affect image contrast as a function of the viewing angle. Therefore, it is important for the viewer to sit directly in front of the monitor when viewing and interpreting mammographic images, instead of at an off-axis angle. In the past few years, newly improved LCD designs, such as molecular alignment in sub-regions within each individual pixel, in-plane switching, and other technologies to compensate for optical anisotropy, have dramatically minimized such angular dependence in LCD monitors.

Classification and quality standards for monitors in digital mammography

Medical image display monitors can be mostly categorized based on their clinical usage. Depending on their primary purposes in the clinical setting, monitors at various workstations may differ in quality and cost. There are usually two classes of monitors used in digital mammography workstations according to the purpose of their primary usage.

Class 1 monitors are designated to be used for medical image interpretation and for making primary diagnoses. The two or more high-resolution, high-brightness monitors commonly used in a mammography workstation are class 1 monitors, since they are designated for viewing and interpreting digital mammography images. Class 1 monitors are usually 5 MP monitors with matching high-performance graphics cards. These monitors require stringent and routine QC checks to ensure they meet the highest performance specifications and conform to Digital Imaging and Communications in Medicine (DICOM) standards, and they are mostly located in reading rooms with well-controlled ambient light and viewing conditions.

In digital mammography, class 2 monitors are mainly used for textual and other nondiagnostic uses. Depending on the specific task, the class 2 monitors are sometimes replaced with simple desktop color monitors designed for general consumer use. These monitors typically do not require any QC measures. A typical mammographic workstation is equipped with at least one such color monitor.

The performance characteristics of the monitors that are used for display and viewing of images in digital mammography should be evaluated and monitored routinely, because the characteristics may deteriorate over time or be changed by the ambient environment. Routine QC/QA is important because such deterioration may be subtle and occur over a long period of time, meaning that the user may not be aware of such changes. The American Association of Physicists in Medicine (AAPM) Task Group 18 (TG18) has developed a set of comprehensive guidelines and procedures that can be used for QC purposes [1,2].

Until several years ago, medical-grade display devices were mostly monochromatic. This was due to the fact that the luminance level and spatial resolution requirements for medical applications were much higher than consumer grade monitors could attain at that time. Today, a typical consumer-grade color monitor can have a maximum luminance level of 300 candelas per square meter (cd/m^2) or higher, with a spatial resolution matrix of approximately 1920×1080. A typical medical-grade monitor, however, usually requires a luminance level of $400 \ cd/m^2$ or higher and a spatial resolution matrix of at least 1500×2000. In the past two years, color monitors with high spatial resolution (3 MP and higher) and high luminance levels ($> 400 \ cd/m^2$) have become available, and they are popular for medical use. As more medical images are presented in color, such as those obtained by Doppler ultrasound, functional magnetic resonance imaging (MRI), nuclear medicine, and positron emission tomography (PET)/computed tomography (CT), medical-grade color monitors with adequate spatial resolution, luminance levels, and contrast will find increasing demand in PACS. Additionally, since most of the interfacing software on a PACS workstation and other text-based software such as radiology information system and hospital information system programs are in color, there will be a need for medical-grade color monitors for fully integrated PACS workstations in the future. Therefore, it is foreseeable that in the future all medical-grade monitors on PACS workstations will be color monitors, except in some very special cases.

An image display system consists of two major components: the image display devices (monitors) and the graphics control cards. Characteristics of both these components directly determine the displayed image quality. In fact, in order to guarantee optimal quality settings for display systems, many medical display device vendors either sell their monitors with their matching graphics cards or strongly recommend that customers use one specific graphics card that has been validated. Because of the multiple conversions that occur on the graphics card and the monitor itself, the final image's appearance and contrast can be altered by any one of these conversions (the LUTs). In other words, the final appearance of a digital mammographic image depends on the configurations of the LUTs on the graphics card and in the monitor. It is possible that identical display systems may have different image appearances depending on the devices' specific setups or configurations.

Because of the possibility of inadvertent change in a monitor's configuration, which may result in nonoptimal image quality, most monitor vendors "lock" the adjustment functions for their display devices, with access to those functions controlled by special passwords or service keys. Furthermore, although unlikely, a sudden power surge or corruption of software may cause the configuration to change. Therefore, it is imperative for users to routinely perform QC on all image display devices throughout a PACS to ensure consistency in quality and performance. AAPM Task Group 18 has developed a detailed guideline and recommended procedures for routine QC for image display devices. DICOM part 14 also specifies a standard luminance conversion table or curve. The DICOM LUT or DICOM luminance conversion table (DICOM Gray-Scale Display Function [GSDF]) is a standard with which all medical display devices should comply.

A GSDF is a conversion table that dictates the relationship between each input pixel value and the corresponding output luminance level of a display system. This table covers the entire range of input pixel values that the display system can sustain and the corresponding output luminance levels from darkest to brightest. The GSDF was selected by the DICOM standard committee because it was believed that when all image display devices satisfy these conditions (or are "in compliance with the DICOM standard GSDF"), identical images displayed on various devices have a similar appearance (that is, the image will be "equalized" on all display devices that conform to the standard LUT). The DICOM GSDF promises equal perceived relative contrast at all luminance levels that a display device is capable of producing, or "perception linearization."

One important aspect of the DICOM GSDF and compliance with the GSDF is that the GSDF is dependent upon both the minimum and the maximum luminance levels the image display spans, or the dynamic range of the display system, which also determines the contrast ratio described above. However, the contrast ratio may be changed depending on the ambient light conditions where the display systems are located. For instance, a system may need to be recalibrated if it is moved to a different location with different ambient light conditions.

Most high-end medical-grade display monitors are calibrated to conform to the DICOM GSDF either at the factory or at the customer's site on demand. The monitors should be verified regularly and recalibrated if needed to ensure compliance to the DICOM standard GSDF.

QC and QA for image display devices in PACS

Just as in traditional film-based mammography, where regular QA and QC on film processing and light-box luminance are important to ensure the quality of patient imaging studies, QA and QC processes on all monitors in digital mammography are vital to ensure the highest quality and consistency in image display, which may have a direct impact on diagnostic accuracy and patient care.

Digital image display devices or monitors deteriorate gradually over time, mainly because the brightness of these display devices gradually decreases as they age. This will cause a reduction in contrast resolution. Without a routine QC check, the deterioration may not be noticed. If low-contrast lesions or other pathological conditions are present in an image but the image display device is of low quality or is not configured properly, these abnormalities may be invisible to the physician, potentially resulting in misdiagnosis. In addition, the quality of digital images on PACS display devices is strongly affected by the ambient environment or viewing conditions (e.g., excessive light in the reading room where the workstation is located). Therefore, it is critical to check the displayed image quality in these devices' actual ambient environment to ensure optimal image quality.

AAPM TG18 recommends QC procedures involving tests and the use of sophisticated equipment to measure display devices' physical characteristics. To make the tests more practical for routine QC checks in the clinical environment, the TG18 report also provides test pattern images that assess particular aspects of device quality [3]. The ultimate goal of routine QC and QA for image display devices is to detect subtle and gradual deterioration in the quality of displayed images, so that corrective actions can be taken before misdiagnosis or other medical errors occur.

There are two major categories of routine QC procedures: routine qualitative checks and less frequent quantitative checks. Quantitative checks require the use of sophisticated measurement tools such as calibrated luminance meters and colorimeters. AAPM TG18 has published detailed guidelines and descriptions for these test procedures. Among these QC tests, some need to be done more frequently than others. Although there is not yet a specific regulatory requirement for soft-copy display system QC in PACS, as a good clinical practice and in the spirit of the Joint Commission guidelines, users of PACS should perform necessary QC and implement QC measures regularly to ensure high-quality patient care. Table 4.1 lists QC measures that we believe should be assessed quantitatively and/or qualitatively, with recommended frequency of such testing.

Ideally, QC checks for these monitors should be performed daily before radiologists start interpreting images. However, depending on time constraints and other factors, daily QC on the monitors may not be practical; therefore, it is recommended to perform QC on the display devices at least weekly or more frequently as recommended by the vendor.

Table 4.1 Frequency of monitor QC checks.

Daily QC

Use the AAPM TG18-QC pattern to look for main features as a quick qualitative check of the monitors before daily image reading. Users should stop using the monitor for primary diagnosis if the main features on the test pattern are not visible.

Monthly QC

Clean the display monitor surface following the vendor's recommendation.

Visually check the ambient environment in the reading room.

Annual QC

Review the previous QC record for the display device.

Check the ambient environment and positioning of the display device.

Measure and document the luminance level of the ambient environment.

Measure and document the minimum and the maximum luminance of the display device and compare them with previous QC test results. If changes are found, the display device should be recalibrated.

Check for spatial resolution using test patterns.

Check for contrast resolution by measuring the detectability of low-contrast objects in the test pattern.

Verify the LUT either by measuring it following the procedure discussed earlier in this chapter or by taking the post-calibration LUT provided by the display device vendor and verifying its conformance to the DICOM standard GSDF.

Load the TG18-QC test pattern on the display monitor for a final review after LUT recalibration, making sure all important features are still visible.

Document QC test results.

Analyze and compare recent QC test results with previous ones and results obtained during acceptance testing.

Check the reflective characteristics of the display devices.

Check for excessive noise.

Check for bad pixels or defects in monitors using a magnifying glass.

One needs to understand that the recommended frequencies for QC checks shown above are not regulatory requirements but rather are based upon the idea of good clinical practice. Digital mammography users should decide which specific items to include in QC checks and how frequently to perform such tests, based upon their own unique situations and available resources [1–3].

AAPM TG18, American Association of Physicists in Medicine Task Group 18; DICOM, Digital Imaging and Communications in Medicine; GSDF, gray-scale display function; LUT, look-up table; QC, quality control.

Some third-party, vendor-independent PACS display device QC program tools also are available; these tools are designed for ease of use and automated documentation for QC management. Mostly, these program tools generate test patterns following the general principles of AAPM TG18 and interact with the user. Additionally, most high-end medical-grade image display device vendors provide their proprietary QC tools as an option when their display device hardware is purchased. However, such vendor-specific QC software is not a replacement for a general QC program implemented by the user because multiple vendor products may be used at the healthcare institution's clinical sites. Nevertheless, the vendor-specific QC tools can make the overall QC program easier and less labor-intensive.

References

1. American Association of Physicists in Medicine (AAPM) Task Group 18. *Assessment of Display Performance for Medical Imaging Systems*, 2005. AAPM On-Line Report No. 03. www.aapm.org/pubs/reports/OR_03.pdf (accessed January 2012).

2. Samei E, Badano A, Chakraborty D. Assessment of display performance for medical imaging systems: executive summary of AAPM TG18 report. *Med Phys* 2005; **32**: 1205–25.

3. American Association of Physicists in Medicine (AAPM) Task Group 18. Test patterns. www.aapm.org/pubs/reports/OR_03_Supplemental (accessed January 2012).

PACS, storage, and archiving

Stamatia Destounis, Valerie Andolina, Shannon DeMay, Diana Kissel, Stephen Switzer, and Nancy Wayne

Introduction

When considering a transition to digital imaging, there are a number of issues that must be investigated before implementation. Time spent planning is a worthwhile investment and will alleviate additional cost, frustration, and time spent in the future. This chapter will give some background of the necessary components for image storage and retrieval within the picture archiving and communication system (PACS), and how these components affect the availability of the images. It is highly recommended to have an information technology (IT) specialist or consultant involved in planning the system right from the outset. See Table 5.1 for acronyms and abbreviations used in this chapter.

If you will be initiating a digital workflow for the first time, everything must be considered, including the hardware and software that will work best for your facility's volume and workflow. If you will be adding to an environment that is already established, compatibility must be examined. Cost is always a consideration that cannot be ignored. Most importantly, planning for the size and volume of your images into the future is key. Large image files such as those obtained with full-field digital mammography (FFDM) require enhanced hardware solutions to maintain a smooth workflow.

Languages and communication

In order for the many different components of an imaging system to work together and communicate effectively, they need to speak the same language. That is the mission of the IHE initiative – Integrating the Healthcare Enterprise (IHE) [1]. Set up by end users in healthcare imaging and the healthcare industry, IHE works to improve the way computer systems in health care share information. Imaging and display systems developed in accordance with IHE communicate with one another better, are easier to implement, and enable care providers to use information more effectively.

IHE promotes the use of established standard computer languages and standards such as Health Level 7 (HL7) and Digital Imaging and Communications in Medicine (DICOM) to address specific clinical needs.

Health Level 7 (HL7)

The accepted standard computer language used in information systems is HL7. This is not a language that a receptionist or scheduler needs to know to be able to input patient information; it is the universal language that allows the radiology information systems (RIS) to communicate with the PACS and with other RIS systems. HL7 is a protocol that can take the patient information that has been typed into a patient scheduling and billing software program, and encode it in a format that can be accepted by the PACS. It could be considered a translation tool, rather than a language.

Digital Imaging and Communications in Medicine (DICOM)

DICOM is the industry standard for transmission of digital medical images and their related information using query, retrieve, and send commands. The DICOM header attached to the electronic image stores and relates the parameters of the image for display. These parameters are linked to the image at the acquisition station and contain tagged files to convey patient demographics (name, date of exam, date of birth, etc.), imaging information (view, laterality, kVp, compression thickness, degree of obliquity, etc.), and display parameters for the image.

A piece of equipment that is said to be "DICOM compatible" uses the DICOM language and should be able to communicate and interact with other pieces of DICOM-compatible equipment. For instance, a digital mammography unit from manufacturer A should be able to communicate with a hard-copy film laser printer from manufacturer B.

Unfortunately, as in any language, sometimes there are disparities in the interpretation, and information can be lost in translation – in this instance, from one manufacturer to another, within the DICOM header. In addition, DICOM does not mandate how to apply the standard and it leaves room for

Digital Mammography: A Practical Approach, ed. Gary J. Whitman and Tamara Miner Haygood. Published by Cambridge University Press.
© Cambridge University Press 2013.

Table 5.1 Acronyms and abbreviations.

Acronym	Stands for	Means
ASP	Application service provider	A company that takes on the job of long-term storage of others' data
ATNA	Audit trail and node authentication	Authentication mechanism that maintains security and privacy
CD	Compact disk	Data storage device usually used for long-term storage or as backup for disaster recovery
CT	Computed tomography	Imaging method that generates 3D images from 2D x-rays
DAS	Direct access storage	Data storage device attached to and available to a single computer
DICOM	Digital Imaging and Communication in Medicine	A standard computer language
DLT	Digital linear tape	Previously called compac tape, a magnetic tape storage device
DVD	Digital video disk	Data storage device usually used for long-term storage or as backup for disaster recovery
EHR	Electronic health record	Computerized, shared medical information
Gbps	Gigabits per second	Refers to bandwidth robust enough to allow the transfer of 1 gigabit of information every second
HIPAA	Health Insurance Portability and Accountability Act	American federal legislation that governs privacy with respect to medical information
HL7	Health Level 7	A standard computer language
HVAC	Heating, ventilation, and air conditioning	As a practical matter for radiology data storage, this usually just means air conditioning, as computers must be kept cool to function well
IHE	Integrating the Healthcare Enterprise	An initiative promoting use of established computer languages to facilitate communication among diverse pieces of healthcare equipment
IP	Internet protocol	An IP address identifies a specific computer
IT	Information technology	Usually used as an adjective, e.g., IT department, meaning one's in-house computer experts
LUN	Logical unit number	Identifies a device that supports read/write operations
MB	Megabyte	See Table 5.2
Mbps	Megabits per second	Refers to bandwidth robust enough to allow the transference of 1 megabit of information every second
MOD	Magneto-optical disk	Data storage device usually used for long-term storage or as backup for disaster recovery
MQSA	Mammography Quality Standards Act	American federal legislation governing performance and interpretation of mammography
MRI	Magnetic resonance imaging	Imaging method that uses a magnetic field to align the body's atoms
NAS	Network attached storage	Data storage attached to and available to several computers that are linked in a network
NIC	Network interface card	An expansion board inserted into a computer so it can be connected to a network
PACS	Picture archiving and communication system	The integrated system of data storage and transport that allows radiologists to read mammograms at a comfortable workstation instead of at a light box
PDA	Personal digital assistant	Small handheld computer for storing personal information, often combined with a cell phone
PHI	Personal health information	A medical record kept by an individual
RAID	Redundant array of independent (or inexpensive) disks	Data storage method that places data on more than one disk and allows rapid communication between the disks, with the redundancy adding security regarding data loss
RFP	Request for proposal	An invitation to companies to bid on desired services
RIS	Radiology information systems	Data systems used in radiology to address non-image-related issues such as reporting and scheduling
SAN	Storage area network	A means of communicating between NAS servers
TB	Terabyte	See Table 5.2
VPN	Virtual private network	A secure network connection method

optional variations. For instance, a DICOM tag from a modality vendor may be present, but ignored by a third-party workstation vendor, causing inconsistency in the display of the images between vendors. In another instance, certain DICOM tags may not even be included in the header of the images, which are necessary for a different vendor to both display images correctly and load at optimal speed. These DICOM incompatibilities can interfere with archiving or display. This possible lack of communication is almost as frustrating and vexing to the manufacturers as it is to the users of the equipment. Improvement in equipment communications was the driving force behind the establishment of the IHE, as vendors (at the insistence of healthcare end users) worked to produce equipment that could be used in conjunction with equipment from other vendors.

Hardware

Network infrastructure

The network infrastructure is the cable and wiring that ties the modalities and workstations together through hardware called the network switch (sometimes called the network backbone). The bandwidth of the infrastructure indicates the amount of traffic that is capable of passing through the network from one device to another at a single point of time: the larger the bandwidth, the more information can pass through simultaneously. Bandwidth represents the "information highway"; more traffic can travel down the road in a shorter time if the road is large enough to accommodate the size and additional number of vehicles (or images) (Figure 5.1) [2].

Within a PACS, sufficient bandwidth is needed for query and retrieval of databases, and for DICOM images. The industry standard at the current time is 1 gigabit per second (Gbps) Ethernet for PACS and medical image transfers, and 100 megabits per second (Mbps) for everything else (for example, RIS).

It is important to note that even with a large bandwidth, images can move slowly depending upon the "traffic" at a certain time. For instance, if a number of large MRI and CT files are being moved along with the large digital mammography files, there may be some additional delay in viewing the images. To help avoid high-traffic situations that can slow image transfer, and consequently the radiologist who is reading cases, archiving

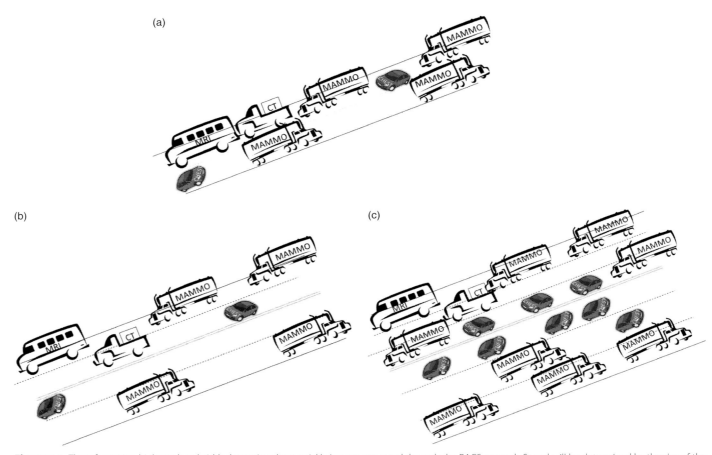

(a)

(b)

(c)

Figure 5.1 The information highway bandwidth determines how quickly images can travel through the PACS network. Speed will be determined by the size of the image and the volume of the traffic. The larger the bandwidth, the faster images can travel, even with a higher volume of large images and traffic: (a) a small bandwidth allows images to travel, but the speed may be slow, depending on traffic within the network; (b) a larger bandwidth allows the same traffic to travel a bit more smoothly; (c) a minimum 1 GB bandwidth will allow larger images, and more of them, to travel faster through the network. Reproduced with permission from Andolina V, Lillé S. *Mammographic Imaging: a Practical Guide*, 3rd edn. Baltimore, MD: Lippincott Williams & Wilkins, 2011 [2].

and pre-fetching of images is often done during the evening hours rather than during the hours when patients are being imaged and exams are being interpreted. The images can only be delivered at the speed of the slowest component of the system at any given point, therefore the speed of computer hardware and back-end storage equipment (i.e., NAS, SAN, etc. – see below) should also be considered.

Storage infrastructure

There are several types of storage hardware that can be used within the PACS. The decision concerning which type to use should be based on usage and volume, and always with a thought to future expectations and needs.

Direct access storage (DAS) refers to a device that is directly coupled or tightly connected to the computer. This would appear as a different partition or drive (such as drive C, D, etc.). Given enough physical space, disks can be added to increase an existing server's capacity. DAS can be configured with an appropriate RAID level (defined below) to add redundancy, but this can make it more difficult to increase capacity. Generally, DAS is available only to the computer it is attached to; however, it may become part of the network if the computer is configured to share to the network. At that point, it becomes network attached storage (NAS).

Network attached storage (NAS) is a method of providing storage to multiple computers over a network, often as an alternative to DAS. Multiple NAS servers can be used within a single network. Additional storage capacity is added with each NAS server, usually without the need for configuration changes within the network. However, as a facility increases its volume of digital images and the number of NAS servers, it can become difficult to manage the images and the NAS servers efficiently. In addition, physical space, electrical load, and cooling also need to be considered. Each time a NAS server reaches its storage capacity, a new NAS server must be purchased and installed, which requires more physical space, more power, and an increased load on air conditioning (HVAC) equipment within the facility's data center. On the positive side, NAS is a relatively cost-effective option.

A **storage area network (SAN)** provides high performance with high availability. This makes SANs a desirable option for online/short-term storage when multiple PACS workstations are in use, since simultaneous users create a demand for faster storage. This may happen in a mammography environment where multiple radiologists are reviewing images concurrently. SANs add another layer of devices between the user and the data, but contrary to what you might expect, this allows for faster data transfer, given the efficiency of typical SANs. Although SAN devices often appear to be the most cost-effective solution, additional conversion software/hardware may be necessary to access the images. SANs are often configured with fiber channel cable between the PACS server and the storage device. Fiber cabling is a high-speed technology that provides high-speed transmission of the images. In comparison to NAS, storage area networks can be a costly option given the technology that is used to create high-speed access to the data. However, this is highly recommended for busy offices in order to keep up with the demand and keep patients moving through the facility.

Removable media provides an economical option for long-term storage. These can be in the form of tape libraries, magneto-optical disks (MOD), CD, or DVD technology. However, accessing images from these media is time-consuming, and they can be unreliable. These are often not recommended for day-to-day storage or archiving in a busy practice, but can be used as backup storage for a disaster recovery plan. This type of media is becoming obsolete, so it may be a poor choice for someone who is planning into the future.

Redundant array of independent (or inexpensive) disks (RAID)

You will often hear "RAID" referenced when discussing the topic of storage. RAID configuration uses multiple hard drives to replicate data. There are different levels of RAID as well. It can vary between RAID 0, 1, 5, 6, 10, or a combination [3]. Each level provides a different degree of fault tolerance, disk space, and performance, and should be very carefully thought out for an appropriate balance. For example, RAID 0 is very fast and provides the most space but significantly increases the likelihood of data loss. When using a RAID level with redundancy, data is stored over several disks. If a disk in the RAID should fail, the data can be regenerated using data stored on another disk within the RAID. However, this should not be considered to be a backup method, as deleting a file on a single hard drive is no different than deleting a file on any RAID – it's still deleted.

Storage tiers

There are usually several tiers of storage within the PACS network. These tiers divide patient studies into cases that are likely to be accessed soon (online or short-term storage), and those that may be accessed at some time in the near future (offline or long-term storage).

Online or short-term storage provides immediate access to the images, with no time delay. Patient studies are pre-fetched from offline long-term storage prior to a patient's appointment and saved into short-term storage. This helps to avoid delays when the radiologist needs to access the studies for comparison when the new images are being read. Once cases are brought into short-term storage, they are available for quick access; keeping them here for a period of time helps to ensure they will be available if the patient is recalled for additional studies or follow-up. As the short-term storage becomes full, the cases that have not been recently accessed "drop off" the short-term archive. This is not a concern, because these studies already have been archived to long-term storage (Figure 5.2).

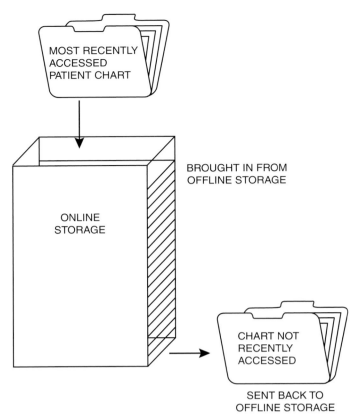

Figure 5.2 As the short-term storage becomes full, the cases that have not been recently accessed "drop off" the short-term archive.

For online storage, the preferred hardware is often a SAN, depending on the image volume and workflow. The SAN allows images to be available with higher transfer rates. In a facility where two-doctor reads are common, the amount of traffic is inherently doubled, and this increases the likelihood that a SAN is required for acceptable performance.

Offline or long-term storage is a holding area for prior patient studies that do not need immediate access. There is a time delay to retrieve data from this storage area; so if possible the images must be fetched in advance of the radiologist's need to access them. At our facility, once the patient makes an appointment, a message is sent via HL7 from the RIS to the PACS. This message makes PACS aware of when the patient will be visiting the office, and it then knows when to pre-fetch the patient's prior images. The patient's prior exams are pulled into the online storage the night before the patient is scheduled to come in.

Offsite backups are often used as a precautionary system to protect the patient data in the event of physical damage to the offline storage. The importance of this was well learned in the wake of Hurricane Katrina, which caused widespread flooding and destruction in New Orleans, Louisiana, and elsewhere along the United States Gulf Coast in 2005 and destroyed the medical records of thousands of patients. It is a Health Insurance Portability and Accountability Act (HIPAA) requirement to have some form of backup of patient files as part of a facility's disaster recovery plan. Some facilities may back up their data to tape, MOD, or DVD and remove it from the facility to protect it. There is also the option of backing data up to disk, which is probably the most reliable option. This can be done by having a second storage device somewhere within the facility where all data files are copied. Some facilities will have their offline storage and backup in two separate parts of the same building. This is not a very secure option, given the possibility of disasters such as a large fire or natural disaster, where both the long-term archive and backup data would likely be lost. In this case, the plan would fail and there can be no disaster recovery, since no backups survived. Therefore, it is best to locate backup copies in separate facilities, preferably miles away from their origin. In fact, it is desirable for the offsite storage to be hundreds or thousands of miles away from the site where the original data are stored. This safely stores the copy, because it is unlikely that a disaster, either natural or man-made, will affect both locations.

Rather than storing data in DVDs or other, similar, finite storage units, you may also use an offsite data center, with the data being sent through a telecommunication line. If your facility's IT department would be responsible for the data, hardware, and software, the device would most likely have to be within a reasonable distance of the facility. This again presents the possibility of a natural disaster affecting that data as well. When considering that option, it is a good idea to research data centers in the area. Look for an up-to-date, highly resilient facility with appropriate security, physical access, and monitoring, as well as its own disaster recovery plan.

Another option is to send data electronically to a third-party vendor known as an application service provider (ASP). The idea of the ASP model is to have the vendor provide the hardware and software in their own secure location and keep everything secure and up to date. This model is attractive to many end users because it takes the main responsibility out of their hands, and provides a single predictable expense for the service. They contract with an ASP vendor who is guaranteeing monitoring and assuming responsibility for their data. When investigating an ASP, it is important to consider the following:

- Security – compliant with HIPAA or other relevant laws, utilizing encryption and access controls for personnel at different levels.
- Service – networking with the ASP should be as simple as changing to a different phone or cable service.
- Open Standard support – be certain that there are no proprietary components that will make switching ASP vendors difficult.
- Standard media guarantee – images should be available to the facility in DICOM format on a standard media such as tape.
- Uptime guarantee – is there one? How big is the risk of downtime?
- Data ownership – who owns the data once it has been transferred to storage?

- Proof of concept – be certain that the product is available, tried, and true. Many vendors offer products that are not yet on the market, or as beta-versions [2].

The archiving and backup process

We have already defined short-term/online storage, long-term/ offline storage, and offsite backup, but it is important to explain how they interact. When images are initially acquired they are sent to the PACS server and stored on the short-term archive. At some point the image is sent on to the long-term archive. Within our own facility, the "archiving" takes place each evening. Even though the image is now stored on the long-term archive, this is not an indicator that it is no longer stored on the short-term archive. The exam will continue to reside on the short-term archive until more space is needed for more recent exams. The older and least accessed exams will then begin "falling off" the online storage (Figure 5.2). The short-term archive is just a temporary storage area, but the long-term archive is where the exams will permanently reside. If an exam is needed for viewing, it can be retrieved from the long-term storage and brought onto the online storage.

All facilities need some form of backup as part of disaster recovery planning. Every night, any new data that is acquired should be backed up. We have already discussed that this could be multiple types of media: tape, DVD, disks. Of course, your facility will be in a much better position following a disaster if you use a more reliable medium. If some sort of disaster occurred, having to restore from media such as tape can be a long process with unfavorable results. Tape degrades over time, and it may be more difficult to access the data. It is also important to remember that disasters can be as small as a hardware failure, human error, or electrical outage, but the consequences can be just as devastating as those of a large disaster such as an earthquake or fire.

Parameters that play a significant role in image archival/retrieval

Image size

Storage space of digital images is measured in megabytes (MB). Digital mammography images are some of the largest digital images. A single digital mammography image is approximately 50 MB; multiply that by four views per patient and the average digital mammogram requires approximately 200 MB of storage space. By comparison, a single-view chest x-ray is only about 1 MB in size. Table 5.2 gives several comparisons for digital image sizes and text file sizes. In addition, it can help calculate and plan the amount of storage space your facility will need, based on the number and type of digital exams you perform.

Processed versus raw images

Due to space constrictions, there is often a discussion as to which image should be saved in the archive: the raw or processed image. **Raw images** consist of the actual data that is captured, pixel by pixel, from the imaging detector. **Processed images** have mathematical algorithms applied to the information captured by the pixels. Image processing optimizes the radiograph for output display, either on a soft-copy workstation or on a printed laser film. These processing parameters are passed in the DICOM header.

The applied algorithms are designed to optimize the visualization of the image in a manner which is pleasing for the radiologist to view. Some algorithms apply a processing operation to each individual pixel, but others adjust the values of pixels based on information in the pixels that are surrounding it. Other algorithms average the pixels within a group.

The controversy surrounding these two types of images is this: the raw image has all of the original information from acquisition, but the processed image is the one that is viewed. If both images are saved, there is additional expense involved. If only processed images are saved, some of the original information may be lost forever. If only the raw images are saved, it is possible that when the image is processed again at another time, there may be a difference in what is visualized, causing possible medico-legal repercussions. It is a decision that each facility must make for itself based on its own use of the archived images. At this time, most facilities save only the processed images that have been interpreted.

Growth and new technology

Planning for storage requirements should involve thought on the expected growth rate of the patient volume and additional technologies that may become integrated into the practice. This would include additional digital mammography units, other imaging modalities such as MRI, CT, and ultrasound, as well as newer technologies that may soon become available, such as breast tomosynthesis or breast CT. Newer technology may mean an increase in the size of each study, as more information is captured. The size of a breast tomosynthesis exam is on average 2 GB, while the minimum size of a cone-beam breast CT exam is approximately 400 MB (D. Conover, personal communication).

To determine the amount of storage space needed, multiply the average number of studies for a period of time by the average number of images in each study. For instance, a facility sees approximately 20 000 mammography patients each year and each patient has an average of four views; that equals 80 000 images per year. Due to the closing of a competing breast imager, we expect the patient volume in this facility to increase by about 30%; therefore we will need storage space for 104 000 mammography images per year. Each image is approximately 50 MB, so the facility needs to store about 5.2 million MB, or 4.96 TB of data next year just for mammograms.

Data compression

Data compression reduces data volume by eliminating redundancies in the image without perceived loss of image quality. This allows data to be stored in a smaller package, thus

Table 5.2 Visualizing data and storage space. Adapted from Andolina V, Lillé S. *Mammographic Imaging: a Practical Guide*, 3rd edn. Baltimore, MD: Lippincott Williams & Wilkins, 2011 [2].

Abbreviation		Bit	Nibble	Byte	Kilobit	Kilobyte	Megabit	Megabytes	Gigabyte	Terabyte
b	bits in a	1	4	8	1 024	8 192	1 048 576	8 388 608	8 589 934 592	8 796 093 022 208
	nibbles in a		1	2	512	2 048	262 144	2 097 152	2 147 483 648	2 199 023 255 552
B	bytes in a			1	128	1 024	131 072	1 048 576	1 073 741 824	1 099 511 627 776
Kb	kilobits in a				1	8	1 024	8 192	8 388 608	8 589 934 592
KB	kilobytes in a					1	128	1 024	1 048 576	1 073 741 824
Mb	megabits in a						1	8	8 192	8 388 608
MB	megabytes in a							1	1 024	1 048 576
GB	gigabytes in a								1	1 024
TB	terabytes in a									1
PB	petabytes									
EB	exabytes									
ZB	zettabytes									

Approximate size of several digital radiography exams	
1 MB	One view chest x-ray
5 MB	One view cervical spine
10 MB	One view lumbar spine exam
50 MB	One view of a digital mammogram

Some useful comparisons	
5 B	The average English word
2 KB	One typewritten page
5 MB	Complete works of Shakespeare, 1 typical mp3 song, 30 seconds of broadcast-quality video
100 MB	8 minutes of broadcast video, 20 King James Bibles
3 GB	200 000 telephone book pages

The chart above represents data sizes in true binary values, but it should be noted that most hard disk manufacturers use a decimal value to calculate storage. For example, a 100 GB drive is actually only 1 000 000 000 bytes, or 100 GiB (gibibytes), which is really only 94 GB.

requiring less space, and space is money. A smaller package also improves transmission performance, allowing images to travel faster over the network. There are two ways to compress data: lossy and lossless.

Lossy compression allows a greater degree of compression, requiring much less space, and allows images to be transferred much faster. This can be performed at ratios of up to 30 : 1. However, when an image is compressed this much, some data will be lost and the image quality can never be fully recovered. Therefore, to be in compliance with MQSA regulations, lossy compression cannot be used to archive digital mammography images or to recreate an image for final interpretation. This may change as image compression technology advances.

Lossless compression is typically performed at approximately a 2 : 1 ratio. Though this seems insignificant compared to lossy compression, the gain in storage space is still important. It means that a 200 MB digital mammography study can

be stored as 100 MB, and can travel faster through the network. This type of compression is allowable within MQSA standards, as the viewing quality of the image is unaffected.

Data transmission/telecommunications

Whether you are considering the ASP model or self-hosting at an offsite data center and managing it yourself, you need to consider what type of line will be transferring data from your facility to the offsite facility. This line will determine the speed at which you archive and retrieve your data. You will have to ask how quickly you "need" this data. Submitting a request for proposal (RFP) to multiple telecommunication vendors is a wise idea when choosing who will be providing the data transfer service. This will be an added expenditure for your facility and should get much consideration before you make a final choice.

One of the most important factors in designing the PACS network is the smooth and efficient transfer of data and images. Often this is a compromise between cost and usage. Within a facility, standard Ethernet cabling with a bandwidth of 1 gigabit per second (Gbps) is generally used. Offsite image retrieval speed is measured at megabits per second (Mbps). An example speed used in a digital mammography facility is 10 Mbps. The speed is obtained by contract through the telecommunications carrier. The highest speed and shortest contract within your budget should be chosen. Contracts generally range from 2–5 years, with longer contracts usually allowing for lower monthly costs. However, technology may eventually outpace your capabilities; leave open the possibility of renegotiating the terms. As an example, we use standard T1 service with a speed of 1.544 Mbps for Internet access. For archiving images, we use 10 Mbps fiber cable for offsite long-term storage. This works fine for us and is within our budget, but the configuration may not work well for everyone.

Telecommunications carrier considerations

Selection of the telecommunications carrier is as important as the archival solution. There must be sufficient bandwidth to support the amount of data being transferred. You may wish to include "burstable service" performance characteristics to help facilitate system recovery when necessary in case of a problem. "Burstable service" is a term for a connection that is allowed to temporarily speed up data transmission beyond the guaranteed rate, "as available." For implementation of a telecommunications carrier service there is an initial setup fee and monthly recurrent charges. There will be a contract, with terms of the agreement usually lasting between three and five years. Be sure to include flexibility within the contract to change the bandwidth requirements if necessary.

Security

Data security is always a major concern, whether the records are kept on film and paper, or whether they are kept electronically as digital images in an electronic health record (EHR). All of this medical information is known as personal health information (PHI). When kept electronically, it is known as ePHI. This includes not only the images, but the patient demographics, billing information, signed consent forms for procedures, medical history forms, and physician notations – anything that can be linked directly to an individual patient and his or her care.

Since the inception of the HIPAA in 1996, patient privacy and data security are more than just a matter of ethical standards; they are law in the United States. Other countries are likely to have similar provisions, although the details may vary. In this age of computer hackers, it is even more important to be on guard and vigilant about data safety. The HIPAA security rule has been an invaluable guideline for security best practices.

Evaluating and assessing a current or future archive system

When evaluating an archive system, there are a number of considerations that should be examined. The answers to the following questions will help find the system that will work for the facility and its needs, and will help determine if a facility has outgrown its current system. Each facility must determine its own tolerance levels to the answers, and this can help when preparing an RFP for an archiving and image storage system.

Availability

To what degree is the system operable? Are all images available to all workstations at all times, or are only certain images available to different workstations? How will this affect the workflow? If an image is opened in one workstation, can it also be accessed simultaneously at another workstation? Are there times when the system is not accessible? If so, when and why does this occur? Does service or repair of a component within the system force the entire system to shut down? Within a PACS, usually all images are accessible at all workstations at all times. However, this depends on the PACS vendor and how the network was designed. Workstations may need to request images that are on long-term storage, and wait for them to be retrieved, while images on short-term storage are available immediately.

Scalability

How well will the system age? What can it handle in terms of data size and transmission speed? Can it be enlarged easily? What will enlargement of the system entail? Will there be downtime when it is enlarged? How will we know when we need to enlarge? Will we lose any data if we don't enlarge in time?

Fault tolerance

Is the system able to withstand failure at hardware and software levels without losing service and data? Have data replication, data redundancy, and diversity in telecommunications been addressed? In a fault-tolerant system, if its operating quality decreases at all, the decrease should be proportional to the severity of the failure, as compared to a naively designed system in which even a small failure can cause total breakdown. Fault-tolerant systems are able to deal with both planned and unplanned service outages. The fault-tolerance measurement is called **availability**, and it is expressed as a percentage. For example, a "five-nines" system would statistically provide 99.999% availability (Table 5.3). It is important when considering an archive vendor to inquire about their uptime guarantee. Table 5.3 represents how much downtime a facility may experience per year, dependent upon the vendor. In any healthcare facility, the end user must decide how much downtime is acceptable.

Table 5.3 Typical availability for a range of applications, expressed as percentage (number of nines) and downtime per year.

Number of nines	Downtime/ year	Typical application
3 (99.9%)	9 hours	Desktop application
4 (99.99%)	1 hour	Critical hospital information systems
5 (99.999%)	5 minutes	Intensive care units, power plants
6 (99.9999%)	31 seconds	Nuclear power plant monitoring

Fault-tolerant systems are typically based on the concept of redundancy. **Data redundancy** is a property of some disk arrays (most commonly in RAID systems), so that all or some of the data stored in the array can be recovered in the case of disk failure. The cost typically associated with redundancy is a reduction of disk capacity available to the user, since the implementations require either a duplication of the entire dataset, or an error-correcting code to be stored across the array. **Replication** is the process of sharing information so as to ensure consistency between redundant resources, such as software or hardware components. Backup is different from replication, since it saves a copy of data unchanged for a long period of time. Replicas are frequently updated and quickly lose any historical data.

Security

Are the data within the system secure? How can you be certain that information is not accessed by people who do not need to see it, while at the same time have it available quickly and easily to those who do require access? PACS vendors are required to sell products that are HIPAA compliant and have the ability to protect data privacy and system integrity. Features such as password protection and standby modes are basic standards. The implementation of security is generally divided into four categories:

- Authentication – identifying the user who is accessing the information.
- Authorization – once the system has determined the identity of the user, the next step is to identify which information the user has access to, based on a user profile or role.
- Confidentiality – once the user has access to the information, who can that user share this information with?
- Integrity – once the information is accessed, what information can be changed by the user? Who is allowed to change which information within the patient record? [3]

Data encryption is one method used to provide security as information is sent, but the software for encrypting and decrypting the data could cause significant increases in transmission time. Another solution is to use a private connection, such as a virtual private network (VPN), but this limits transmission to the members of the secure network. Information sent outside the VPN would still need to be encrypted.

Integrating the Healthcare Enterprise (IHE) has defined a security profile. The Audit Trail and Node Authentication (ATNA) Integration Profile establishes security measures which, together with the Security Policy and Procedures, provide patient information confidentiality, data integrity, and user accountability. ATNA contributes to access control by limiting network access between nodes and limiting access to each node to authorized users. Network communications between secure nodes in a secure domain are restricted to only other secure nodes in that domain. Secure nodes limit access to authorized users as specified by the local authentication and access control policy. A **node** is any device connected to a computer network. Nodes can be computers, personal digital assistants (PDAs), cell phones, or various other network appliances. On an internet protocol (IP) network, a node is any device with an IP address. A secure node is a system that validates the identity of any user and of any other node to determine whether system access and information exchange are allowed.

Integration

Will the system integrate easily with other systems? Compliance with IHE profiles increases the credibility of a claim of integration, particularly in a case where the vendor has successfully passed the IHE "Connectathon" requirements. There are many profiles detailed to specific functions, including workflow, patient information reconciliation, consistent presentation of images, and many more. When considering a RIS, PACS, or modality purchase, it is strongly recommended to specify compliance with the appropriate IHE profiles within the RFP. Obtaining a copy of the product's DICOM conformance statement from the vendor is also a wise request. This will inform the consumer exactly which DICOM classes/tags are supported by the product.

System management

What will be the cost and complexity of managing the system? The work of a PACS administrator is challenging and comprises numerous and varied tasks. It requires technical skills as well as people skills, and a PACS administrator is often someone who can multi-task, be a forward thinker, and handle crisis management well. The system and network configurations for each facility are unique, and so therefore are the duties of the PACS administrator at each facility. Some facilities find that a PACS administrator with an IT background is most beneficial; others find that someone with a radiology background is better suited.

PACS administration encompasses duties within three main areas: (1) project management, (2) system maintenance, and (3) image and information management. Each of these areas contains tasks:

- Project management – Within the scope of project management, the PACS administrator will be involved in planning and implementing the system, from the beginning or as additions are made. Depending on the status of the current PACS, this may involve factors such as training, location, space assessment, monitor placement, and environmental factors such as air conditioning and power requirements. Understanding the workflow directly impacts project management. Workflow mapping helps plan the necessary interactions that will define system placement, configuration, routing, testing, and maintenance. The introduction of software upgrades, new modalities, workstations, interfaces, and users, as well as staff training, must be carefully planned and is important for smooth daily operations.

- System maintenance – Whenever an issue surfaces, the PACS administrator is the first line of defense. He or she must troubleshoot the problem and decide on an action plan. Preventive maintenance and quality-control checklists, managing configurations within the system as changes are made, performing general system maintenance, and acceptance testing as new modalities are added are among the ongoing maintenance tasks that will help reduce the occurrence of surprise issues.

- Image and information management – Image quality, data integrity, image communication, image compression, and offline storage management are some of the many details that need to be overseen and monitored. Are the correct monitors being used for the applications of that workstation, and are they correctly calibrated? Is the DICOM header of each image configured correctly? Are images being transferred using lossy or lossless compression, and is this acceptable for each application?

Performance

Can the system maintain/improve productivity? Are images transmitted quickly enough for the workflow? If not, how can this be remedied? Is it a matter of bandwidth or volume? Each link of the imaging "chain" will affect the overall performance of the system.

Data migration

This is the process of transferring data from one storage medium or computer system to another. Migration addresses the possible obsolescence of the data carrier. When updating to a new system or software, or when systems merge, data from the old system must be mapped to the new system. This relates old data formats to the new system's formats and requirements, so that the data will remain accessible. Therefore it is important to know how the images on the system are stored: in a proprietary format or standard DICOM? How easily can the images be transferred, particularly onto a different vendor's system? Data migration is a key element to consider when adopting any new system.

The archiving history of our facility: a case study

Our facility began performing digital mammograms in 2003 as participants in the American College of Radiology Imaging Network (ACRIN) Digital Mammographic Imaging Screening Trial (DMIST) study [4]. We began with three digital units from three separate vendors and read from three separate vendor-specific workstations. It was quite a headache. We stored one vendor's images to MODs, and the others were stored on CDs. Not a very efficient way to store images.

In June of 2004, we came in contact with a Company A, which was marketing its PACS. Having a PACS meant that we would have the ability to send all our digital images to one server and sit at any PACS workstation to view images from any of our acquisition stations. Company A provided us with a server, a short-term storage device, and three one-terabyte NAS devices (Figure 5.3). Our facility was not educated in archiving/retrieving and we depended on Company A's expertise for guidance. To back up our images for disaster recovery purposes, we used a tape library and stored our data to DLT tapes. As we slowly eased our way into digital mammography, it took us nearly two years to fill those three NAS devices to capacity.

In 2006, our facility saw the importance of backup for disaster recovery first-hand. Our short-term archive was RAID 5 configured and could stand to lose two drives before there needed to be

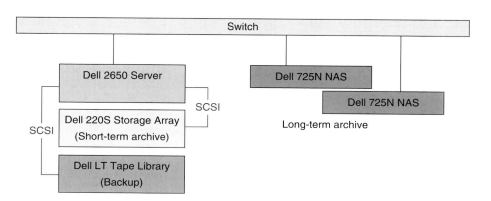

Figure 5.3 Original archive configuration installed in 2004.

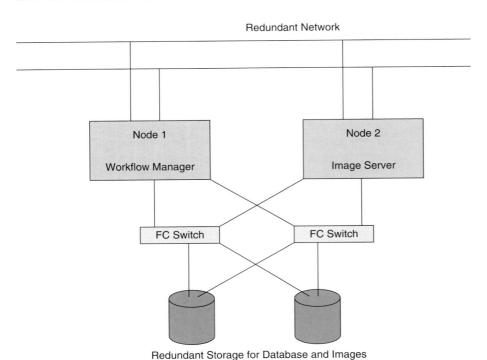

Redundant Network

Figure 5.4 Cluster architecture: high-availability solution.

Node 1

Workflow Manager

Node 2

Image Server

FC Switch

FC Switch

Redundant Storage for Database and Images

any concern for data loss; it is very rare to lose three drives at once. However, we had three drives fail on our short-term storage and the PACS was down for a full week. We were unable to send any images to PACS. To correct the situation we had to replace the drives, rebuild the volume (which is an area of storage on a hard disk), and restore data from tape. Luckily, we were not fully digital at that time, so we were able to stay in operation by performing all exams on our film-screen equipment.

Following this incident, we decided to put in a high-availability system with clustered servers (Figure 5.4), which meant that if one server failed, the other would continue to run, and workflow would not be interrupted. A storage array was purchased and installed, creating a new SAN for the short-term (online) storage. This assured more reliability for our system. Again, it was RAID 5 configured and was equipped with both dual power supplies and network interface cards (NIC). Having dual NICs meant that if we lost the network connection to one server due to a faulty NIC or bad network cable, the other would continue to function, and there would be no interruption in workflow (Figure 5.5).

By the end of 2007, we were able to image exclusively with digital technology and had filled 12 one-terabyte NAS devices (Figure 5.6). The NAS devices were becoming difficult to manage in terms of physical space and maintenance. We began considering new options for both our long-term archive and our method of disaster recovery.

Two consultants were brought in, and they each brought separate solutions. RFPs were submitted to multiple vendors. The RFP is usually a lengthy document stating the needs of the facility and a request for vendors to submit their proposal for a

solution. The RFP process allows the consumer to read through the offered proposals and narrow down the choices to those that best fit the needs. Usually, two or three vendors are interviewed to systematically make a decision based on the information the vendors have provided.

Our first consultant knew that we preferred having control and responsibility for our archived images, and suggested that we purchase more disks for our storage array and have the SAN act as our short-term, as well as our long-term, archive. Using the same piece of hardware, the storage array would be sectioned and LUNs (logical unit numbers) would be created with separate technologies. Faster disks with fiber connections would be used for the short-term archive, while the long-term archive could use less expensive, slower disks. This was a cost-effective option, but did create some risk by using only one device for both the short- and long-term archives. In the event that the storage array was somehow damaged, there would be a possibility of both the short- and long-term archives being affected.

For the disaster recovery portion of the solution, the proposal was to purchase another storage array to house at a local data center. With the data being stored off site, yet locally, it would be possible for our IT department to easily access the hardware in the event of an emergency that could not be handled remotely. Of course, it also posed the threat of losing all our data if a major disaster were to occur in our area.

The second consultant had a different solution. He believed that the right idea for our facility was to go with the ASP model and allow another company to take the responsibility

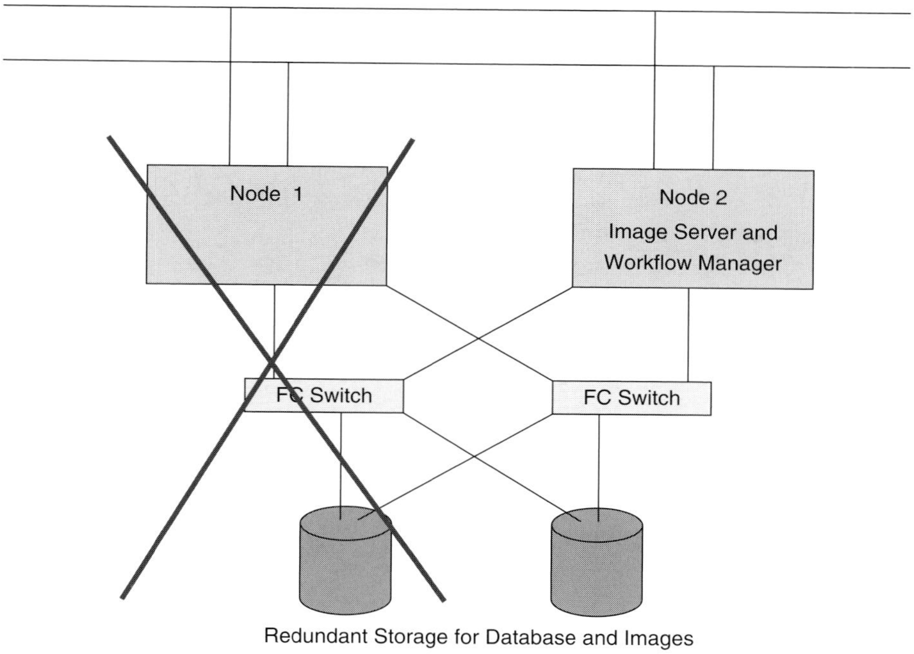

Figure 5.5 Redundant network.

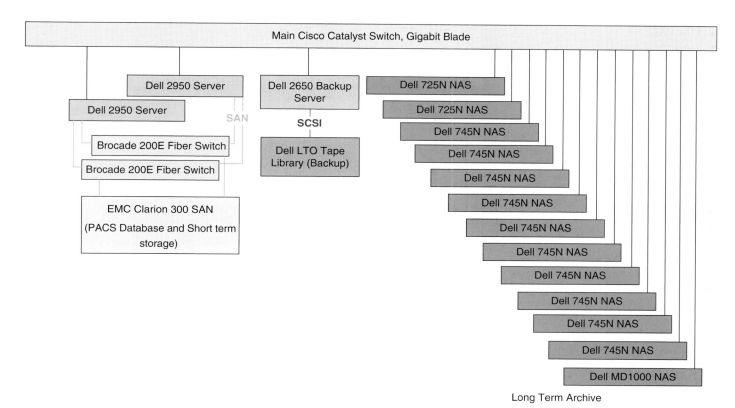

Redundant Storage for Database and Images

Figure 5.6 High-availability solution added to existing hardware.

out of our hands. The vendor would provide all of the hardware and monitor our facility's data 24/7 for any problems that might occur with either the hardware or the software. We would be immediately notified if any issues occurred. The vendor that was most highly considered wanted to place both the long-term archive and disaster recovery at two separate offsite locations.

We were not comfortable with having the entire long-term archive placed off site. Our ideal solution was to have the full offline archive on site. Having it off site would mean added time to retrieve images. It was also important to consider how the PACS and ASP would integrate. We asked questions regarding whether they had ever worked with our PACS vendor, and if they had a successful track record. We also needed to know how they planned to integrate the two systems and what testing would be performed prior to commencement of the new solution.

After much consideration, management decided the best option for our facility was to use the ASP model. We would hand responsibility over and let them manage our long-term archive as well as our disaster recovery. We would be using the offsite location for all of our backups, including disaster recovery for the images and databases in our PACS. In regards to the long-term archive, it was realized

that having all the data kept within the facility would be very costly. However a compromise was reached, where five years' worth of studies are kept on site to expedite retrieval of these cases as needed. The entire long-term archive would be stored on spinning disk in Connecticut, approximately 300 miles away, and the disaster recovery archive data would be stored at a second location in Arizona using DVD jukeboxes.

This decision has had both pros and cons for our facility. We no longer have to concern ourselves with the safety of our long-term and disaster recovery archives, since it is being continuously monitored by our vendor. If an issue occurs, we will be notified by the vendor before we even notice that it has occurred. One disadvantage to using an ASP vendor is that when an issue does crop up, our PACS department has to address both the PACS vendor and the ASP to discover the root of the issue. There is usually not a simple way to distinguish on which side the issue is occurring. In cases such as this, the "blame game" can become an issue and slow down resolution of the problem. Often, vendors will want to point fingers at each other while the customer is left in the middle to deal with the fallout. Therefore, it is important to establish that all the vendors involved have a good working relationship

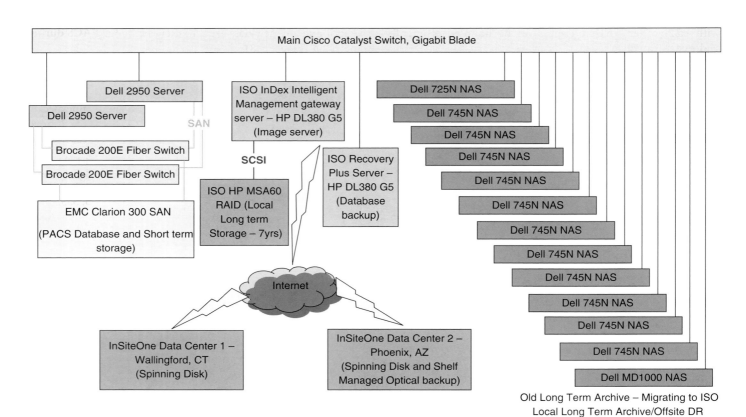

Figure 5.7 Archive solution during migration process.

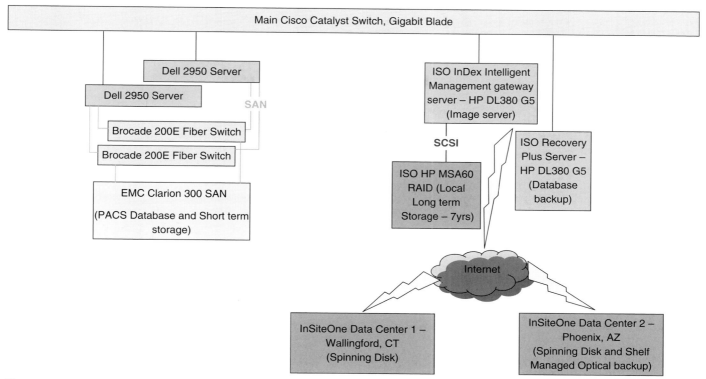

Figure 5.8 Current archiving.

with each other so that issues can be handled efficiently and expeditiously.

Once we decided on our archive solution, we needed to migrate all of our images from our NAS over to the new vendor (Figure 5.7). This was nearly 13 terabytes of compressed data. Our PACS and archive vendor worked together to set up the migration, which took over a year to complete. Today all our prior images are stored to our new archive vendor and any new data are sent there from our PACS during archiving (Figure 5.8).

In conclusion, the path from film to digital with a PACS, archiving, and storage solution takes time, patience, funding, and key IT/PACS personnel to make the transition as seamless as possible. No matter how well prepared one may be, unexpected issues may arise daily, and the radiologist needs to be as educated as possible in order to offer some guidance and support as need be.

References

1. Integrating the Healthcare Enterprise. *IHE Radiology User's Handbook*, 2005. www.ihe.net/Resources/upload/ ihe_radiology_users_handbook_ 2005edition.pdf (accessed April 2012).

2. Andolina V, Lille S. *Mammographic Imaging: a Practical Guide*, 3rd edn. Baltimore, MD: Lippincott Williams & Wilkins, 2011.

3. Oosterwijk H. *PACS Fundamentals*. Dallas, TX: OTech, Inc, 2004; pp. 53; 60–61; 205.

4. Pisano E, Gatsonis C, Hendrick E, *et al.* Diagnostic performance of digital versus film mammography for breast-cancer screening. *N Engl J Med* 2005; **353**: 1773–84.

Interpretation of digital screening mammography

Tamara Miner Haygood and Basak E. Dogan

Introduction

Digital and film-screen screening mammography are fairly similar in their ability to detect cancer. Depending on which paper one is reading, this might be measured by sensitivity and specificity or by comparing other measures including cancer detection rate, recall rate, and positive predictive value. Because it is not the mammogram itself that may exhibit a certain accuracy but rather the radiologist interpreting the mammogram, it follows that radiologists' interpretation of digital screening mammograms is similar in accuracy to their interpretation of film-screen screening mammograms. There are, however, differences in the approach that may be taken. These are addressed here, and we will provide some suggestions.

Digital mammograms may be of two types, either computed radiography (CR) or digital radiography (DR). To make it more interesting, digital mammograms may be printed on film for interpretation or interpreted using soft copy on a computer monitor. Film-screen mammograms are normally interpreted on film, but they can be digitized and viewed on a computer screen, usually to serve as a comparison study to a mammogram that will be interpreted on the computer. The main focus of this chapter will be interpretation of DR-type digital mammograms on computer monitors.

Time utilized

Time used for soft-copy interpretation of digital mammograms may be considerably greater than time expended in interpretation of film-screen screening mammograms. Pisano *et al.* in 2002 found that speed of interpretation of digital screening mammograms on the computer monitor was not significantly different from interpretation of the same images printed on film [1]. Their digital mammograms were displayed on an in-house workstation, however, which limits applicability of the study to ordinary practice, and also neither the time to hang the films nor the time needed to close one study on the computer and bring up the next was included. Another study conducted in Malaysia compared film-screen, computed

radiography, and digital mammography and found interpretation time to be 5 minutes for all of them. It was not clear, however, how this was measured or how the images were presented for interpretation. In particular, the time required for interpreting film-screen mammograms seemed rather long. Double reading was used, and if the time for each radiologist to read the images was included, that could account for some of the time. The images were specified to be interpreted on alternators, but it was not mentioned whether the radiologists had to hang the films themselves or whether the films were hung for them [2].

Four other studies have found that interpretation time is nearly twice as great for digital screening mammograms displayed on a monitor as for film-screen screening mammograms. Berns *et al.* directly measured the speed of interpretation of seven radiologists as they interpreted digital screening mammograms and film-screen screening mammograms and found that it took significantly longer to interpret digital than film-screen studies, an average of 2.0 minutes per mammogram for digital mammograms compared with 1.2 minutes per mammogram for film-screen mammograms by experienced radiologists [3]. We also performed a timed reading study that confirmed the findings of Berns *et al.* and discovered by direct comparison that the increased interpretation time for digital screening mammography was independent of other variables including the presence or absence of comparison studies, the number of images in the study, whether the study was interpreted as normal or abnormal, and whether or not the radiologist selected and hung additional films [4]. Another study performed in Japan and one performed in Italy also found that it took about twice as long to read soft-copy digital screening mammograms as to read film-screen screening mammograms [5,6]. A survey of members of the Society of Breast Imaging confirmed that it was the opinion of the majority of 396 respondents that it takes longer to read digital than film-screen screening mammograms [7]. Longer interpretation times for soft-copy digital images put digital mammography at an economic disadvantage compared with film-screen mammography, although one

Digital Mammography: A Practical Approach, ed. Gary J. Whitman and Tamara Miner Haygood. Published by Cambridge University Press.
© Cambridge University Press 2013.

saves technologist time [3,4,6]. Wang *et al.*, conducting an analysis of anticipated economic impact of switching from film-screen to digital screening mammography in Australia, estimated that the personnel cost involved per screening mammogram would be $21.87 per patient with digital mammography and $21.39 per patient with film-screen mammography, expressed in Australian dollars at 2007 prices. It was assumed that radiologists would average 5 minutes to double-read a digital mammogram versus 3 minutes to double-read a film-screen mammogram, and that technologists would require 10 minutes to obtain a digital mammogram versus 15 minutes to obtain a film-screen mammogram. In addition, it was proposed that each film-screen mammogram would require 5 minutes' time from an assistant whose duty it was to develop films, while this assistant could be dispensed with entirely for digital mammography [8].

Choice of image size and hanging protocols

If digital images are viewed on a monitor, one challenge that contributes to lengthening of interpretation time for digital screening mammograms is that for many digital systems, the resolution of the detector is higher than the resolution of the usual 5-megapixel (5 MP) monitors on which these images are typically viewed. These monitors are generally arrayed with approximately 2000 pixels laterally by 2500 pixels vertically for 5 million pixels total. If the detector has more than 5 million picture elements, then the resulting image will not fit when viewed in such a way that one pixel on the detector corresponds with one pixel on the monitor. This method of viewing goes by various names depending on the preferences of the vendor. It may be called 1 : 1, full resolution, or 100% resolution. When mammograms are viewed at any other resolution, the information obtained in each detector element of the detector must be altered to allow the image to fit into the allotted space on the monitor. Exactly how this alteration is accomplished is normally considered proprietary information and presumably varies from one workstation manufacturer to another. When mammograms are viewed at a lesser resolution than that at which they were obtained, then at a minimum information must be combined so that information from more than one detector element on the detector is used to create the appropriate gray-scale rendering for each pixel on the monitor that is allotted to that particular image. The amount allotted to the image may be the entire monitor, but it may also be only a part of the monitor. For example, if the images are displayed using a 4-on-1 hanging protocol, then the image will have to be adjusted to fit only one-fourth of the monitor. As the allotted part of the monitor becomes smaller, the amount of adjustment of the original image becomes greater, and eventually averaging of pixels may be abandoned for the dropping of data. The loss of data is not permanent, and the data will come back in when the image is again displayed at a larger physical size.

The amount of adjustment therefore depends on the number of pixels on the monitor, the portion of the monitor allotted to the image, and the number of detector elements in the detector (Table 6.1). For a detector of any specific physical size, the number of detector elements will be inversely proportional to the width of the detector elements. Therefore if an image obtained with an 18 × 24 cm Hologic detector having 70 μm detector elements is displayed on a Dome E5 monitor (and allowed to occupy the entire monitor), there will be roughly 1.5 times as many detector elements as monitor pixels, and the information coming from individual detector elements will have to be adjusted accordingly. On the other hand, if an image acquired with a General Electric 19 × 23 cm detector having 100 μm detector element size is displayed on the same monitor (again being allowed to occupy the whole monitor), the monitor will have more pixels than the detector had detector elements, and the entire image can be displayed in 100% resolution without the need for averaging or dropping of data. Indeed, there will be the opposite situation in which the data need to fill more pixels than there are detector elements. This readjustment of information to accommodate the allowed space on the monitor is called rebinning. It occurs both when the image accommodates a smaller space and also when it accommodates a physically larger space, in other words one with more pixels than the number of detector elements. If the image is zoomed to 200%, then 2 × 2 or 4 pixels will be allotted to each detector element, so in that case, as with viewing at 100%, the information from each detector element can be viewed without any recombination with information from other detector elements.

The American College of Radiology in 2007 published guidelines recommending that all digital mammographic images should be viewed for interpretation at the resolution at which they were acquired [9], in other words, at 100% resolution. Because of the mismatch between the resolution of many detectors and the resolution of the monitor, as discussed above, digital mammographic images may need to be enlarged beyond the physical size of the monitor (Figures 6.1, 6.2). If the image is of a relatively small breast, it is often possible, particularly on the craniocaudal (CC) view, to position the image so that the entire breast is visible at one time. This is because the periphery of the image will be occupied by blank space containing no anatomy. That area may be safely excluded from view. In all other situations in which there are more picture elements in the detector than pixels available on the monitor, however, to see the entire breast requires additional manipulation. Depending on the options available on the workstation and the preferences of the radiologist, this can include either dragging the image around the monitor, looking at it in tiled portions (a technique often called quadrant zooming) or using a magnifying-glass function built into the workstation in which a small portion of the screen is dedicated to 100% resolution viewing, the image is displayed in "fit-screen" mode, and that magnifying portion is dragged around the image to include the whole breast. These manipulations allow the image to be viewed at the resolution at which it was acquired.

The recommendations of the American College of Radiology appear to be based on the desire to avoid rebinning, but there is

Table 6.1 The number of detector elements available using five different commercially available digital mammography detectors, and the number of pixels available on four different commercially available 5 MP monitors. Whenever the number of detector elements exceeds the number of pixels, the image will be too large to fit the entire image at one time on the monitor at 100% resolution. This is the case for every possible combination except when using the General Electric Senographe, in which case the image is smaller than each monitor and therefore can be fitted on the monitor at 100% resolution without rebinning.

Detector specifications

Detector brand	Hologic	Hologic	General Electric	Fujifilm	Fujifilm
Style	Selenia	Selenia	Senographe	Amulet	Amulet
Field size (cm)	18 × 24	24 × 30	19 × 23	18 × 24	24 × 30
Rows	3328	4096	2294	4800[a]	6000[a]
Columns	2560	3328	1914	3600[a]	4800[a]
Detector element size (μm)	70	70	100	50	50
Number of detector elements	8.5 M	13.6 M	4.4 M	17.3 M[a]	28.8 M[a]

Monitor specifications

Monitor brand	Dome	Barco	Barco	Eizo
Style	E5	Coronis	Nio (MDNG-6121)	RadiForce GS521 CLP
Screen size		42.2 × 33.8	43.2 × 32.4	42.2 × 33.8
Rows	2048	2048	2100	2048
Columns	2560	2560	2800	2560
Number of pixels	5.24 M	5.24 M	5.88 M	5.24 M
Pixel width (mm)		0.165	0.154	0.165

[a] These values are calculated from the detector element size and field size assuming no pixel overlap. Other values are taken from manufacturers' specifications. M indicates 1 000 000. Thus 8.5 M means 8 500 000 pixels or 8.5 megapixels.

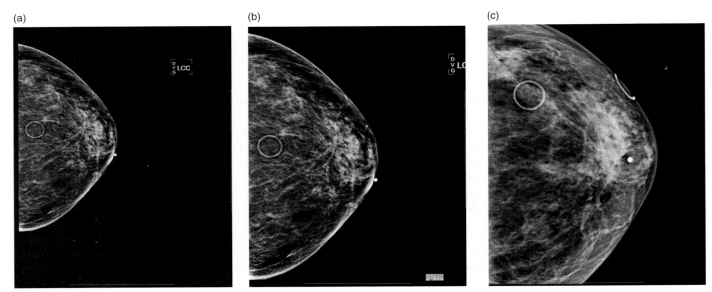

Figure 6.1 Monitor displays with small field-of-view detector sizes. (a) CC view obtained with the smaller detector size on Hologic Selenia equipment and displayed on a Dome 5 MP monitor using the fit-screen viewing mode in which the entire image is rebinned to fit the monitor. (b) The same view displayed using 100% resolution: note that the image has been positioned on the monitor so that the entire breast can be seen; all that is missing is some of the blank space around the breast. (c) CC view of the same woman obtained 2 years earlier on Fischer equipment using a 50 μm pixel size and displayed at 100% resolution: with this pixel size, it is not possible to display the entire breast at one time on the monitor at 100% resolution.

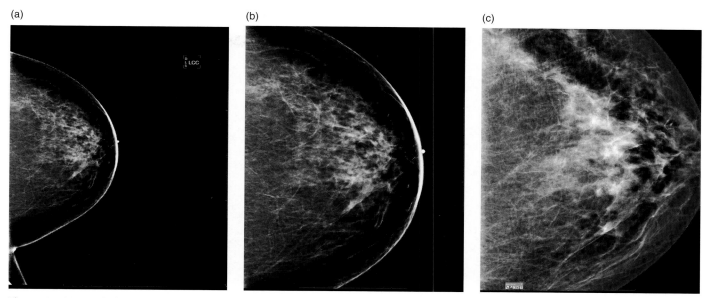

(a)   (b)   (c)

Figure 6.2 Monitor displays with larger field-of-view detector sizes. (a) CC view obtained with the larger detector size on Hologic Selenia equipment and displayed on a Dome 5 MP monitor using the fit-screen viewing mode in which the entire image is rebinned to fit the monitor. (b) The same view displayed using 100% resolution: note that the image cannot be positioned on the monitor so that the entire breast can be seen. (c) CC view of the same woman obtained 2 years earlier on Fischer equipment using a 50 μm pixel size and displayed at 100% resolution. It can be compared with Figure 6.1c: this woman's breast is larger than that of the woman portrayed there, and the larger field-of-view detector was used. Therefore, proportionately even less of the breast tissue will fit on the monitor at one time when displayed at 100% resolution.

little information available in the literature as to whether this is truly a practical concern. We tested the ability of radiologists to find malignant microcalcifications using various degrees of monitor zooming. The digital images were obtained on a Hologic system with 70 μm detector element size. We tested images obtained with the larger field-of-view (24 × 29 cm) detector. We tested the 100% resolution images, fit-screen images (61%), images obtained with 4-on-1 hanging (30%), a size midway between fit-screen and 100% (88%), and a size slightly larger than 100% (126%). We were unable to discover any statistically significant advantage to any of these image sizes over the others, although the 4-on-1 image did not perform quite as well as the others. We next tested images obtained with the smaller field-of-view (18 × 24 cm) detector using the 100% resolution images, fit-screen images (74%), and sizes midway between fit-screen and 100% (88%) and slightly larger than 100% (124%). We were again unable to find any significant difference between the tested sizes. In this study, the fit-screen images did not perform quite as well as the others, and in the first study they had also performed just a little less well. Therefore, based on this research, we suggest that it may not be prudent to search for microcalcifications on the 4-on-1 or fit-screen images alone or on other images displayed at similar proportional reductions in size compared with 100% resolution [10,11]. This would, of course, be likely to vary depending on one's equipment. With 100 μm detector elements, the fit-screen images will portray the image at 100% resolution or larger on a 5 MP monitor.

Although 5 MP monitors are recommended at the present time [9], some literature suggests that digital mammography may be interpreted accurately with the same 3 MP monitors that are typically used for other digital imaging examinations. In 2007 Kamitani *et al.* compared detection of masses using film, 3 MP monitors, and 5 MP monitors, using deliberately assembled sets of images. They found similar accuracy with all three modalities. When they compared detection of calcifications, these authors found that film and 5 MP monitors performed similarly, but there was a slight trend (not statistically significant) for less accurate detection with 3 MP monitors [12]. In 2008 Uematsu and Kasami compared the performance of a 5 MP cathode ray tube (CRT) monitor to that of a 3 MP liquid crystal display (LCD) monitor. They used a single radiologist as their observer and 100 cases, 46 with masses representing proven cancer and the remainder normal or with benign findings. There was no significant difference in detection of cancers between the two monitors [13]. Also in 2008 Yamada *et al.* compared the performance of six radiologists and six breast surgeons interpreting an experimental grouping of 100 cases, 32 of which had biopsy-proven breast cancer and the remainder of which did not. The images were interpreted using hard copy, 3 MP, and 5 MP LCD monitors. There was no statistically significant difference in performance between the three modes of image display [14]. Further studies of the efficacy of digital mammography interpretation on 3 MP monitors would be useful.

Zooming images to fill the whole screen or even larger may be expected to hamper radiologists' ability to compare views side by side with other views from the current study or with comparison images from earlier studies. It may also interfere with the gestalt overview that has, in gaze-tracking studies, been shown to allow radiologists to fixate on cancers within 1–3 seconds of laying eyes on a mammogram [15,16]. Further, they contribute to the previously described near doubling of

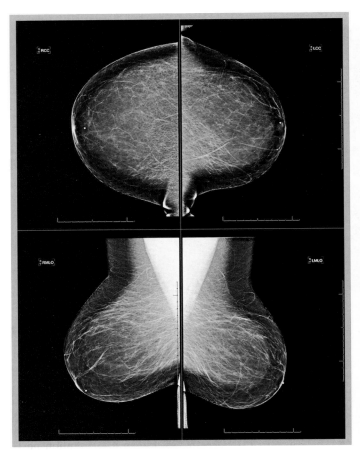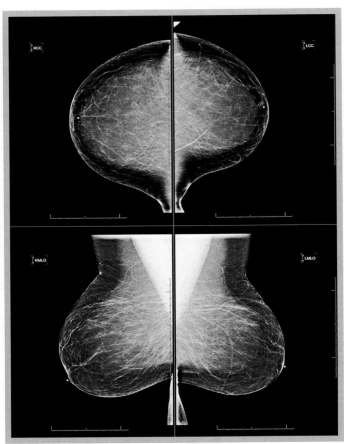

Figure 6.3 Opening hanging protocol. This is the hanging protocol with which we begin our interpretation of each screening mammogram. On the left side monitor are displayed the new CC images on top and the new MLO images on bottom. On the right side monitor are displayed the comparison films in the same arrangement. This arrangement allows for easy comparison from side to side and between old and new images. After viewing this set of images, we enlarge each new image in turn.

interpretation time for screening mammograms interpreted on a monitor versus for films prehung on an alternator [3,4,17].

Other than for the American College of Radiology's suggestion of including 100% images in one's viewing strategy, choice of hanging protocols is largely a matter of individual preferences. Because of the desirability of comparing with other views and old images, consider starting with a 4-on-1 display. This can be organized in various ways depending on the radiologist's desires and the limitations of the workstation. Using two monitors, we place the new images on the left monitor and any comparison study on the right monitor, with the CC images on top and the mediolateral oblique (MLO) images on the bottom row (Figure 6.3). In our experience it is more common in film-screen reading to have the new images on the bottom row of a set of light boxes and the old images on the upper row, and many radiologists may prefer to imitate that hanging protocol on a monitor. After looking at the images in the 4-on-1 display, enlarge each image to fill the screen and then zoom up from there using the trackwheel in the middle of the mouse. This works very well, in our opinion,

for the picture archiving and communication systems (PACS) system that we use (Philips iSite 3.4), but other methods may work better with different systems. In our survey of members of the Society of Breast Imaging, we asked about preferred hanging protocols for digital images and found that responding radiologists had a wide variety of preferences [7]. The most common preference was for a combination of 4-on-1 and 2-on-1 hanging, preferred by 66 (34.2%) of respondents. The combination of 2-on-1 and 1-on-1 hanging was preferred by 41 (21.2%) respondents. Thirty-eight responding radiologists used 1-on-1 hanging only, and 25 (13%) used only 2-on-1 hanging. Other combinations were also chosen, but none by more than 9% of respondents. Articles in the medical literature that discuss the efficacy of digital screening mammography rather seldom mention the hanging protocols used during interpretation. Suggested hanging protocols from four such articles that did mention this topic are given in Table 6.2.

During the first two or three years after a practice begins converting from film-screen screening mammography to digital screening mammography, newly acquired images will

Table 6.2 Suggested hanging protocols from four articles in the literature. All of these articles left any further manipulations up to the judgment of the interpreting radiologists.

Article	Hanging protocol	
	1st	**2nd**
Hambly *et al.* [43]	Four views on one monitor	Each view at full resolution
Skaane *et al.* [21]	Two CC on one monitor, two MLO on the other	Each view at full resolution
Skaane and Skjennald [44]	Two CC on one monitor, two MLO on the other	Each view at full resolution
Karssemeijer *et al.* [45]	Four views on one monitor	Each view fit-screen

be digital and the older studies with which the reader will want to compare will be film-screen. There are three possible approaches. One can place an alternator next to the workstation, usually at right angles, and then read the digital images on a monitor and compare with film – effective but awkward because of the need to turn at least the head and perhaps the torso back and forth, and it can increase the time needed for interpretation [4]. It is also problematic due to the relatively bright light emitted by the viewboxes. One can print the digital images on film and interpret them that way until a few years' worth of digital images have been stored away and then abandon film – more convenient perhaps but more expensive, and one loses the ability to manipulate the images. Finally, one can digitize the film images and then do the comparison as well as the interpretation on the monitor. This has been shown in 2009 by Taylor-Phillips *et al.* to be effective, but those researchers did not indicate how many of the abnormal cases in their test set were evidenced by microcalcifications [18], and we personally find that display of microcalcifications, an important finding that may be associated with breast cancer, is suboptimal on digitized film, although this may be variable depending on the type of digitizer used. Therefore we believe that if this option is chosen, it is important to keep the films handy so they may be made available in selected cases. Use of digitized film comparison studies may counteract the increase in interpretation time occasioned by use of analog comparison images printed on film. Garg *et al.* compared interpretation time for four radiologists reading a set of 100 digital screening mammograms using analog comparison studies printed on film versus use of the same comparison studies after digitization. The digitized images were displayed on the same monitors as the images being interpreted, while the printed images were displayed on viewboxes located at a 90-degree angle to the monitors. They found a 32.1% improvement in interpretation time for the use of digitized comparison studies. Interpretation times ranged from 17 to 186 seconds (average 59 seconds) when the comparison studies were printed on film. Interpretation times ranged from 11 to 109 seconds (average 40 seconds) when the prior studies were digitized. These interpretation times apparently did not include the time to report a case or to transition from one set of images to the next [19].

Post-processing at the monitor

If the digital images are displayed on a monitor, the radiologist will have the option to perform any of numerous post-processing techniques in addition to zooming to modify the image according to the viewer's individual opinion of what is most helpful or pleasing. For example, the gray scale can be reversed (Figure 6.4), and the window and level can be changed to make the image appear lighter or darker overall or to adjust the contrast between the darkest and lightest portions of the image. Use of contrast-limited adaptive histogram equalization (CLAHE) may also be an optional function (Figure 6.5).

Unfortunately there is very little information available in the medical literature as to how helpful any of these options are, and all of them require extra time for interpretation. In many reader performance studies, the authors mention post-processing functions that were available but do not indicate whether they were used or not. A 2008 study by Skaane *et al.* of observer variability in mammographic interpretation is typical. The authors mentioned that a magnifying glass was available for use with film-screen mammograms. Post-processing including zooming, adjustment of display window and level, and gray-scale inversion were recommended but not required. The authors did not report on usage of these tools [20].

In our survey of Society of Breast Imaging members, we asked which of various means of enlarging the image, minification (sometimes called "true size," in which the image is adjusted to appear the same physical size as it would if it were obtained as a film-screen study), and computer-aided detection (CADe) a respondent would use on an occasional basis after examining the screening images in the respondent's usual fashion, when deciding whether or not to call a patient back for diagnostic evaluation. If all methods of enlarging the physical size of the image were lumped together, 94% of respondents reported using one or another of these methods to make the decision whether to call back a patient. Forty-two of the 187 respondents who answered that question reported using only zooming of the image. Our respondents were allowed to indicate as many different methods as they wished, but no one checked more than two. The most commonly reported combination was use of the 100% resolution images with CADe [7].

(a)

(b)

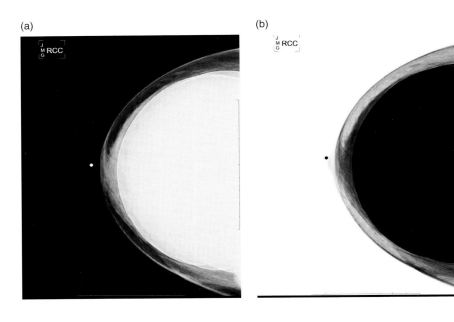

Figure 6.4 Right CC view of a patient with breast implants. In (b) the gray scale has been reversed so that areas that were previously light are now dark and vice versa. In our opinion, this can be helpful to allow improved visualization of the breast tissue immediately next to the implant.

(a)

(b)

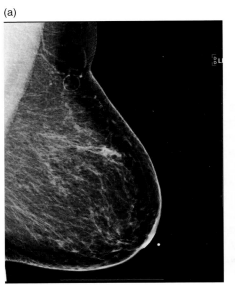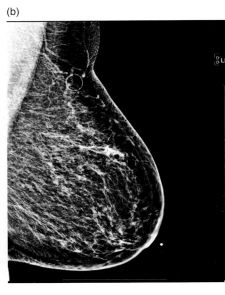

Figure 6.5 Demonstration of CLAHE function. (a) Left MLO mammogram displayed in fit-screen mode using default window and level settings. (b) The CLAHE function has been turned on, resulting in a more contrasty image, in which the bright areas appear brighter, and the dark areas appear darker than in the standard image in (a).

In their first study of digital screening in Oslo, Norway, Skaane *et al.* had two radiologists who had not previously been involved in interpretation of the mammograms evaluate the conspicuity of known cancers as seen on the digital screening images and determine whether the conspicuity of these cancers was improved by any of several post-processing manipulations including quadrant zooming, free continuous zooming using the mouse, free continuous adjustment of window and level using the mouse, or image inversion. They found that most post-processing other than quadrant zooming contributed little to enhancing the conspicuity of their known cancers. Out of 31 cases that were examined in this way, two cancers were better demonstrated using a combination of what they termed "extensive zooming" and free windowing. One of these

was a case of pure ductal carcinoma in situ (DCIS), presumably manifested by microcalcifications alone, and the other was an invasive ductal carcinoma manifested by an ill-defined mass together with microcalcifications. They noted that one cancer was considered less conspicuous when subjected to extensive zooming [21].

In 1997 Pisano *et al.* studied the effect of intensity windowing on detection of simulated microcalcifications. They used background images taken from normal dense breasts, superimposed an artificial cluster of microcalcifications in one quadrant of each image, and asked their observers to decide in which quadrant the microcalcifications lay. They tested 10 different intensity windows and four different contrast levels. They showed the resulting 800 images to 20 observers, all graduate students. The images were printed on film, so the tested window levels were fixed, and the observers could not manipulate them. They did find significant differences in performance of their student observers depending on the tested window level [22]. A very similar experiment by essentially the same group of investigators studied the effect of intensity windowing on detection of simulated masses and also found that windowing affected the performance of their 20 student observers [23]. Because the observers could not manipulate the windows, these experiments highlight the importance of choosing carefully the default window and level that will be used to present digital mammograms for interpretation, but they do not directly predict what result may be expected with free windowing.

Eight years later, Elizabeth Krupinski and coworkers studied use of image post-processing tools by three experienced attending radiologists who read mammograms routinely versus three inexperienced radiology residents. The radiologists examined 160 mammograms, 100 of which were digitally acquired, 46 using the Trex system from Hologic (Danbury, CT) and 54 using the General Electric Senographe system (Waukesha, WI). The remaining 60 were digitized film-screen mammograms originally acquired with the Kodak Lumiscan 85 (Rochester, NY). Half of the images contained masses and half contained microcalcifications, all of which were biopsy-proven, with half of each type being benign and half being malignant. There were no normal cases. The tools available to the readers were (1) manual alteration of window and level, and (2) activation of a window that both brought the area of interest up to full resolution and applied an image-processing technique called gray-level stretching to maximize brightness and contrast. If they wished, while using the window, the radiologists could also activate a modulation transfer function compensation algorithm intended to improve detectability of image details. Krupinski *et al.* found differences in the use of these tools between the experienced mammographers and the radiologist residents. The experienced readers used window/level manipulation more often than the inexperienced readers; in fact, on practically every image. Use of the zoom window also varied considerably. With calcifications, the inexperienced readers magnified the images 55% of the time, compared with 46% of the time for the experienced readers. With masses, the inexperienced readers used the zooming tool almost twice as often as the experienced readers, 60% of the time compared with 38% of the time. Performance did improve when the cases on which zooming was performed were compared with cases on which it was not used. It is not clear, however, whether detection improved because the tool was used or whether the zooming tool was used because an abnormality or potential abnormality had already been noticed and the radiologist wished to examine it more closely. Most likely the latter contributed at least partly. The attending radiologists were both more accurate and faster in their interpretations than the residents, even though they used zooming less often [24].

Optical magnification with a magnifying glass or similar tool is frequently used in reading film-screen mammography. Of 199 members of the Society of Breast Imaging who participated in our survey and who answered the question concerning use of optical magnification for film-screen mammograms, 174 (87.4%) responded that they grab their magnifying glass 75% of the time or more when reading film-screen mammograms [7]. Use of optical magnification is less common for digital screening mammograms. Of the 193 radiologists who answered the question concerning use of optical magnification for mammograms displayed on a monitor, 84 (43.5%) said that they never do. The majority (56.5%) responded that they do use optical magnification at least occasionally, and 42 of them (21.8%) said they do so 75% of the time or more [7]. Optical magnification may help compensate for any remaining defect in vision after glasses or contact lenses are used. Also, depending on how close one sits to the monitor, the size of the pixels can be small enough that optical magnification will increase one's ability to obtain all the available information with digital mammography at 100% resolution in the same way that it does with film-screen mammography, and therefore can be a viable and perhaps quicker alternative to zooming.

CADe or double reading

CADe refers to computer-aided detection; it is a method of allowing a computer program to apply predetermined criteria to scan a screening mammogram and identify features that suggest that an area of the mammogram may have a heightened likelihood of harboring a cancer. These areas are then pointed out so that the radiologist can give them some extra attention. Commercially available systems are carried by several vendors for both analog and digital mammography.

Double reading refers to the practice of interpretation of screening mammograms by two radiologists. Double reading is used infrequently in the United States but is common in Europe and is also used in Australia [25]. It can be performed in several different ways, and the method used can be expected to influence the outcome. For example, a method in which women are called back for diagnostic evaluation if either of the two readers suspects a cancer would be expected to increase cancer detection (sensitivity) at the price of a higher recall rate (therefore lower specificity). On the other hand, a method in which all cases with suspected cancer are subjected to a consensus panel before recall might decrease recall rate. Methods used in several papers in the medical literature are summarized in Table 6.3. Several methods are used, with the most common shared feature being the use of a consensus meeting before patients are called back for further imaging.

Because digital screening mammography has gained popularity relatively recently and because of the lag time of a few years that occurs between a researcher having an idea for a project and a paper generated from that project actually being published, most published articles on efficacy of either CADe

Table 6.3 Double-reading techniques employed in eight papers in the screening literature.

Article	Double reading?	How performed?	Consensus meeting?
Hambly et al. [43]	Yes	Unblinded	Yes
Skaane et al. [21]	Yes	Independent	Yes
Del Turco et al. [46]	Yes	Unblinded	No
Sala et al. [47]	Variable	Variable	Not specified
Skaane and Skjennald [44]	Yes	Not specified	Yes
Karssemeijer et al. [45]	Yes	Independent	Yes
Heddson et al. [48]	Variable	Not specified	Yes
Juel et al. [49]	Yes	Independent	Yes

or double reading at the time of this writing are based on analog rather than digital mammography.

Independent double reading can increase the sensitivity of screening mammography. In the Norwegian Breast Cancer Screening Program screening mammograms are independently graded on a scale of 1 to 5. A score of 1 is considered normal and encompasses both entirely normal breasts and those with clearly benign abnormalities that in the Breast Imaging Reporting and Data System (BI-RADS) system might be scored a 2. A score of 2 in Norway is a probably benign lesion. Each reader enters into a computer a score for each breast. Hofvind et al., writing about the Norwegian Breast Cancer Screening Program's experience with double reading of screening mammograms, utilized case material from 1 033 870 screening mammograms, 97% of which were analog images and 3% of which were digital images [26]. A pair of readings was considered concordant if both radiologists gave a score of 1 or if both radiologists gave a score of 2 or higher to the same breast, even if for those scored 2 or higher the two radiologists did not give exactly the same score. A pair of readings was considered discordant if one radiologist gave a score of 1 and the other gave a score of 2 or higher. 1326 out of 5611 (23.6%) screening-detected cancers were found in women with discordant independent double interpretations [26]. It would follow logically that with single readings about half of these cancers, 663 of them, might have been missed.

The cancers detected among discordant readings were smaller (12.9 mm average versus 14.9 mm) and more often node-negative (78.4% versus 73.2%) than the cancers detected among concordant readings [26]. This is to be expected, since larger and more advanced cancers would be more visually obvious and therefore less likely to be missed by either reader. These results also suggest that the value of double reading in this study was greater than the mere discovery of additional cancer would imply, because the additional cancers were at an earlier and more curable stage.

Independent double reading alone would be expected as suggested above to improve sensitivity, but if every study considered potentially abnormal by either radiologist is recalled for diagnostic evaluation, the improved sensitivity

would come at the price of an elevated recall rate. Among the readings in this study, a score of 1 was entered concordantly by both radiologists for each breast in 957 495 (92.6%) of 1 033 870 readings. All other mammograms, those with scores of 2 or higher by either radiologist, were discussed in the consensus meetings. At the consensus meetings 36 380 (66.8%) of 54 447 discordant screenings and 3932 (17.9%) of 21 928 concordant screenings were dismissed. The ultimate recall rate was 3.5%. Inevitably there were some interval cancers at follow-up among the dismissed cases. One hundred seventeen (6.5%) of 1791 interval cancers occurred among women whose previous screening mammograms were dismissed at consensus. This does not seem like a sufficiently high percentage to suggest that an inordinate number of visible cancers were being dismissed. In addition, details as to the location within the breast of the originally suspected lesion and of the later cancer were not available, so it is not known how often the findings that were dismissed were in the same area as the subsequent cancer [26].

CADe can be used for both film-screen and digital mammography. Its use with film-screen images requires that the images be digitized, so one advantage for its use with digital examinations is that this step is not required. The effectiveness of CADe in improving the accuracy of screening mammography is unclear. One of the largest and most recent studies of CADe, performed with analog images, studied the effect of ImageChecker M1000, version 2.2 (R2 Technologies, Sunnyvale, CA) on cancer detection rate, recall rate, and the positive predictive rate of biopsy. These authors found that before consulting CADe their radiologists found potential abnormalities in 2101 patients out of 21 349, for a recall rate of 9.84%. This led to 256 breast biopsies and 105 cancer diagnoses, for a cancer detection rate of 0.49% and a positive predictive value of biopsy of 41.0%. With CADe an additional 199 patients were recalled, for a recall rate of 10.77%. Among these 199 patients there were 21 additional breast biopsies, and eight additional breast cancers were diagnosed. This raised the cancer detection rate from 0.49% to 0.53% and minimally lowered the positive predictive value of biopsy from 41.0% to 40.8% [27]. In general, it can be expected that use of CADe will increase the recall rate

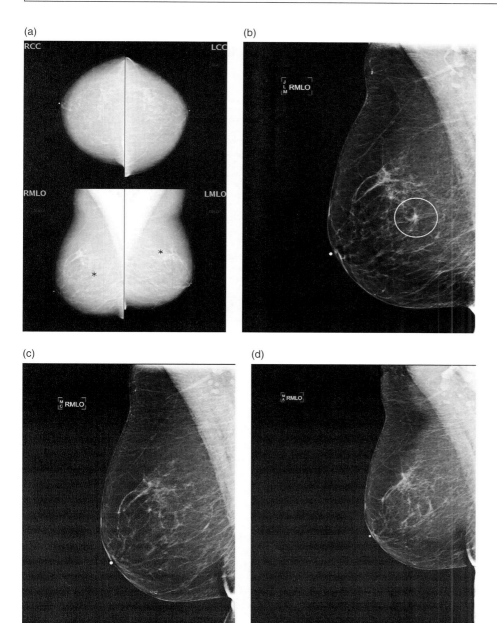

Figure 6.6 False-positive callback with CADe. (a) CADe prompted two areas of concern, one in the left breast, which the interpreting radiologist chose to dismiss, and one in the right breast, both on the MLO views. (b) The right MLO from the corresponding screening mammogram was sufficiently suggestive of a small spiculated opacity in the area of the CADe prompt (circle) that the interpreting radiologist decided to call the patient back. (c) As the first step for the resulting diagnostic mammogram, the left MLO was repeated, and the area of concern disappeared. The diagnostic mammogram was interpreted as negative. (d) Follow-up mammography 2 years later was still negative.

(Figure 6.6), and one can hope that it will increase the cancer detection rate and therefore the sensitivity of the test (Figure 6.7, Table 6.4). It functions to call attention to suspicious areas that might otherwise be overlooked and therefore helps prevent perceptual errors, but it does not prevent judgment errors in the same way that a human second reader might [28].

Two studies have compared CADe versus human double reading. The first drew on experience with the United Kingdom National Breast Screening Programme. These authors compared the effect of single reading alone versus single reading with CADe and double reading. They studied 6111 women undergoing analog screening mammography. All examinations were double-read, and after an initial opinion was entered, each reader then viewed CADe images and entered a new opinion.

The relative sensitivity for each of the three tested conditions was calculated by comparing the number of cancers found with each method against the total number found by all methods. Relative sensitivity was 90.2% for single reading, 91.5% for single reading with CADe, and 98.4% for double reading without CADe. For this practice, double reading was a better method of increasing sensitivity than CADe [29].

The second paper comparing CADe with human double reading also dealt entirely with analog images, 6381 film-screen screening mammograms. These authors also compared the results obtained with a single reader alone, the same reader with CADe, or two human readers. In this study, the first reader marked areas of concern on the mammograms using a wax pencil, so the second reading was not entirely

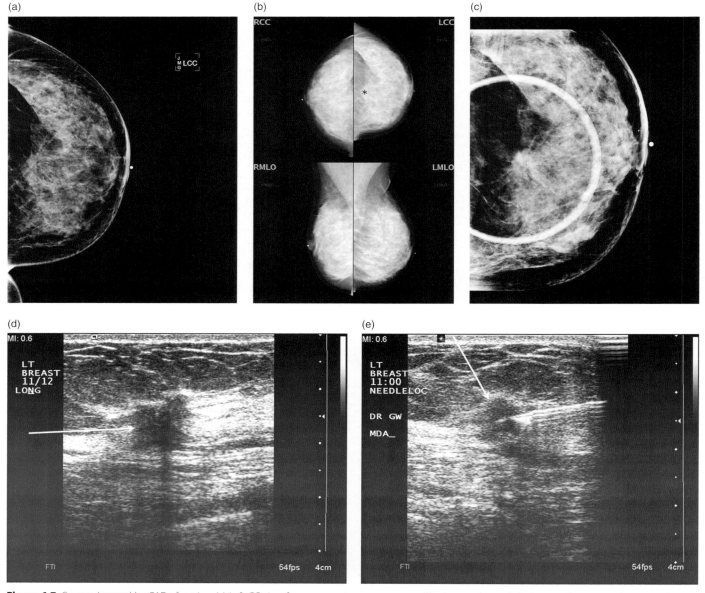

Figure 6.7 Cancer detected by CADe function. (a) Left CC view from a screening mammogram. The interpreting radiologist was about to render a negative interpretation when a look at the CADe image (b) called attention to a nodular area of increased density in the posterior breast with associated tenting of the posterior parenchymal border. (c) The patient was called back for diagnostic study, where spot compression view confirmed an area of architectural distortion with a small central mass. (d) Ultrasound was then performed, showing a hypoechoic lesion with irregular margins and long axis perpendicular to the skin. (e) Ultrasound-guided core biopsy was performed. Pathology revealed invasive ductal carcinoma.

independent, as that reader had access to the wax-pencil marks. In this study, the first reader had a recall rate of 7.4%, which was increased slightly by both CADe (an additional 0.47%) and the second reader (an additional 0.53%). The human second reader called back two women for what proved to be cancers missed by the first reader. These cases had also been marked by CADe, but the first reader dismissed the marks. Overall there was no significant difference in the performance of CADe and the human second reader [30].

In the same way that some actual cancers may be dismissed at consensus meeting with human double reading, cancers correctly prompted by CADe may be dismissed by the interpreting radiologist. Khoo *et al.* noted that CADe correctly prompted nine of the 12 cancers missed on single reading, but only two of these prompts were followed by the reader, while the other seven were dismissed. They estimated that their readers would have had to dismiss 180 false CADe prompts for every CADe prompt actually pointing to a cancer [29]. Freer and Ulissey found that readers in a community-based practice dismissed 97.4% of CADe prompts [31]. Therefore, dismissal of some CADe prompts that later prove actually to have been pointing to a cancer is not terribly surprising, nor should

Table 6.4 Incremental increase in cancer detection and recall rates of combined single reader and CADe as compared with single reader alone.

Study	Incremental increase in cancer detection with CADe (%)	Incremental increase in recall with CADe (recall rate %)
Ciatto et al. [50,51]	85/617 (+13.7%)	245/703 (+35.5%)
Freer et al. [31]	8/41 (+19.5%)	34/344 (+9.8%)
Helvie et al. [52]	1/10 (+10.0%)	57/487 (+11.7%)
Gur et al. [34]	4/206 (+1.9%)	214/1163 (+18.4%)
Khoo et al. [29]	2/61 (+1.3%)	18/372 (+5.8%)
Birdwell et al. [53]	2/27 (+7.4%)	73/887 (+8.2%)
Cupples et al. [54]	17/101 (+16.8%)	164/2100 (+7.8%)
Ko et al. [55]	2/45 (+4.4%)	100/602 (+16.6%)
Morton et al. [27]	8/105 (+7.6%)	191/1996 (+9.5%)
Dean et al. [56]	10/104 (+9.6%)	152/590 (+25.7%)

dismissal of such CADe prompts be taken as evidence that a radiologist is performing below the standard of care [30].

There is some concern among US radiologists that dismissing a CADe prompt on a cancer may be considered negligence. In the only North American legal case involving CADe that we know of to have reached the appellate court, however, CADe was used in support of the radiologist. In this case, a radiologist missed subtle calcifications; CADe also did not prompt this feature. This was accepted as powerful evidence by the court that the finding was so subtle that the radiologist was not negligent in failing to diagnose the cancer on that film, and the case was dismissed [32].

Double reading and CADe, therefore, can both increase the sensitivity of screening mammography. Which one to use is not a clear choice, and in fact it is not entirely clear that one needs to use either. Radiologists vary significantly in their intrinsic sensitivity and specificity in finding breast cancer; in other words, they vary in their performance in the role of a single reader. Beam et al., studying a group of 108 radiologists gathered from a random sampling of US mammography practices, found that those radiologists varied as much as 40% in their sensitivity [33]. Other authors have also found variability in performance at screening mammography. It seems reasonable, then, that the performance of different radiologists may be affected in varying ways by the use of either CADe or double reading.

Gur et al. studied the effect of CADe (R2 Technologies, Los Altos, CA) on recall rate and cancer detection rate for a group of 24 academic radiologists. Recall rates both for the group as a whole and for the subset of seven highest-volume readers, each of whom read more than 8000 mammograms over a 3-year period, were very similar before and after introduction of CADe. Recall rate for the group as a whole was 11.39% without

CADe and 11.40% with CADe. Cancer detection rate was 0.35% without CADe and 0.36% with CADe. Values for the higher-volume readers were similar to those of the group as a whole, and for neither group was there a statistically significant difference after the introduction of CADe [34].

Gur et al. did not directly discuss the effect of CADe on the lower-volume readers, but if one simply subtracts the figures for the higher-volume readers from the total, then it follows that without CADe 17 lower-volume readers found 36 cancers in 11 803 mammograms, for a cancer detection rate of 0.31%. With CADe, the 17 lower-volume readers found 79 cancers in 21 639 mammograms, for a cancer detection rate of 0.37%, so the apparent affect on the cancer detection rate of the lower-volume readers was greater than on that of the higher-volume readers, although still not statistically significant [34,35]. This may indicate that CADe will be more helpful to lower-volume mammographers, and by implication perhaps less experienced mammographers, than to higher-volume, more experienced individuals.

A further consideration for CADe is that not all systems are created equal. Gur et al. compared the performance of three different CADe systems – ImageChecker M1000, version 3.1 (R2 Technologies, Los Altos, CA; Second Look, version 6.0 Beta Cadx Systems, Beavercreek, OH); and a system that the authors developed in-house. The performance of these systems was tested on 219 digitized film examinations which included 58 known and prospectively identified cancers appearing as masses, 39 images obtained the previous year on these same women, 22 known cancers that had received false-negative readings at initial interpretation, 50 verified negative or benign examinations, and 50 false-positive examinations which had resulted in the recall of a patient for a finding that ultimately was considered negative or benign after workup [36]. There were no large differences in performance among the three tested systems. The two commercial systems correctly cued 72% and 71% of known malignant masses. The false-positive cuing rate, however, was a bit higher with Second Look than with ImageChecker [36]. Because systems are rapidly altered by manufacturers, the important point of this paper is not to understand the performance of these specific systems in this study but to realize the need to recognize the strengths and limitations of any system with which one may be working or which one may consider buying.

Just as the effect of CADe may vary depending on the system being used and the radiologist using it, so may the effect of double reading vary not only with the style of double reading used but also depending on which pair of radiologists is participating together. Beam et al. invited radiologists from a nationwide sampling of American mammography practices to attend an experimental session in which they interpreted a set of 79 screening mammograms. The investigators then compared readings of pairs of radiologists who came from the same practice, to answer the question of what would happen if that pair were double reading the mammograms and called back each patient that either one of them thought should be recalled. In this way, they were testing pairings that would truly have been possible in the real world of radiology as practiced in the United States in the mid-1990s. They found that there was considerable variation in the changes that would occur in the individual radiologists' readings based on adding the partner's callbacks to his or her own. They offered in detail the results for three pairs as examples. For the first pair, double reading would have produced an increase in the sensitivity of both radiologists at the expense of an increase in each radiologist's false-positive rate (callbacks of patients who will prove not to have cancer), for one radiologist a 35.7% increase in false positives, for the other a 69.7% increase. For the second pair, one of the two readers would have benefited greatly from the pairing via an increase in sensitivity of 39.2% with minimal increase in the false-positive rate for either radiologist. For the third pair, double reading would not have increased the sensitivity of one of the pair at all, nor would it have had much effect on his false-positive rate, as he had a high recall rate already. For the other partner, an increase in sensitivity of just under 10% would have come at the cost of a near tripling of his false-positive rate, which the authors noted that radiologist would probably have found unacceptable. Thus, the effectiveness of double reading may vary a great deal depending on the characteristics of the individual radiologists involved [37]. One limitation of this study was that it was not designed to evaluate the effect of a consensus meeting, which may have mitigated the tendency towards increasing false positives.

Double reading of screening examinations is recommended by the European guidelines for quality assurance in breast cancer screening and diagnosis, which specifically suggest independent double reading with arbitration by a third expert in the case of discordant original opinions [38]. According to these guidelines, in smaller screening centers, where the radiologists may not interpret as many as the recommended number of 5000 examinations per year, the second reading should be done in larger centers where the radiologists read at least 5000 annual cases [38]. This recommendation is probably the main reason why it is so common for European practices to use double reading. Most of the studies that have explored the efficacy of digital mammography in European practices have employed double reading.

In American practices, double reading is less common. This difference probably relates to economics. In the United States, one can typically bill and collect more money for an interpretation performed with CADe than for one performed without it, while there is no monetary reward for double reading despite a presumed doubling or near-doubling of time invested by radiologists. In countries that require double reading, however, the cost of that service is built into and provided for in funding for the screening program, so that not only is double reading required, but there is no economic disadvantage to the radiologists to do it [28]. In a survey of radiologists participating in the United States Breast Cancer Surveillance Consortium to which 257 radiologists responded, 41% of respondents reported using CADe for all of their screening mammography interpretations, and 37% said they used CADe for some but not all of their screening mammography interpretations. Fewer than 2% of the respondents reported double reading all screening mammograms, although more than a fourth reported double reading at least some screening mammograms [28]. It was not clear in what context this limited double reading was considered to take place. For example, if an academic radiologist interpreted mammograms with a resident, might that have been counted as double reading? Or was limited double reading performed as part of a peer-review activity?

Despite the greater use of CADe than of double reading in the survey by Onega et al., the respondents generally had a more favorable view of double reading than of CADe in several ways. They were more likely to believe that double reading is reassuring to radiologists, improves cancer detection, and provides some protection from malpractice suits. They thought it was less likely to increase the recall rate. The differences in these perceptions between CADe and double reading, however, were small, while there was a much larger difference in the radiologists' economic perceptions. One hundred nine of the respondents (43.8%) thought that CADe improved the profitability of breast imaging, while only four (1.7%) thought that double reading did so. Forty respondents (15.9%) thought that CADe took too much time, while 166 (70.6%) thought that double reading took too much time [28].

How much time does CADe take? Two studies have timed radiologists' use of CADe. One study used digital screening mammograms and was performed in the United States. The other used film-screen screening mammograms and was performed in the United Kingdom. Both came up with similar results. Tchou et al. found that five mammographers interpreting digital images used an additional 23 seconds average per case to review CADe as opposed to interpreting the images without CADe, a difference of 19% [39]. Khoo et al. found that with film-screen mammograms the use of CADe increased reading time from 25 seconds on average to 45 seconds, a difference of 20 seconds and 80% [29]. Thus the absolute time for CADe review was remarkably similar between these two papers – 23 seconds versus 20 seconds – with the difference in percentage being accounted for by initially faster interpretation time of the film-screen mammograms as opposed to the digital mammograms. Khoo and co-authors also assumed the time spent on double reading to be an extra 25 seconds per case over that needed for CADe; in other words, they assumed that the second reader would require on average the same amount of time as the first reader. If that is true, then the slower reader times for digital mammography would also be reflected in equally slow second reader interpretation. In Khoo's study there was also time needed for arbitration of double readings, which they calculated as a total of 9.43 hours of radiologist time over the course of the study, in which mammograms of 6111 women were interpreted [29].

Reading environment

Radiology reading rooms can be quiet and peaceful or full of hectic activity, depending on how many people are sharing the room and what occurs there. Burnside *et al.* compared recall rate, cancer detection, and tumor size for 7984 screening mammograms interpreted in the midst of frequent interruptions for the other activities of a busy mammography practice – phone calls, online interpretation of diagnostic examinations, and procedures – with the same results for 1538 screening mammograms interpreted during uninterrupted batch reading. The readings were performed by five radiologists and included 7261 analog images and 2271 digital images. For both analog and digital interpretations, the recall rate decreased following institution of batch reading. Recall rate with analog images went from 19.9% before to 16.1% after the beginning of batch reading, while recall rate with digital images went from 21.0% before to 16.3% after the beginning of batch reading. This was a statistically significant drop for both types of imaging, and this drop was observed in the recall rate of each individual radiologist, although the decreases for three of the individual radiologists did not reach statistical significance. It was not stated whether the digital examinations were interpreted from printed film or on monitors. Cancer detection rate and the characteristics of those cancers identified were not separately analyzed for digital versus film-screen mammography, but for the practice as a whole there was no significant difference between images interpreted before and after batch reading was started, and the trend was for an improvement in cancer detection rate [40]. This research suggests that batch reading of screening mammograms in a calm environment should be advantageous. One question that was not addressed was what mixture of images should be interpreted in this quiet, calm reading room. For radiologists in general practices it might be reasonable to set aside uninterrupted reading time for one radiologist, who may handle a variety of image types, while another handles procedures, telephone calls, protocoling, and similar tasks. This makes intuitive sense, but to our knowledge it has not been tested.

The maximum light intensity emitted by a computer monitor is less than that emitted by a viewbox. Therefore, according to the fourth edition of the European guidelines for quality assurance in breast cancer screening and diagnosis, ambient light present in the reading room should be less than 10 lux as measured with a light meter placed at the center of the monitor, facing outward, and with the monitor turned off [38,41]. American College of Radiology 2007 guidelines suggest that ambient light should be approximately equal to the average luminance of the clinical image being displayed [9]. This is sound advice [42] but a bit difficult to carry out in practice because the luminance given off by the image can vary from one image to the next. It is easy enough to get a general idea of how much light is about right. Take a handheld light meter and hold it horizontally, parallel to the floor at about eye-height with the room lights turned off and the monitors turned on and displaying a fairly representative mammogram – one that would have a breast of typical size and density for your practice. Record the light level in lux. Turn off the monitors, and then adjust the room lights until they are producing about the same amount of light. More subjectively, it should simply not require noticeable dark or light adaptation when looking from the monitors out into the room or vice versa.

Conclusions

In conclusion, there are many variables that radiologists can choose among when interpreting digital screening mammograms. Some are entirely a matter of personal preference. Among those that we may recommend are that images be viewed both with a 4-on-1 or 2-on-1 protocol that allows side-to-side and temporal comparison and, if not at 100% resolution, then at least at a resolution near 100%, screening mammograms be interpreted in batches in a calm and uninterrupted environment, practices consider whether CADe or double reading may be helpful (if the latter is not required by local law), and that reading-room lighting be similar to the light coming from the monitors and be positioned to minimize glare on the monitor surfaces.

References

1. Pisano ED, Cole EB, Kistner EO, *et al.* Interpretation of digital mammograms: comparison of speed and accuracy of soft-copy versus printed-film display. *Radiology* 2002; **223**: 483–8.

2. Ranganathan S, Faridah Y, Ng KH. Moving into the digital era: a novel experience with the first full-field digital mammography system in Malaysia. *Singapore Med J* 2007; **48**: 804–7.

3. Berns EA, Hendrick RE, Solari M, *et al.* Digital and screen-film mammography: comparison of image acquisition and interpretation times. *AJR Am J Roentgenol* 2006; **187**: 38–41.

4. Haygood TM, Wang J, Atkinson EN, *et al.* Timed efficiency of interpretation of digital and film-screen screening mammograms. *AJR Am J Roentgenol* 2009; **192**: 216–20.

5. Ishiyama M, Tsunoda-Shimizu H, Kikuchi M, Saida Y, Hiramatsu S. Comparison of reading time between screen-film mammography and soft-copied, full-field digital mammography. *Breast Cancer* 2009; **16**: 58–61.

6. Ciatto S, Brancato B, Baglioni R, Turci M. A methodology to evaluate differential costs of full field digital as compared to conventional screen film mammography in a clinical setting. *Eur J Radiol* 2006; **57**: 69–75.

7. Haygood TM, Whitman GJ, Atkinson EN, *et al.* Results of a survey on digital screening mammography: prevalence, efficiency, and use of ancillary diagnostic aids. *J Am Coll Radiol* 2008; **5**: 585–92.

8. Wang S, Merlin T, Kreisz F, Craft P, Hiller JE. Cost and cost-effectiveness of digital mammography compared with film-screen mammography in Australia. *Aust N Z J Public Health* 2009; **33**: 430–6.

9. American College of Radiology. ACR-AAPM-SIIM practice guideline for determinants of image quality in digital mammography 2007. www.acr.org/SecondaryMainMenuCategories/

quality_safety/guidelines/breast/ image_quality_digital_mammo.aspx (accessed April 2012).

10. Haygood TM, Arribas E, Brennan PC, et al. Conspicuity of microcalcifications on digital screening mammograms using varying degrees of monitor zooming. Acad Radiol 2009; 16: 1509–17.

11. Haygood TM, Arribas E, Liu QMA, et al. Detection of microcalcifications on digital screening mammograms using varying degrees of monitor zooming. AJR Am J Roentgenol 2011; 197: 761–8.

12. Kamitani T, Yabuuchi H, Soeda H, et al. Detection of masses and microcalcifications of breast cancer on digital mammograms: comparison among hard-copy film, 3-megapixel liquid crystal display (LCD) monitors and 5-megapixel LCD monitors: an observer performance study. Eur Radiol 2007; 17: 1365–71.

13. Uematsu T, Kasami M. Soft-copy reading in digital mammography of mass: diagnostic performance of a 5-megapixel cathode ray tube monitor versus a 3-megapixel liquid crystal display monitor in a diagnostic setting. Acta Radiol 2008; 49: 623–9.

14. Yamada T, Suzuki A, Uchiyama N, Ohuchi N, Takahashi S. Diagnostic performance of detecting breast cancer on computed radiographic (CR) mammograms: comparison of hard copy film, 3-megapixel liquid-crystal-display (LCD) monitor and 5-megapixel LCD monitor. Eur Radiol 2008; 18: 2363–9.

15. Koontz NA, Gunderman RB. Gestalt theory: implications for radiology education. AJR Am J Roentgenol 2008; 190: 1156–60.

16. Kundel HL, Nodine CF, Conant EF, Weinstein SP. Holistic component of image perception in mammogram interpretation: gaze-tracking study. Radiology 2007; 242: 396–402.

17. Haygood TM, Wang J, Lane D, et al. Why does it take longer to read digital than film-screen screening mammograms? A partial explanation. J Digit Imaging 2010; 23: 170–80.

18. Taylor-Phillips S, Wallis MG, Duncan A, Gale AG. The effect of digitising film prior mammograms on radiologists' performance in breast screening: a JAFROC study. Proc SPIE 2009; 7263: 726311. DOI: 10.1117/12.810902.

19. Garg AS, Rapelyea JA, Rechtman LR, et al. Full-field digital mammographic interpretation with prior analog versus prior digitized analog mammography: time for interpretation. AJR Am J Roentgenol 2011; 196: 1436–8.

20. Skaane P, Diekmann F, Balleyguier C, et al. Observer variability in screen-film mammography versus full-field digital mammography with soft-copy reading. Eur Radiol 2008; 18: 1134–43.

21. Skaane P, Young K, Skjennald A. Population-based mammography screening: comparison of screen-film and full-field digital mammography with soft-copy reading: Oslo I Study. Radiology. 2003; 229: 877–84.

22. Pisano ED, Chandramouli J, Hemminger BM, et al. Does intensity windowing improve the detections of simulated calcifications in dense mammograms? J Digital Imaging 1997; 10: 79–84.

23. Pisano ED, Chandramouli J, Hemminger BM, et al. The effect of intensity windowing on the detection of simulated masses embedded in dense portions of digitized mammograms in a laboratory setting. J Digital Imaging 1997; 10: 174–82.

24. Krupinski EA, Roehrig H, Dallas W, Fan J. Differential use of image enhancement techniques by experienced and inexperienced observers. J Digit Imaging 2005; 18: 311–5.

25. Australia and New Zealand Horizon Scanning Network. National Horizon Scanning Report. Computer aided detection systems in mammography. Commonwealth of Australia, 2004. www.health.gov.au/internet/horizon/ publishing.nsf/Content/58685F8B48 CC9EE7CA2575AD0080F340/$File/ CAD%20HS%20Report%20Final.pdf (accessed April 2012).

26. Hofvind S, Geller BM, Rosenberg RD, Skaane P. Screening-detected breast cancers: discordant independent double reading in a population-based screening program. Radiology 2009; 253: 652–60.

27. Morton MJ, Whaley DH, Brandt KR, Amrami KK. Screening mammograms: interpretation with computer-aided detection – prospective evaluation. Radiology 2006; 239: 375–83.

28. Onega T, Aiello Bowles EJ, Miglioretti DL, et al. Radiologists' perceptions of computer aided detection versus double reading for mammography interpretation. Acad Radiol 2010; 17: 1217–26.

29. Khoo LAL, Taylor P, Given-Wilson RM. Computer-aided detection in the United Kingdom National Breast Screening Programme: prospective study. Radiology 2005; 237: 444–9.

30. Georgian-Smith D, Moore RH, Halpern E, et al. Blinded comparison of computer-aided detection with human second reading in screening mammography. AJR Am J Roentgenol 2007; 189: 1135–41.

31. Freer TW, Ulissey MJ. Screening mammography with computer-aided detection: prospective study of 12,860 patients in a community breast center. Radiology 2001; 220: 781–6.

32. Brenner RJ, Ulissey MJ, Wilt RM. Computer aided detection as evidence in the courtroom: potential implications of an appellate court's ruling. AJR Am J Roentgenol 2006; 186: 48–51

33. Beam CA, Layde PM, Sullivan DC. Variability in the interpretation of screening mammograms by US radiologists: findings from a national sample. Arch Intern Med 1996; 156: 209–13.

34. Gur D, Sumkin JH, Rockette HE, et al. Changes in breast cancer detection and mammography recall rates after the introduction of a computer-aided detection system. J Natl Cancer Inst 2004; 96: 185–90.

35. Feig SA, Sickles EA, Evans WP, Linver MN. Re: Changes in breast cancer detection and mammography recall rates after the introduction of a computer-aided detection system. J Natl Cancer Inst 2004; 96: 1260–1.

36. Gur D, Stalder JS, Hardesty LA, et al. Computer-aided detection performance in mammographic examination of masses: assessment. Radiology 2004; 233: 418–23.

37. Beam CA, Sullivan DC, Layde PM. Effect of human variability on independent double reading in screening mammography. Acad Radiol 1996; 3: 891–7.

38. Perry N, Broeders M, de Wolf C, et al. European guidelines for quality assurance in breast cancer screening and diagnosis 4th ed: summary document. Ann Oncol 2008; 19: 614–22.

39. Tchou PM, Haygood TM, Atkinson EN, et al. Interpretation time of computer-aided detection at screening mammography. *Radiology* 2010; **257**: 40–6.

40. Burnside ES, Park JM, Fine JP, Sisney GA. The use of batch reading to improve the performance of screening mammography. *AJR Am J Roentgenol* 2005; **185**: 790–6.

41. Perry N, Broeders M, de Wolf C, et al. European guidelines for quality assurance in breast cancer screening and diagnosis, 4th edn. Brussels: European Communities, 2006. screening.iarc.fr/doc/ND7306954ENC_002.pdf (accessed April 2012).

42. Brennan PC, McEntee M, Evanoff M, et al. Ambient lighting: effect of illumination on soft-copy viewing of radiographs of the wrist. *AJR Am J Roentgenol* 2007; **188**: W177–80.

43. Hambly NM, McNicholas MM, Phelan N, et al. Comparison of digital mammography and screen-film mammography in breast cancer screening: a review in the Irish breast screening program. *AJR Am J Roentgenol* 2009; **193**: 1010–18.

44. Skaane P, Skjennald A. Screen-film mammography versus full-field digital mammography with soft copy reading: randomized trial in a population-based screening program: the Oslo II Study. *Radiology* 2004; **232**: 197–204.

45. Karssemeijer N, Bluekens AM, Beijerinck D, et al. Breast cancer screening results 5 years after introduction of digital mammography in a population-based screening program. *Radiology* 2009; **253**: 353–8

46. Del Turco MR, Mantellini P, Ciatto S, et al. Full-field digital versus screen-film mammography: comparative accuracy in concurrent screening cohorts. *AJR Am J Roentgenol* 2007; **189**: 860–6.

47. Sala M, Salas D, Belvis F, et al. Reduction in false-positive results after introduction of digital mammography: analysis from four population-based breast cancer screening programs in Spain. *Radiology* 2011; **258**: 388–95.

48. Heddson B, Rönnow K, Olsson M, et al. Digital versus screen-film mammography: a retrospective comparison in a population-based screening program. *Eur J Radiol* 2007; **64**: 419–25.

49. Juel IM, Skaane P, Hoff SR, et al. Screen-film mammography versus full-field digital mammography in a population-based screening program: the Sogn and Fjordane study. *Acta Radiol* 2010; **51**: 962–8.

50. Ciatto S, Rosselli Del Turco M, Risso G, et al. Comparison of standard reading and computer aided diagnosis (CAD) on a national proficiency test of screening mammography. *Eur J Radiol* 2003; **45**: 135–38.

51. Ciatto S, Brancato B, Rosselli Del Turco M, et al. Comparison of standard reading and computer aided diagnosis (CAD) on a proficiency test of screening mammography. *Radiol Med* 2003; **106**: 59–65.

52. Helvie MA, Hadjiiski L, Makariou E, et al. Sensitivity of noncommercial computer-aided detection system for mammographic breast cancer detection: pilot clinical trial. *Radiology* 2004; **231**: 208–14.

53. Birdwell RL, Bandodkar P, Ikeda DM. Computer-aided detection with screening mammography in a university hospital setting. *Radiology* 2005; **236**: 451–7.

54. Cupples TE, Cunningham JE, Reynolds JC. Impact of computer-aided detection in a regional screening mammography program. *AJR Am J Roentgenol* 2005; **185**: 944–50.

55. Ko JM, Nicholas MJ, Mendel JB, Slanetz PJ. Prospective assessment of computer-aided detection in interpretation of screening mammography. *AJR Am J Roentgenol* 2006; **187**: 1483–91.

56. Dean JC, Ilvento CC. Improved cancer detection using computer-aided detection with diagnostic and screening mammography: prospective study of 104 cancers. *AJR Am J Roentgenol* 2006; **187**: 20–8.

Efficacy of digital screening mammography

Tamara Miner Haygood

Introduction

Screening mammography, whether performed using digital or analog technique, is the best method available of finding breast cancer at an early, potentially curable, stage. This has been demonstrated in numerous articles. One study from 2009 combined information from several large databases to study Texas women. These authors compared women living in a county with a mammography facility to those living in counties adjacent to a county with a facility and to others living in counties with no mammography facility either in that county or in an adjacent county. They discovered that merely living in a county with a mammography facility made women significantly more likely than women living in counties without mammography facilities to undergo screening and, even more importantly, more likely to have a breast cancer diagnosed at an early stage rather than a more advanced stage [1]. Diagnosis of cancer at earlier stages does translate into prevention of death from breast cancer [2–4]. Berry *et al.* used seven different statistical models to investigate causes of a drop in the breast-cancer death rate from 49.7 per 100 000 women aged 30–79 in 1990 to 38.0 per 100 000 in 2000. Depending on the model employed, the estimated contribution of screening to this drop in the breast-cancer death rate ranged from 28% to 65%, with the remainder of the drop being attributed to improvements in treatment [5].

Most of the literature regarding the benefits of screening mammography utilizes data from film-screen technique. There is every reason, however, to suppose that these benefits would also apply to digital mammograms. Weigel *et al.* studied the epidemiology of breast cancer in the Műnster/Coesfeld/Warendorf area of Germany, comparing the years 2002–04, before screening mammography was routinely offered, and 2005–07, following the introduction of a digital screening program [6]. Before screening was implemented, the average breast-cancer detection rate was 297.9 cases per 100 000 women. After screening was implemented, the detection rate jumped to 532.9 cases per 100 000 women, presumably due to earlier discovery of cases that would otherwise have lain hidden until being found clinically at a later date. Without screening, 15% of breast cancers were ≤ 10 mm in diameter and 64% were node-negative. Of cancers detected through the screening program, 37% were ≤ 10 mm in diameter and 75% were node-negative [6].

It is difficult to discuss even briefly the benefits of screening without bringing up the issue of the timing of screening mammography and related controversy spurred by the release in November 2009 by the United States Preventive Services Task Force (USPSTF) of guidelines for performing screening mammography, although it is beyond the scope of this chapter to discuss this controversy fully. The USPSTF guidelines suggest that screening mammograms should be performed every two years for women aged 50–74 and provide little encouragement for screening either before age 50 or after age 74 [7]. USPSTF guidelines contradict the recommendations of other American organizations. The American Cancer Society, for example, recommends annual mammography beginning at age 40 and continuing as long as a woman is in good health [8]. The American College of Surgeons supports the American Cancer Society's recommendations [9], and the American College of Radiology, which also backs the American Cancer Society's views, termed the USPSTF guidelines "ill advised and dangerous" [10]. In other countries, however, biennial screening in the 50- to 74-year-old age group is common. In addition, the USPSTF guidelines are supported by research by Mandelblatt *et al.* These investigators used six different statistical models to test the expected results of different screening intervals. All six models produced results favoring biennial screening. If the intent is primarily to reduce mortality from breast cancer, then biennial screening beginning at age 50 and continuing until age 69, 74, or 79 would be efficient. If the main intent is to maximize the number of life-years saved, then biennial screening should start at age 40 [11]. The USPSTF itself took notice of this article, published in November 2009, and at the time of this writing has a link to it on its own website. No matter what screening interval one favors, an important point concerning the USPSTF guidelines is that they do not question the basic value of screening mammography, but rather address the optimal frequency of screening.

Digital Mammography: A Practical Approach, ed. Gary J. Whitman and Tamara Miner Haygood. Published by Cambridge University Press.
© Cambridge University Press 2013.

Statistical modeling by Tosteson et al. has suggested that the most cost-effective approach in terms of cost per quality-adjusted life-year saved may be to use film-screen mammography in women aged 50 and over and reserve digital mammography for those aged 40 to 49 [12]. This study, however, was based on data from the Digital Mammographic Imaging Screening Trial (DMIST), which found an accuracy benefit for digital mammography in women younger than 50 years, premenopausal or perimenopausal women, and those with dense breasts [13]. The latter two groups so greatly overlap the first group, of course, as to have little practical difference. Not all other studies of the efficacy of screening mammography have found similar results with regard to age-related differences among patients, and therefore different conclusions might have been reached with different input assumptions regarding accuracy of interpretation. In addition, Tosteson et al. used cost data based on a $50 greater payment by Medicare for digital than for film-screen screening mammography. This differential would be expected to vary from place to place and over time, which would also cause the validity of these investigators' conclusions to vary.

Analog film-screen mammography has been the gold standard for breast cancer screening for decades, so digital mammography had to be tested against film-screen technique. Because economic and convenience factors balance out in favor of digital mammography for many practices, digital mammography did not have to be better than film-screen mammography in terms of accuracy, but it needed to be comparable. There is now a large body of literature comparing the interpretive accuracy of film-screen and digital screening mammography. The salient points of several such articles are summarized in Table 7.1. The methodologies of these studies vary, and so do their conclusions, but the consensus is that digital screening mammography is roughly similar in its efficacy to that of film-screen screening mammography and may be slightly better.

Equipment

Various different types of equipment have been used in tests of digital screening mammography. One article compared the accuracy of digital mammography to that of film-screen screening mammography according to the acquisition platform used [14]. The types of equipment examined were those manufactured by Fischer (no longer on the market), Fuji, and General Electric. A set of mammograms was constructed containing all cancer cases imaged with the relevant equipment during the American College of Radiology Imaging Network (ACRIN) Digital Mammographic Imaging Screening Trial (DMIST) together with some normal and benign cases. Because of differential accrual to the study, the number of cases available for each manufacturer varied. For Fischer, there were 42 cancer cases and 73 normal or negative cases; for Fuji, 27 cancer cases and 71 normal or negative cases; and for General Electric, 48 cancer cases and 72 normal or negative

cases. Truth was established by biopsy for the cancer cases and by follow-up for the normal or negative cases. Hologic equipment had also been used in the original DMIST trial, but too few cases were available for it to be included in this subsequent analysis. Each set consisted of the paired digital and film images. Twelve radiologists interpreted both the digital and analog studies for the Fuji and General Electric equipment, while six were recruited to review the studies for the Fischer equipment. The digital images were interpreted on soft copy using each manufacturer's recommended workstation. Sensitivity, specificity, and area under the ROC curve were compared for the digital versus the film-screen images for each manufacturer, and in no case was any significant difference detected. The manufacturers were not compared directly against one another, but as there was no difference noted between any of them and film, it suggests that accuracy of interpretation would also be about the same between the various manufacturers [14]. In a later reader-performance study using a subset of images from the DMIST trial and 22 readers, Nishikawa et al. found no significant difference in accuracy between interpretations of paired digital images printed on film versus those displayed on monitors [15].

Study methodology

Among studies of the efficacy of digital screening mammography, it is fairly unusual for each woman participating to have had both digital and film-screen mammograms, as was the case in the DMIST trial. Other researchers who have used this approach were Skaane et al. in the Oslo I trial [16,17] and Lewin et al. [18]. Because obtaining both digital and film-screen mammograms requires the woman to undergo two procedures and therefore be exposed to twice the radiation dose, specific consent to participate would generally be needed from each woman. Ordinarily, for a study of this sort, researchers would also need specific funding. Governmental screening organizations and insurance carriers will want to pay for only one examination, not two. Presumably for these reasons, most large evaluations of digital mammography study the technique in comparison with historical film-screen controls [19,20] or in comparison with contemporaneous film-screen mammography obtained in a similar but not identical population [21–26]. Weigel et al., addressing the German experience with digital mammography, compared its performance with a historical control at a time when no systematic screening at all was offered to German women, and also with performance parameters found in the literature [6,27].

Measures of efficacy: sensitivity and specificity

Another fairly unusual feature of the DMIST trial is that the researchers had established truth for each case. This is particularly unusual for the negative patients because the only way to determine accuracy of negative readings is to follow the patients at least until the next screening mammogram, with the assumption that if that mammogram is also interpreted as negative, the likelihood that an undetected cancer was lurking on the initial mammogram is extremely low. For European practices, where screening is normally accomplished every two years, one could not begin to process follow-up data until two years following the date of the last mammogram included in the study. Skaane *et al.* found a unique solution to this problem by publishing first on their preliminary data [16,28] and then following those publications two or three years later with new articles including the follow-up data for negative cases [17,23], and, like the authors of the DMIST trial, Juel *et al.* simply waited until follow-up examinations were available before venturing into print [20].

Alternative measures of efficacy

Presumably because of the delay inherent in waiting to have follow-up for thousands of women, most large studies of the efficacy of screening mammography use measures other than sensitivity and specificity to evaluate the effectiveness of this technique. These surrogate measures include the rate of cancer detection, callback rate, and the positive predictive value of a callback referral.

Cancer detection rate

For the 14 articles in Table 7.1 that provided these data, the overall cancer detection rate with digital screening mammography averaged 0.59%, range 0.4–0.98%, median 0.61%. Thirteen articles in Table 7.1 provided this information both for digital and for film-screen mammograms, for which the cancer detection rate averaged 0.5%, range 0.31–0.76%, median 0.47%. This calculation does not include two articles that broke cancer detection rates into separate figures for first and subsequent screenings and did not give a combined, overall figure [24,29]. For those studies, the cancer detection rates were 0.77% and 0.63% at first screening and 0.55% and 0.57% for subsequent screenings with digital mammography. They were 0.62% and 0.69% at first screening and 0.49% and 0.47% at subsequent screenings with film-screen mammography. As compared with film-screen mammography, the cancer detection rate was slightly higher for digital mammography in seven studies, equal in one study, and slightly lower in five studies. Although both the original and the follow-up articles for the Oslo I and Oslo II studies are listed in Table 7.1, their data are counted once for Oslo I and once for Oslo II in this and subsequent calculations.

Recall rate

Callback or recall rate measures the frequency with which patients are requested to return after screening mammography for additional imaging to evaluate an abnormality suspected on the screening examination. It serves as an inverse surrogate measure for specificity, as one would expect a low callback rate to correspond to a high specificity. In looking at figures, it is important to note that there are relevant differences between European practices, from which most of these studies of digital

mammography originate, and American practices. First, the legal environment is different, with worries about lawsuits [30] possibly stimulating a higher callback rate in the United States. Second, many European practices use human double reading, which, although uncommon in American practices, is actually recommended by the European guidelines for quality assurance in breast-cancer screening and diagnosis [31]. Double reading can be organized in various ways, but a typical method is for two radiologists to read through the studies separately, neither knowing the other's conclusions. Afterward any study that either radiologist thought suspicious is brought to a consensus meeting at which the radiologists who are present vote, and the finding may either be referred for callback or dismissed [20,24,28]. When double reading is applied in this or similar fashion, it can reduce the callback rate [32,33]. For digital screening mammography, recall rates for the European studies in Table 7.1 averaged 3.92%, range 1.00–6.89%, median 4.15%. For film-screen screening mammography, recall rates for the European studies in Table 7.1 averaged 3.59%, range 1.40–8.10%, median 3.40%. Six of the European studies found that recall rates were higher with digital screening mammography than with film-screen mammography, and five found them higher with film-screen screening mammography than with digital mammography. In the one Asian study [34], recall rates were within the range of those in the European studies, 2.19% for digital mammography and 1.31% for film-screen mammography. In one outlier European study (not included in the above pooled figures), the recall rate was 16.2% for digital mammograms and 13.7% for film-screen mammograms. The authors speculated that these high figures might be because of the influence of a particular reader [35]. In the sole American study [18], callback rates were also higher than for the typical European studies, 11.8% for digital mammography and 14.9% for film-screen mammography. A study published in 2009 by the members of the American Breast Cancer Consortium found an average recall rate of 9.3% and range of 6.3–13.2% among 205 radiologists in 111 geographically varied facilities who interpreted 1 036 155 screening mammograms [36]. Hofvind *et al.* also compared screening practices in Norway and Vermont and found that the recall rate was nearly four times higher in Vermont than in Norway, and that this difference was independent of the screening interval [37]. Despite this difference, the cancer detection rate and prognostic status of screening-detected cancers was similar in the two locations [37].

Positive predictive value

Another surrogate measure related to specificity is the positive predictive value of the test. The positive predictive value for screening mammography may be considered to be the percentage of studies with positive findings that actually lead to a diagnosis of breast cancer. For the articles in Table 7.1, the average positive predictive value for digital screening mammography was 18.14%, range 3.4–47%, median 15.7%.

Table 7.1 Summary of information from articles that discuss the performance of digital screening mammography, either alone or in comparison with film-screen screening mammography. Information is included as available in each article. When a piece of data was not included, no attempt has been made to infer it from other information. Numbers in brackets in the reference column refer to the relevant entry in the bibliography.

Reference	Location	Number digital	Number film-screen	Digital mammography acquisition equipment	Cancer detection rate (digital/film-screen)	Recall rate (digital/film-screen)	Positive predictive value among recalled cases (digital/film-screen)
Lewin et al. 2002 [18]	Denver, Colorado, and Worcester, Massachusetts	6736	6736	Senographe 2000D, General Electric Medical Systems, prototype model	0.4%/0.49%	11.8%/14.9%	3.4%/3.3%
Comments				6736 women underwent both digital and film-screen mammography. 42 cancers were detected. 18 were found on both digital and film-screen images, 9 were found only on digital mammography, and 15 were found only on film-screen mammography. The difference in cancer detection was not statistically significant.			
Skaane et al. 2003 (Oslo I) [16]	Oslo, Norway	3683	3683	Senographe 2000D, GE Medical Systems, Milwaukee, WI	0.62%/0.76%	4.6%/3.5%	not specified
Comments				3683 women aged 50–69 years had both digital and film-screen screening mammograms. There was no statistically significant difference in cancer detection rate or lesion conspicuity between the two modalities.			
Skaane and Skjennald 2004 (Oslo II) [28]	Oslo, Norway	6944	16 985	Senographe 2000D, GE Medical Systems, Milwaukee, WI	0.59%/0.38%	4.2%/2.5%	13.9%/15.1%
Comments				Women aged 45–69 years were randomized to digital or film-screen screening mammography. A higher cancer detection rate in the women aged 50–69 with digital mammography (0.83%) versus film-screen mammography (0.54%) approached statistical significance. No comparison studies available at initial interpretation, but they were available at the consensus meeting. Median size of screen-detected invasive cancers was 14 mm for digital and 13 mm for film-screen screening mammography.			
Skaane et al. 2005 (Oslo I follow-up) [17]	Oslo, Norway	3683	3683	Senographe 2000D, GE Medical Systems, Milwaukee, WI	0.62%/0.76%	4.6%/3.5%	13.9%/15.1%
Comments				Follow-up to the Oslo I Study primarily to look at false negatives. Digital mammography was noted to have had more false-negative reports than film-screen mammography, particularly for cancers presenting as spiculated masses or as microcalcifications alone.			
Pisano et al. 2005 [13]	33 different sites in the US and Canada. Study conducted under the auspices of the American College of Radiology Imaging Network	42 760	42 760	SenoScan (Fischer Medical), Computed Radiography System for Mammography (Fuji Medical), Senographe 2000D (General Electric Medical Systems) and Selenia Full Field Digital Mammography System (Hologic)	not specified	not specified	not specified
Comments				This study is best known as the DMIST trial. Analysis was of 42 760 women (more began the study but dropped out before analysis) who underwent both digital and film-screen screening mammography. Accuracy was judged by biopsy or follow-up study. Overall accuracy was similar, but digital mammography was slightly yet statistically significantly more accurate in women under 50 years, those with dense breasts, or those who were premenopausal or perimenopausal (largely overlapping groups). Accuracy was expressed as an area under the curve using ROC-type analysis.			
Del Turco et al. 2007 [21]	Florence, Italy	14 385	14 385	General Electric Healthcare 2000D	0.72%/0.58%	4.56%/3.96%	15.9%/14.7%
Comments				Early-stage cancer was more frequent among those detected with digital mammography (41.3%) than with film-screen mammography (27.3%).			
Skaane et al. 2007 (Oslo II follow-up) [23]	Oslo, Norway	6944	16 985	Senographe 2000D, GE Medical Systems, Milwaukee, WI	0.59%/0.38%	4.2%/2.5%	13.9%/15.1%
Comments				23 929 women from the Oslo II Study were followed up at 1.5–2 years. Interval cancer rate was 17.4/10 000 for digital mammography and 23.6/10 000 for film-screen mammography.			

Table 7.1 (cont.)

Reference	Location	Number digital	Number film-screen	Digital mammography acquisition equipment	Cancer detection rate (digital/film-screen)	Recall rate (digital/film-screen)	Positive predictive value among recalled cases (digital/film-screen)
Ranganathan et al. 2007 [34]	Singapore	200	2534	Novation DR, Siemens, Erlangen, Germany	not specified	2.19%/1.31%	not specified
Comments				Radiologists were accustomed to soft-copy interpretation of other images and found no increase in time to report digital mammography as opposed to film. The film images were obtained with CR.			
Heddson et al. 2007 [25]	Helsingborg Hospital, Sweden	9841	25 901	For CR – Siemens Mammomat 2 and Siemens Mammomat 3000 Nova with Fuji Imaging Plate HR-BD with Fuji Image Reader FCR 5000MA-plus, changed later to Fuji Image Reader FCR PROFECT. For DR – Sectra MicroDose Mammography (Sectra)	0.49%/0.38%/0.31%	1.0%/1.0%/1.4%	47%/39%/22%
Comments				The authors compared film-screen mammography with both DR and CR. 16 430 patients were included in the CR arm of the study. Figures are given in the following order: DR, CR, film-screen.			
Vigeland et al. 2008 [41]	Vestfold County, Norway	18 239	324 763	Lorad Selenia (Hologic, Inc., Danbury, CT)	0.77%/0.65%	4.09%/4.16%	16.6%/13.5%
Comments				This was a prevalence screen, as screening had not previously been offered in this county. Comparison with film-screen mammography was done using historical data from the first prevalent 2-year round in the other 18 counties of Norway. There was no statistically significant difference in the size or stage of diagnosed breast cancers.			
Vinnicombe et al. 2009 [26]	London, England	8478	31 720	3 Senographe DS units (GE Healthcare, Slough, England) and 1 Selenia unit (Lorad, London, England)	0.68%/0.72%	3.2%/3.4%	14.29%/14.60%
Comments				Reported performance of digital and film-screen screening mammography in the UK 2006–7. There was no significant difference in cancer detection rate (on adjustment for age, ethnicity, type of referral, and area of residence), recall rate, or characteristics of detected tumors. Digital mammograms were printed on film for interpretation.			
Sala et al. 2009 [19]	Barcelona, Spain	6074	12 958	DM1000, Agfa, Greenville, SC, and Lorad, Danbury CT	0.4%/0.4%	4.2%/5.5%	9.7%/7.5%
Comments				Study in Barcelona, Spain, compared 12 958 women screened with film-screen mammography to 6074 women screened subsequently after introduction of digital mammography. Recall and cancer detection rates were higher for first-round screenings than for subsequent rounds with digital mammography, as would be expected based on prior experience with film-screen mammography. No significant difference in cancer detection rate between modalities.			
Karssemeijer et al. 2009 [24]	Utrecht, the Netherlands	56 518	311 082	Lorad Selenia (Hologic, Inc., Danbury, CT)	Initial screening 0.77%/0.62%. Subsequent screenings 0.55%/0.49%	Initial screening 4.4%/2.3%. Subsequent screenings 1.7%/1.2%	Initial screening 17.4%/26.8%. Subsequent screenings 30.4%/43.1%
Comments				No significant difference in overall cancer detection rate between film-screen and digital mammograms, but the recall rate was significantly higher with digital mammograms (rates still lower than in most US practices). Digital images were especially likely to result in recall for microcalcifications. Detection rate, recall rate, and positive predictive value were quoted for initial and subsequent screenings separately, with no data pooling the two screening rounds.			

Weigel et al. 2009 [6]	Münster/Coesfeld/Warendorf, Germany	35 961	Not applicable	0.98%	6.89%	not specified	MicroDosis Mammography, MDM, Sectra Medical Systems; Mammomat 3000 Nova, Siemens Healthcare, DirectView CR975 EHR-M2, Carestream Health; Mammomat 3000 Nova, Siemens Healthcare, FCR Profect CS, Fuji and Senographe DMR+, General Electric with DirectView CR975, Carestream Health
	Comments						This was a prevalence screen, as systematic screening had not previously been offered in Germany. Therefore there are no comparable numbers available for film-screen mammography.
Lipasti et al. 2009 [40]	Finland	23 440	27 593	0.623%/0.406%	1.71%/1.59%	36.4%/25.6%	Nuance Classic and Sophie Classic (Planmed, Helsinki, Finland) units using CR plates
	Comments						The film-screen cohort was a historical control using the time-period of 1999–2000. Unlike many of the other studies, the digital system tested was CR.
Hambly et al. 2009 [22]	Republic of Ireland	35 204	153 619	0.63%/0.52%	4.0%/3.1%	15.7%/16.7%	Sectra MDM (Sectra), Lorad Selenia (Hologic), or GE Essential (GE Healthcare)
	Comments						The authors broke down their evaluation based on patient age and found a significantly higher cancer detection rate ($p = 0.01$) for digital mammography in patients over 50 years of age.
Juel et al. 2010 [20]	Sogn og Fjordane County, Norway	6932	7442	0.48%/0.39%	2.4%/2.3%	19.6%/16.7%	Sectra MicroDose Mammography, D 40 (Sectra Intec AB, Linkoping, Sweden)
	Comments						The difference in the technical recall rate was statistically significant, 0.01% for digital mammography and 0.3% for film.
Van Ongeval et al. 2010 [29]	Flanders, Belgium	11 355	312 166	Initial screening 0.63%/0.69%. Subsequent screenings 0.57%/0.47%	Initial screening 2.6%/2.8%. Subsequent screenings 1.2%/1.1%	Initial screening 24.1%/25.3%. Subsequent screenings 48.0%/41.3%	Not specified
	Comments						This article compared the performance of digital screening mammography in three regional centers with two different control groups, the historical performance of film-screen screening mammography in those same regional centers, and the performance of film-screen screening mammography in 47 regional centers over a 7.5-year period. The numbers reported here for film-screen mammography come from the larger second control group.
Balu-Maestro et al. 2010 [35]	Alpes-Maritimes region of France	9640	24 036	0.5%/0.7%	16.2%/13.7%	Not indicated	Not indicated
	Comments						This article discusses the experience of the Alpes-Maritimes region during its first year using digital screening mammography. The article is written in French.
Sala et al. 2011 [42]	Spain	71 647	171 191	0.43%/0.45%	6.2%/8.1%	7%/5.6%	2000D (Senographe, GE Medical Systems, Milwaukee WI), DM 1000 (Agfa, Lorad, Danbury Conn)
	Comments						Results are reported from four different Spanish screening programs. Therefore several factors such as reading method (single reading versus double reading) varied from one program to another.

The average positive predictive value for film-screen mammography was 14.12%, range 3.3–25.6%, median 14.7%. Positive predictive value was higher for digital than for film-screen mammography in eight articles and higher for film-screen mammography in three articles. In Karssemeijer et al. [24] the positive predictive value was higher for film-screen mammography than for digital mammography for both initial and subsequent screenings. Van Ongeval [29] found the positive predictive value to be higher for film-screen mammography than for digital mammography in the initial screening only.

Positive predictive value has also been studied in a diagnostic population. Seo et al. studied a cohort of 11 621 women in the area of Chapel Hill, North Carolina. In this study, positive predictive value was defined as the percentage of biopsies that yielded a diagnosis of cancer. A typical path to biopsy would be discovery of a suspect finding on screening mammography followed by diagnostic imaging and then by biopsy. Women presenting with symptoms or signs of cancer, women with personal history of breast cancer, and women who had undergone augmentation skipped screening mammography and went straight to diagnostic mammography, at which time biopsy might be recommended. The positive predictive value was similar between patients undergoing digital versus film-screen diagnostic mammography: 47% and 48%, respectively [38].

Reproducibility

Another factor related to the overall efficacy of a diagnostic test is the consistency or reproducibility of its interpretations. A study published by Skaane et al. in 2008 suggests that inter- and intraobserver variability is similar between film-screen screening mammography and digital screening mammography with interpretation on a monitor [39]. Six radiologists interpreted 232 screening mammograms obtained with both techniques, 20% of which demonstrated cancers, the remainder either being normal or containing benign abnormalities. For interobserver variability, in which readings were compared from one radiologist to another using the same modality, the mean weighted kappa score for film-screen screening mammography was 0.74, and for digital screening mammography 0.71. Regarding intraobserver variability, in which a single observer's interpretations of the two types of screening mammograms were compared, the mean kappa score was 0.54.

Microcalcifications and DCIS

Microcalcifications associated with breast cancer are often small and subtle, and as digital screening mammography was being introduced, there was some worry that it would not adequately display microcalcifications because of the inherently lower spatial resolution accompanying this technique as compared with film-screen screening mammography. This has not been the case. Using computed radiography technique for image acquisition and interpreting mammograms with soft copy, Lipasti et al. discovered that radiologists recalled

significantly more women because of microcalcifications in their digital mammography cohort than among patients imaged with film-screen technology [40]. Despite this, their recall rate remained quite low for both groups, 1.71% for digital mammograms versus 1.59% for film-screen mammograms [40]. Microcalcifications are particularly typical of ductal carcinoma in situ (DCIS), and some studies have noticed a higher proportion of DCIS among cancers detected with digital screening mammography compared with those found with film-screen screening mammography. For example, investigators in Vestfold County, Norway, found that their detection rate for DCIS was 0.21% using digital mammography compared with 0.11% among women screened in the other counties using film-screen mammography [41]. Karssemeijer et al., working in the Netherlands, found that for initial screening examinations detection of DCIS was almost twice as great with digital screening mammography as with film-screen screening mammography [24]. In this study, however, computer-aided detection (CADe) was available for the digital mammograms but not for the analog images. Therefore, the difference in detection of DCIS might have been due either to the difference in modality, the use of CADe with digital but not with film-screen screening mammography, or both. Other authors have also noticed an increased rate of detection of DCIS [22,42].

Of what value is the sensitivity of digital mammography in finding microcalcifications? In other words, what percentage of cancers detected in this way are invasive or will develop into invasive breast cancer and have a chance of killing the patient? Weigel et al. examined this question in conjunction with cancers detected with digital mammography in the German breast cancer screening program [27]. They found that about a third of the cancers found by microcalcifications alone were invasive, and that tumor grade did not differ between cancers detected by microcalcifications and those detected from other signs such as a mass or architectural distortion, either alone or with microcalcifications. Although the grade of the tumors did not differ, the invasive cancers detected by microcalcifications alone were smaller than those detected in other ways. The median diameter of invasive cancers detected because of microcalcifications alone was 7 mm compared with 14 mm for those detected due to masses, 15 mm for those detected due to architectural distortion, and 17 mm for those detected by a combination of microcalcifications with either a mass or architectural distortion. These data suggest that the enhanced ability of digital screening mammography to display microcalcifications may in fact allow earlier detection of potentially lethal cancers [27].

Conclusion

In general, then, there was a tendency for digital screening mammography to have a slightly higher cancer detection rate, slightly lower callback rate, and slightly higher positive predictive value than film-screen screening mammography. Interpreting these figures is a bit problematic. In my opinion they can reasonably be taken to indicate that digital and film-screen screening mammography are fairly similar in their ability to find cancer at a reasonable price in terms of callback of patients who will ultimately prove not to have cancer. These studies dealt with a grand total of 368 037 patients who had digital screening mammograms and 1 446 794 patients who had film-screen screening mammograms. They were obtained in 15 different countries on three different continents using a variety of equipment and a mixture of reading styles and screening intervals. They included both first-time and subsequent screens. These enormous variations between the studies make it problematic to compare them directly, point for point. Indeed, the preceding paragraphs in which I produce average and median numbers for this array of studies would probably be like fingernails on a chalkboard to any statistician who might read them. On the other hand, those numbers make clear that with a few exceptions, such as the distinctly higher recall rate in the American study [18] and in our one outlier European study [35], the performance of digital and film-screen screening mammography in this array of studies is, overall, fairly similar both to each other and from study to study, while the tremendous variation in the settings for these reports does suggest that they may together approach universal truth.

References

1. Elting LS, Cooksley CD, Bekele BN, *et al.* Mammography capacity impact on screening rates and breast cancer stage at diagnosis. *Am J Prev Med* 2009; **37**: 102–8.

2. Hellquist BN, Duffy SW, Abdsaleh S, *et al.* Effectiveness of population-based service screening with mammography for women ages 40 to 49 years: evaluation of the Swedish Mammography Screening in Young Women (SCRY) cohort. *Cancer* 2011; **117**: 714–22.

3. Gøtzsche PC, Nielsen M. Screening for breast cancer with mammography. *Cochrane Database Syst Rev* 2006; (4): CD001877.

4. Smith RA, Duffy SW, Gabe R, *et al.* The randomized trials of breast cancer screening: what have we learned? *Radiol Clin North Am* 2004; **42**: 793–806.

5. Berry DA, Cronin KA, Plevritis SK, *et al.* Effect of screening and adjuvant therapy on mortality from breast cancer. *N Engl J Med* 2005; **353**: 1784–92.

6. Weigel S, Batzler WU, Decker T, *et al.* First epidemiological analysis of breast cancer incidence and tumor characteristics after implementation of population-based digital mammography screening. *Rofo* 2009; **181**: 1144–50.

7. US Preventive Services Task Force. Screening for breast cancer, 2009. www.uspreventiveservicestaskforce.org/uspstf/uspsbrca.htm (accessed April 2012).

8. American Cancer Society. Guidelines for the early detection of cancer 2011. www.cancer.org/Healthy/FindCancerEarly/CancerScreeningGuidelines/american-cancer-society-guidelines-for-the-early-detection-of-cancer (accessed April 2012).

9. American College of Surgeons. College supports American Cancer Society screening mammography guidelines. *Bull Am Coll Surgeons* 2010. www.facs.org/fellows_info/bulletin/2010/mammo0110.pdf (accessed April 2012).

10. American College of Radiology. Detailed ACR statement on ill advised and dangerous USPSTF mammography recommendations. www.acr.org/MainMenuCategories/media_room/FeaturedCategories/PressReleases/UPSTFDetails.aspx (accessed April 2012).

11. Mandelblatt JS, Cronin KA, Bailey S, *et al.* Effects of mammography screening under different screening schedules: model estimates of potential benefits and harms. *Ann Intern Med* 2009; **151**: 738–47.

12. Tosteson AN, Stout NK, Fryback DG, *et al.* Cost-effectiveness of digital mammography breast cancer screening. *Ann Intern Med* 2008; **148**: 1–10.

13. Pisano ED, Gatsonis C, Hendrick E, *et al.* Diagnostic performance of digital versus film mammography for breast-cancer screening. *N Engl J Med* 2005; **353**: 1773–83.

14. Hendrick RE, Cole EB, Pisano ED, *et al.* Accuracy of soft-copy digital mammography versus that of screen-film mammography according to digital manufacturer: ACRIN DMIST retrospective multireader study. *Radiology* 2008; **247**: 38–48.

15. Nishikawa RM, Acharyya S, Gatsonis C, *et al.* Comparison of soft-copy and hard-copy reading for full-field digital mammography. *Radiology* 2009; **251**: 41–9.

16. Skaane P, Young K, Skjennald A. Population-based mammography screening: comparison of screen-film and full-field digital mammography with soft-copy reading. Oslo I Study. *Radiology* 2003; **229**: 877–84.

17. Skaane P, Skjennald A, Young K, *et al.* Follow-up and final results of the Oslo I Study comparing screen-film mammography and full-field digital mammography with soft-copy reading. *Acta Radiol* 2005; **46**: 679–89.

18. Lewin JM, D'Orsi CJ, Hendrick RE, *et al.* Clinical comparison of full-field digital mammography and screen-film mammography for detection of breast cancer. *AJR Am J Roentgenol* 2002; **179**: 671–7.

19. Sala M, Comas M, Macià F, *et al.* Implementation of digital mammography in a population-based breast cancer screening program: effect of screening round on recall rate and cancer detection. *Radiology* 2009; **252**: 31–9.

20. Juel IM, Skaane P, Hoff SR, *et al.* Screen-film mammography versus full-field digital mammography in a population-based screening program: The Sogn and Fjordane study. *Acta Radiol* 2010; **51**: 962–8.

21. Del Turco MR, Mantellini P, Ciatto S, *et al.* Full-field digital versus screen-film mammography: comparative accuracy in concurrent screening cohorts. *AJR Am J Roentgenol* 2007; **189**: 860–6.

22. Hambly NM, McNicholas MM, Phelan N, *et al.* Comparison of digital mammography and screen-film mammography in breast cancer screening: a review in the Irish breast screening program. *AJR Am J Roentgenol* 2009; **193**: 1010–18.

23. Skaane P, Hofvind S, Skjennald A. Randomized trial of screen-film versus full-field digital mammography with soft-copy reading in

population-based screening program: follow-up and final results of Oslo II Study. *Radiology* 2007; **244**: 708–17.

24. Karssemeijer N, Bluekens AM, Beijerinck D, *et al.* Breast cancer screening results 5 years after introduction of digital mammography in a population-based screening program. *Radiology* 2009; **253**: 353–8.

25. Heddson B, Rönnow K, Olsson, *et al.* Digital versus screen-film mammography: a retrospective comparison in a population-based screening program. *Eur J Radiol* 2007; **64**: 419–25.

26. Vinnicombe S, Pinto Pereira SM, McCormack VA, *et al.* Full-field digital versus screen-film mammography: comparison within the UK breast screening program and systematic review of published data. *Radiology* 2009; **251**: 347–58.

27. Weigel S, Decker T, Korsching E, *et al.* Calcifications in digital mammographic screening: improvement of early detection of invasive breast cancers? *Radiology* 2010; **255**: 738–45.

28. Skaane P, Skjennald A. Screen-film mammography versus full-field digital mammography with soft-copy reading: randomized trial in a population-based screening program: the Oslo II Study. *Radiology* 2004; **232**: 197–204.

29. Van Ongeval C, Van Steen A, Vande Putte G, *et al.* Does digital mammography in a decentralized breast cancer screening program lead to screening performance parameters comparable with film-screen mammography? *Eur Radiol* 2010; **20**: 2307–14.

30. Dick JF, Gallagher TH, Brenner RJ, *et al.* Predictors of radiologists' perceived risk of malpractice lawsuits in breast imaging. *AJR Am J Roentgenol* 2009; **192**: 327–33.

31. Perry N, Broeders M, de Wolf C, *et al.* European guidelines for quality assurance in breast cancer screening and diagnosis. Fourth edition: summary document. *Ann Oncol* 2008; **19**: 614–22.

32. Caumo F, Brunelli S, Tosi E, *et al.* On the role of arbitration of discordant double readings of screening mammography: experience from two Italian programmes. *Radiol Med* 2011; **116**: 84–91.

33. Shaw CM, Flanagan FL, Fenlon HM, *et al.* Consensus review of discordant findings maximizes cancer detection rate in double-reader screening mammography: Irish National Breast Screening Program experience. *Radiology* 2009; **250**: 354–62.

34. Ranganathan S, Faridah Y, Ng KH. Moving into the digital era: a novel experience with the first full-field digital mammography system in Malaysia. *Singapore Med* 2007; **48**: 804–07.

35. Balu-Maestro C, Bailly L, Granon C, Namer M. Numérique en dépistage organisé: bilan à 1 an dans les Alpes-Maritimes [Screening digital mammography: one year result for the Alpes-Maritimes region]. *J Radiol* 2010; **91**: 549–53.

36. Elmore JG, Jackson SL, Abraham L, *et al.* Variability in interpretive performance at screening mammography and radiologists' characteristics associated with accuracy. *Radiology* 2009; **253**: 641–51.

37. Hofvind S, Vacek PM, Skelly J, Weaver DL, Geller BM. Comparing screening mammography for early breast cancer detection in Vermont and Norway. *J Natl Cancer Inst* 2008; **100**: 1082–91.

38. Seo BK, Pisano ED, Kuzmiak CM, *et al.* The positive predictive value for diagnosis of breast cancer: full-field digital mammography versus film-screen mammography in the diagnostic mammographic population. *Acad Radiol* 2006; **13**: 1229–35.

39. Skaane P, Diekmann F, Balleyguier C, *et al.* Observer variability in screen-film mammography versus full-field digital mammography with soft-copy reading. *Eur Radiol* 2008; **18**: 1134–43.

40. Lipasti S, Anttila A, Pamilo M. Mammographic findings of women recalled for diagnostic work-up in digital versus screen-film mammography in a population-based screening program. *Acta Radiol* 2010; **51**: 491–7.

41. Vigeland E, Klaasen H, Klingen TA, *et al.* Full-field digital mammography compared to screen film mammography in the prevalent round of a population-based screening programme: the Vestfold County Study. *Eur Radiol* 2008; **18**: 183–91.

42. Sala M, Salas D, Belvis F, *et al.* Reduction in false-positive results after introduction of digital mammography: analysis from four population-based breast cancer screening programs in Spain. *Radiology* 2011; **258**: 388–95.

Chapter 8

Artifacts in digital mammography

William R. Geiser

Introduction

A high-quality mammogram optimizes a radiologist's ability to identify abnormalities with high sensitivity and high specificity [1]. Artifacts reduce the quality of mammograms and may mimic or obscure abnormalities and cause interpretation errors. Recognizing artifacts improves the quality of mammographic interpretation and prevents the characterization of artifacts as breast pathology. It also allows correction of the artifact and may contribute to its prevention on future mammograms. It is even more valuable to prevent artifacts from occurring than to recognize them after they have occurred. In this chapter, we illustrate the appearance of artifacts in digital mammography, review the causes of these artifacts, and discuss methods to eliminate artifacts in digital mammography. We present artifacts that we have encountered at The University of Texas MD Anderson Cancer Center. References to laws and regulations refer to United States laws. Those of other countries may vary. Indeed, United States law can vary over time or from state to state.

Classification of artifacts in digital mammography

Artifacts are grouped into the following five categories according to the origin of the artifact: those related to the detector, the gantry, the patient, the processing algorithm, and the image storage [2–4]. To recognize and properly classify a specific artifact, it is important to be aware of the methods used to obtain, display, and store the image. For example, patient-related artifacts are common to all forms of mammography, including both film-screen and digital mammography, whether acquired with direct digital radiography (DR) or computed radiography (CR). Processing-related artifacts may be seen with all forms of mammography as well, but those occurring with analog and digital acquisition techniques will have distinct differences in form. Storage-related artifacts occur with digital storage of images, no matter how the images were originally acquired.

Detector-related artifacts

Detector-related artifacts can be due to single dead detector elements (DELs), groups of dead DELs, dead or unread lines, banding, or ghosting.

Single dead detector elements

Malfunctioning DELs occur only with DR. They will usually appear as a white dot resembling a microcalcification. Figure 8.1a is a left mediolateral oblique view (LMLO) of the breast with a malfunctioning DEL. The white dot represents the single pixel whose signal should have been provided by the bad DEL. In the absence of input from that DEL, no signal is available, and the pixel shows up as pure white. If the pixel supplied by the bad DEL is over a white background, the image-processing algorithm may cause the associated pixel to appear dark. In Figure 8.1b the pixel supplied by the dead DEL is black in the region of the implant as a result of image processing. The absence of signal from the dead DEL is recognized by the processing algorithm as different from the low signal obtained with the surrounding normally functioning DELs. The processor will then sometimes alter the resulting appearance of the pixel to make it appear different from the surrounding pixels, in this case making it appear dark in this mediolateral view of the augmented left breast. The bad DEL in both these images is the same DEL, overlying different parts of the image with different backgrounds.

To remove the artifact, a service call to the manufacturer needs to be placed. The service engineer downloads a flat-field image from the detector and uses software to map out the bad DEL. The software replaces the signal from the bad DEL with a value that is a weighted average of the signals from the surrounding DELs. Once the DEL is mapped out, a new DEL map is made and loaded onto the imaging system, and the unit is returned to service after testing by the quality-control (QC) technologist or the medical physicist. The DEL that was mapped out is no longer functional and will always have the value assigned by the new DEL map. The information on how

Digital Mammography: A Practical Approach, ed. Gary J. Whitman and Tamara Miner Haygood. Published by Cambridge University Press.
© Cambridge University Press 2013.

(a)

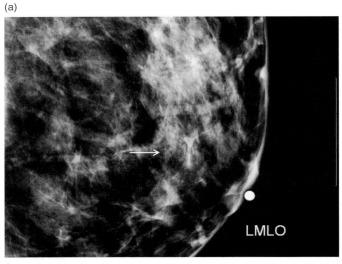

(b)

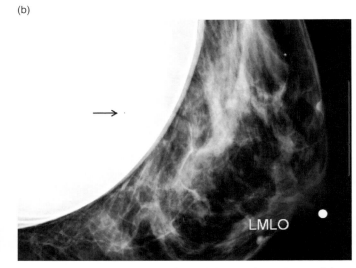

Figure 8.1 (a) Dead DEL (arrow) in the LMLO view. Note that the white dot caused by the dead DEL can be mistaken for a calcification. (b) LMLO view of the augmented breast. Zoomed image shows dead DEL (arrow) projecting over the implant. The pixel supplied by the dead DEL is black in the region of the implant as a result of image processing.

many dead DELs are allowed is proprietary information. The vendors hold this information very closely, and they make the determination as to when to replace a detector due to too many bad DELs.

Multiple dead detector elements

After several thousand exposures, the detector may start to show signs of radiation damage. This damage will show up as DELs that may no longer give any signal or may give 100% signal. Mapping out the bad DELs will not improve image quality as more DELs quickly go bad. Figure 8.2a is a right magnified lateromedial (RMLM) view of the breast where it was noted that there was high noise in the image. Subsequent testing showed that the detector was dying and that DELs were going bad more quickly than they could be mapped out. Figure 8.2b is a right lateromedial (RLM) view taken on the same patient. Note that the processing has turned the missing information from the dead DELs black in the dense areas of the breast.

This system was taken out of service immediately after the artifact was discovered by the radiologist in the reading room. A new detector was ordered, installed, and tested the next day. The system was then placed back into service.

Misread lines

Sometimes an entire line in the image fails or does not get read out. This artifact can manifest in two ways. The first manifestation is as a very fine line across the image, as illustrated in Figure 8.3a. This is a left magnified lateromedial (LMLM) view of the breast. A single line failed to be read out during the readout process. This manifested as a fine black line across the image. The artifact was so faint that the technologist missed it on her review of the image before sending it to be interpreted. The radiologist reading the study noted the artifact on the high-quality 5-megapixel monitors

used for primary interpretation of the images. Figure 8.3b is the left craniocaudal magnification view (LMCC) taken immediately after the LMLM view. There is no longer a missing line of data.

Another manifestation of this phenomenon is shown in Figure 8.4a, with the subsequent retake shown in Figure 8.4b. Figure 8.4a shows an LMLO view that was taken during a screening exam. The technologist failed to note any artifacts on the image at the acquisition station and sent the image to the picture archiving and communication system (PACS). When reviewing the image on PACS, the technologist noted a large band of missing information on the image. The technologist called the patient back into the room and repeated the image (in the same room). The retake shows no artifact.

In both these cases, a service call was placed, and the detector was checked for dead detector rows and columns. Nothing was noted on testing, and the failure could not be reproduced. Technical support from the detector manufacturer recommended that a new readout sequence file be loaded onto the system. This file controls the sequence of events that take place to read out the detector. A new readout sequence file was installed, and the unit was tested. No artifacts were noted. The system was placed back into service.

Banding artifacts

Banding artifacts cause lines of varying brightness across the image (Figure 8.5). This is a common artifact caused by vibration of the detector or a shock to the detector during the readout phase of the image cycle. The artifact in Figure 8.5 was noticed by the radiologist and was seen only on the right craniocaudal (RCC) view. The system was checked, with an emphasis on trying to reproduce the artifact. The artifact could not be reproduced after several test exposures with a phantom. The system was returned to clinical use after testing was complete.

(a)

(b)

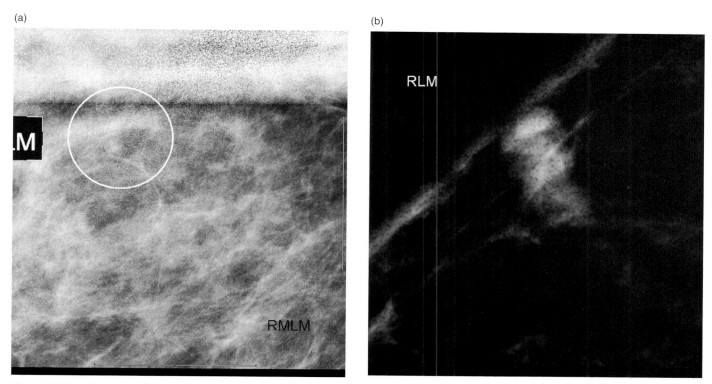

Figure 8.2 Multiple misread or dead DELs. (a) RMLM view demonstrates selenium detector as it begins to fail, with a large number of misread or dead DELs. Misread or dead DELs can look like clusters of microcalcifications (circle). (b) RLM view with digital detector failure. In this contact view, the image processing algorithm has made the information from the dead DELs black for display.

(a)

(b)

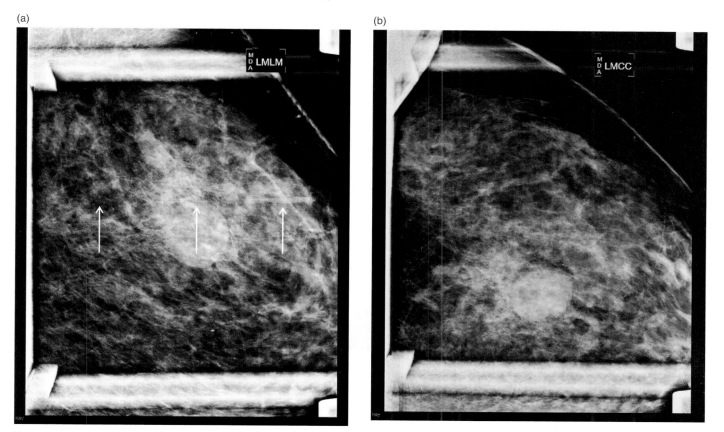

Figure 8.3 (a) LMLM view of the breast, showing a single line of the detector with no information. (b) LMCC view taken immediately after the image in (a): there is no missing information in this image.

(a)

(b)

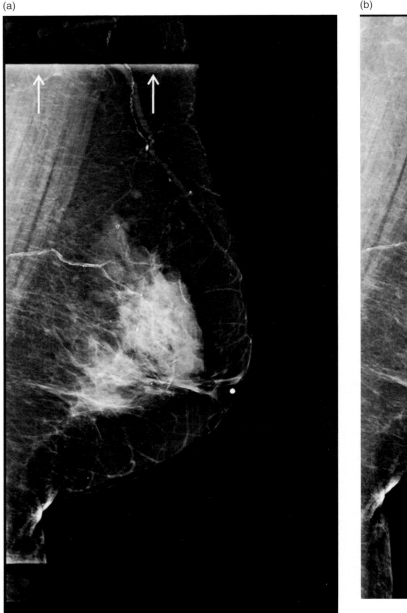

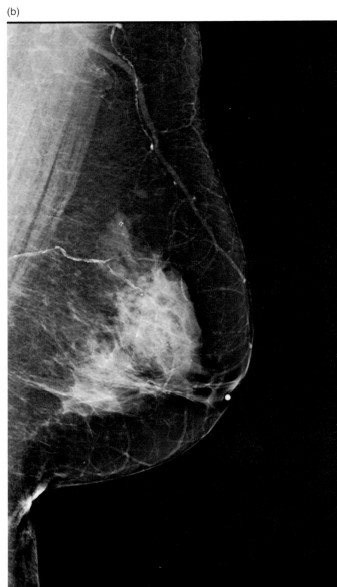

Figure 8.4 (a) LMLO view on a screening mammogram with a large band of missing data across the image (arrows). This artifact was due to a line of data from the detector that had been missed on readout of the detector. (b) Retake of the LMLO view in (a) with the same piece of equipment: the artifact is not present.

Figure 8.6 is another example of a banding artifact, which was noted only on a laterally exaggerated left craniocaudal (LXCCL). Note that there are two sets of banding on the image. The popular term for this artifact is "tire tracks," as it looks like two sets of tire tracks across the image. The room was placed out of service, and a call was placed to the service engineer to come and check the system. The image was downloaded to technical support for evaluation. The artifact was explained as being caused by a mismatch in frequency between the detector power supply and the readout electronics. The service engineer replaced the power supply for the detector. After the power supply was replaced, the

system was tested. No artifacts were noted, and the system was placed back in service.

Ghosting artifacts

Ghosting was an artifact problem that was noted with the first generation of selenium-based detectors. The ghost image is caused when there is residual charge in the detector from the previous image. When a second image is taken, the residual charge adds to the charge collected for the second image, leaving a "ghost" of the previous image superimposed on the

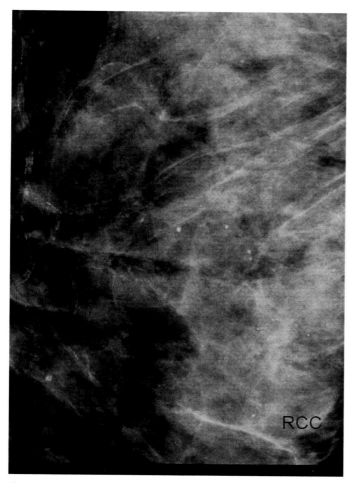

Figure 8.5 RCC view demonstrating a banding artifact across the entire image resulting in numerous linear stripes resembling grid lines.

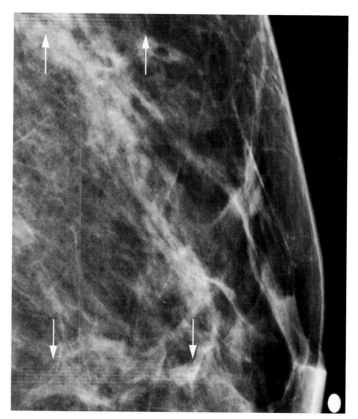

Figure 8.6 LXCCL view with the banding artifact known as "tire tracks" (arrows).

current image. The main reason for ghosting in the early detectors was low detector temperature. Allowing the detector to warm up properly or operating the detector at a slightly higher temperature cleared the problem. With improvements in detector technology and systems to better regulate detector temperature, this problem is becoming less common.

Figure 8.7 shows an LMLO view that demonstrates a ghost of the previous image taken. Proper operating temperature for the selenium detector is 25–35 °C. Detector temperature was found to be at the low end of the allowed temperature range (27 °C). When the operating temperature of the detector rose above 29 °C, the ghosting resolved.

Gantry-related artifacts

Gantry-related artifacts are artifacts that arise from problems with components in the x-ray beam path that are not directly associated with the detector or the patient. These artifacts are associated with the compression paddle, the anti-scatter grid, or the collimation system.

Artifacts from the compression paddle can come from cracks in the compression paddle or foreign material that has accumulated on the compression paddle. Dust or foreign material may also accumulate on components used to filter the x-ray beam, which may cause artifacts similar to those from dust on the compression paddle. Other gantry-based artifacts can arise when the automatic exposure control (AEC) system is not properly adjusted. The image may be well processed and have the correct contrast and gray scale, but improper technique may result in low signal-to-noise ratio, which may obscure small objects or may lead to improper processing of the image.

Foreign material on the compression paddle

Because of its design, the compression paddle can begin to collect dust and other foreign material that may come to rest on it. Highly attenuating foreign material on the surface of the compression paddle can cause artifacts that mimic calcifications in the breast. Figure 8.8a is an LCC view of the breast in which a high-density calcification-like object was noted on the lateral aspect of the image. A similar-looking object was also noted on the RCC view (Figure 8.8b). Because there were similar artifacts on views of two different breasts obtained with the same detector, the technologist recognized that there was an artifact on these two views and that the artifact was most likely caused by a foreign object either on the compression paddle or on the breast support plate. Cleaning of both surfaces removed the object, and the study was completed with no further artifacts.

The Mammography Quality Standards Act (MQSA) requires that there be procedures in place for infection control that allow for "cleaning and disinfecting mammography equipment after contact with blood or other potentially infectious materials" [5]. This is usually interpreted to mean any contact with the patient, even through intact skin. Thus, the

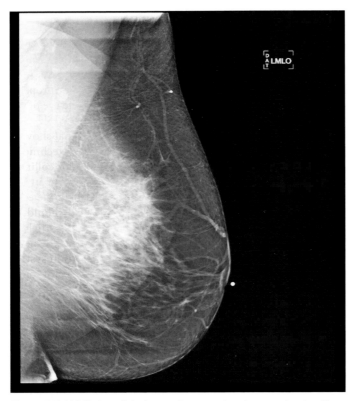

Figure 8.7 LMLO view of the breast, demonstrating detector ghosting. The lines running across the top half of the breast roughly parallel to the image edge are the most obvious sign of this ghost image.

technologist will disinfect any surfaces that the patient's skin contacts. Often the technologist will clean or disinfect the breast support plate and the surface of the compression paddle that comes into contact with the patient's skin (the bottom surface) but not clean the top surface of the compression paddle, which does not touch the patient but where dust can easily accumulate. It is recommended that the technologist clean the entire compression paddle at least once a day, and more often if dust is seen to be accumulating on the compression paddle.

Grid artifacts

Currently, all digital mammography systems approved in the United States by the Food and Drug Administration (FDA) have a moving grid that removes scatter photons and helps to improve contrast, with one exception. That exception is the Sectra MicroDose mammography system. The Sectra MicroDose mammography system is a slot-scan device with a narrow detector, approximately 1 cm wide, that does not require an anti-scatter grid.

Currently, two grid types are used in digital mammography. The most common type is a linear grid, where the lines of the grid are parallel to the anode–cathode axis of the x-ray tube. One manufacturer uses a cross-hatched grid in which the grid septa cross one another at a 45-degree angle to the x-ray tube anode–cathode axis. Both of these types of grid are driven by a small motor and are subject to mechanical failure. A grid artifact may arise if the grid fails to move at all or if there is a problem with the timing of the initial motion of the grid.

Figure 8.9 is an LMLO view where the grid failed to move. An image of the grid is clearly seen overlying the entire breast (cross-hatch pattern). It was found that the mechanism that supported the grid was warped and had caused the grid to become stuck in place. To fix the problem, the entire detector array system had to be replaced, as the grid is an integral part of the detector assembly.

(a)

(b)

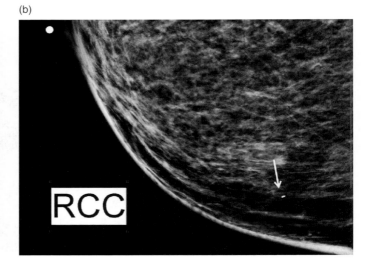

Figure 8.8 (a) LCC view with a linear calcification-like object visualized in the breast (arrow). (b) RCC view with a linear calcification-like object also visualized in the breast (arrow).

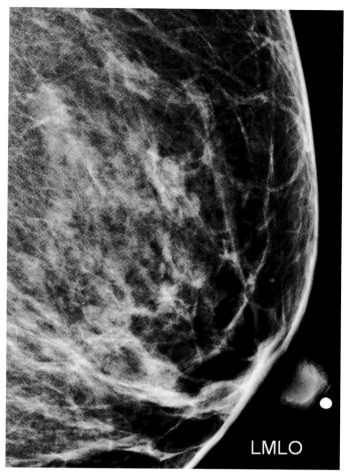

Figure 8.9 LMLO view with severe grid lines.

Improper collimation

Collimation of the x-ray beam serves two purposes. In general radiography, it can be used to limit radiation exposure to body parts that are not relevant to the examination. In both general radiography and mammography, it also ideally serves to ensure that the entire detector (whether film or a digital detector) is exposed to the x-ray beam. Improper collimation can be a problem in mammography. If collimation leaves a portion of the detector unexposed to the x-ray beam, that area will be displayed as an area of intense brightness similar to what would be seen if a film-screen mammogram were taken in a similar fashion and displayed on a bright viewbox or if the film were not properly masked. This stray light can limit the contrast that the eye of the radiologist can perceive in the remainder of the image [6].

Figure 8.10a is an RLM CR image of the breast that shows a large area of over-collimation. Even though this technique satisfies the United States regulatory requirements for collimation, for the radiologist to perceive all of the contrast in the image, the image should be exposed all the way out to the edge of the detector. To achieve this goal, a service call should be made to have the collimation adjusted so that the x-ray field is just slightly larger than the image receptor along each edge.

Figure 8.10b is a LMLO view where the collimation system was misadjusted, leaving a small area of the detector on a digital mammography system unexposed along the right edge of the detector. A call to service the system and a quick adjustment by the service engineer resolved the problem.

Collimation must be checked by the medical physicist on an annual basis. Part of the annual survey is to ensure that the compression paddle is not visible along the chest-wall edge of the image and that the compression paddle is not preventing visualization of all the breast tissue. Figure 8.11 is an image where the compression paddle was not properly adjusted, and the

(a)

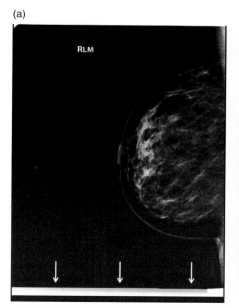

(b)

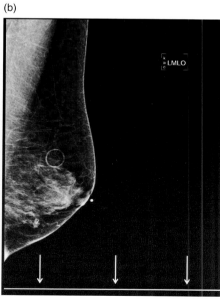

Figure 8.10 (a) RLM view demonstrating over-collimation on a CR-based system (arrows). The image should be exposed all the way out to the edge of the imaging plate. (b) Over-collimation on a DR system on LMLO view (arrows). Although the misalignment is not as severe as the over-collimation on the CR-based system, the collimation needs to be adjusted so that no area of the image detector is unexposed.

chest-wall edge of the paddle is visible in the image. A couple of millimeters of tissue along the chest-wall of this LMLO view are not visualized because the compression paddle obscures the

chest-wall side of the image. MQSA regulations state, "The shadow of the vertical edge of the compression paddle shall not be visible on the image" [5]. This needs to be resolved within 30 days of discovery of the problem. Proper alignment of the compression paddle will ensure that all the tissue along the chest wall is visible to the maximum extent possible.

Patient-related artifacts

Patient-related artifacts have been described for film-screen mammography and digital mammography and have well-known causes [7]. Patient-related artifacts may be caused by motion, by superimposition of objects or substances over the breast parenchyma, or by foreign substances on the skin [2]. The most commonly reported patient-related artifact is patient motion. Other types of artifacts include hair, gowns, or other foreign objects overlying the breast during imaging. The technologist may not notice that the patient has placed a hand on the breast support plate or compression paddle or that there are other undesired objects in the image field.

Patient motion

A look at repeat image rates at MD Anderson Cancer Center showed that patient motion was the second highest reported cause for repeats, after patient positioning errors. Patient motion is more likely to be detected during longer exposure times. Figure 8.12a is a left mediolateral oblique magnification view (LMMLO) image where patient motion is evident. Blurring was not detected by the technologist before sending the image to be viewed by the radiologist as the technologist could not see blurring on the relatively low-quality monitor at the acquisition station. The radiologist viewing the image noted that the edges of the surgical clips were not sharp or well defined, the calcifications visible on the image were blurred, and the other anatomical structures in the breast were not well defined. Also noted by the radiologist were

Figure 8.11 Edge of the compression paddle (arrows) seen in the field of view along the chest-wall edge of the LMLO view.

(a)

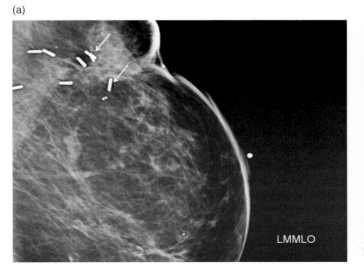

(b)

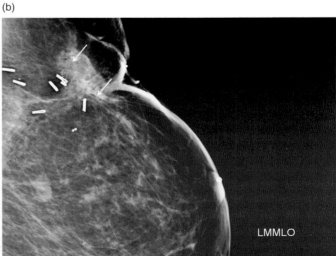

Figure 8.12 (a) Blurring on LMMLO view as a result of patient motion. Edges of clips (arrows) have shadows. (b) Repeat of the LMMLO view without patient motion shows clips sharply defined (arrows).

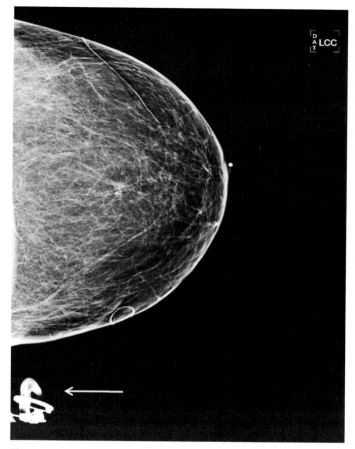

Figure 8.13 LCC view with ear and earring in image field of view (arrow). Making sure that the face shield is in place will prevent this type of artifact.

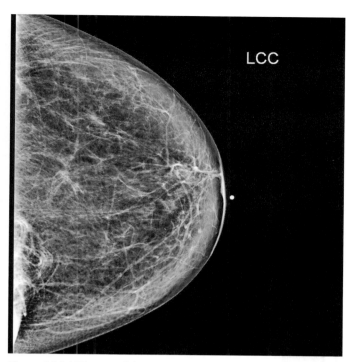

Figure 8.14 LCC view with hair seen over the medial aspect of the breast. This image comes from a slot-scan device that had no light field for the technologist to use in positioning the patient.

the technical factors used to take the image. In this case, the breast was compressed to a thickness of 80 mm with 57.8 newtons (13 pounds) of force, and the AEC system used 33 kVp and 64 mAs to get the proper exposure. At the request of the radiologist, the technologist performed a repeat of the image (Figure 8.12b) to try to eliminate the motion artifact. The repeat image was performed using 80.1 newtons (18 pounds) of force, which resulted in a compressed breast thickness of 71 mm, allowing the technical factors to be reduced to 32 kVp and 61.8 mAs. Because most of this reduction was in mAs rather than in kVp, the time needed for the exposure was shortened, thus reducing the likelihood of patient motion. Note that in the repeated image the edges of the surgical clips have a sharp appearance, and the calcifications in the surgical bed are clearly defined. In this case, the cause for motion was undercompression of the breast, resulting in the need for a prolonged exposure. Proper compression and the use of technical factors to reduce patient exposure time will minimize the number of repeats for patient motion.

Unwanted anatomy

Unwanted anatomy in the image is a common artifact that can be found in digital mammograms. Patients' fingers, chins, and noses have all been seen on mammograms. Hair in the field of view is another common artifact noted. This unwanted anatomy can obscure portions of the breast and lead to missed lesions. It also results in unnecessary radiation exposure to the extraneous body parts (Figures 8.13, 8.14).

The mammogram in Figure 8.13 was taken after the technologist had removed the face shield from the system while performing magnification views of the previous patient. When the technologist set up the mammography system to image this patient, she neglected to place the face shield back on the system. As a result, the patient leaned her head into the x-ray beam, and the projection of her ear and earring ended up in the image field of view.

Figure 8.14 shows what can happen when there is no light field for the technologist to position by. The image was taken using a slot-scan mammography system that had no light field for positioning. The technologist could not see the shadow of the hair overlying the breast and did not remove it from the field of view. The shadow of the hair clearly obscures the breast tissue over the medial aspect of the breast near the chest wall.

To keep unwanted anatomy from showing up in the image of the breast, the technologist should ensure that the face shield that comes with the mammography system is in place when performing contact mammography. This will ensure that no facial anatomy will overlie the breast tissue to be imaged. In addition to this, the technologist should carefully check the light field used for positioning to make sure that there are no unwanted shadows from objects such as the patient's gown or the patient's hair in the field of view.

(a)

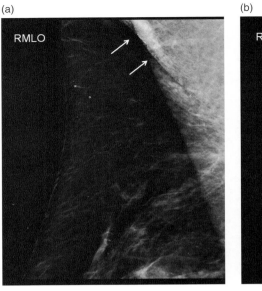

(b)

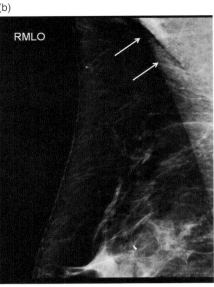

Figure 8.15 (a) Deodorant artifact (arrows) seen in the axillary region on a RMLO view. (b) Retake of RMLO view after having the patient clean under her arms to remove any deodorant residue.

(a)

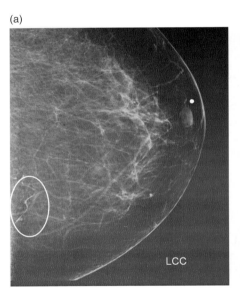

(b)

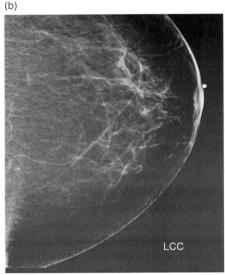

Figure 8.16 (a) Artifact caused by residue left by a cardiac monitor pad (roughly S-shaped bright line in circle) on an LCC view of the breast. (b) Retake of the LCC view of the breast after the patient was asked to clean the breast to remove the residue from the cardiac monitor pad.

Foreign substances on the patient's skin

Foreign substances on the patient's skin can cause a variety of different artifacts that may mimic calcifications, masses, or fiber-like structures of the breast. One common artifact of this type is caused by deodorant. Most deodorants contain aluminum-bearing chemicals that attenuate the x-ray beam in a fashion similar to calcium in the breast. Thus, deodorant can leave an artifact that looks like calcifications. Combine this with the fact that the deodorant may be in skin folds, and the artifact looks very much like a linear grouping of calcifications. Figure 8.15a is an RMLO view of the breast where the patient did not properly clean under her arm before being imaged. The radiologist noted calcifications in the axillary region of the image and assumed they were a deodorant artifact due to their location. After having the patient clean under her arms, the image was repeated to prove that the calcifications were actually from deodorant on the patient's skin (Figure 8.15b).

Another artifact seen is residue left on the patient from tape or other objects that are designed to stick to the patient. Figure 8.16a shows an artifact on the LCC view, created by residue left on the breast from a cardiac monitor pad. The pad had been placed on the patient during a visit to another clinic earlier in the day. The patient had removed the pad but was unaware that some of the adhesive used to hold the pad in place was still on her skin. The technologist taking the image also failed to notice anything on the patient's skin and proceeded to perform the study. Upon review by the radiologist, the artifact was noted on both the LCC and the LMLO views of the study. The technologist was asked to check the patient for foreign substances on her breast. A careful

(a)

(b)

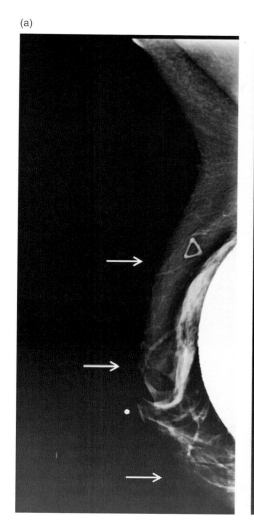
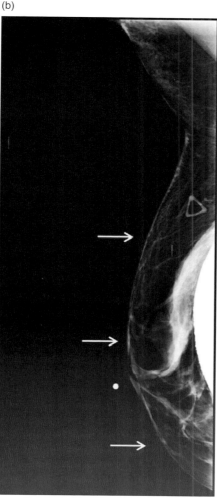

Figure 8.17 (a) RLM view of the breast with image-processing problems due to underexposure of breast tissue. The processing algorithm could not find the skin line and thus could not properly process the image. (b) Retake of the RLM with proper technique, showing the skin line properly processed and displayed.

look at the skin surface revealed the tape residue left on the skin from the cardiac monitor pad. The breast was cleaned, and the LCC and LMLO views were retaken. Figure 8.16b is the repeat LCC view showing that the tape residue had been removed.

Processing-related artifacts

Processing-related artifacts arise when the processing algorithm encounters something in the raw data that it does not know how to process properly. When digital mammography was in its infancy, processing artifacts were encountered quite frequently even though they were rarely of clinical significance. As digital mammography matured and the vendors learned from the artifacts their customers encountered, software patches were designed and installed that enhanced the image-processing algorithms and reduced artifacts caused by the high degree of processing used. Today, artifacts caused by image processing are seldom encountered if the latest version of software is installed on the imaging system.

Examples of processing-related artifacts include loss of the skin line on the displayed image, shading of the detector area

around the skin line, reversal of pixels in high-density objects, and lines in the image due to improper gain and offset calibration of the detector.

Failure of skin-line processing algorithm

One of the advantages of digital mammography over film-screen mammography is the ability to view the breast tissue all of the way out to the skin line without the need for special viewing tools such as hot lights. All of the vendors of digital mammography equipment have a special processing algorithm to find the skin line of breast and enhance it so that it is visible to the radiologist.

Figure 8.17a is an RLM view where the technical factors used (32 kVp and 27.8 mAs) resulted in underexposure of the detector, which caused the skin-line processing algorithm to fail, causing poor visualization of the tissue along the outer portion of the breast. A retake of the image using 32 kVp and 107 mAs (Figure 8.17b) produced enough exposure to the detector that the skin-line processing algorithm could define the skin line and process it properly, resulting in an optimally processed image. The ability of the skin-line processing algorithm to perform properly is

(a)

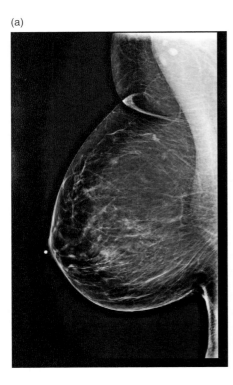

(b)

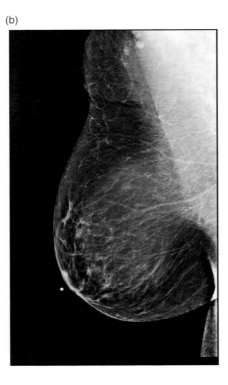

Figure 8.18 Background shading artifact. (a) RMLO view with inappropriate display processing parameters. (b) RMLO view of the same patient a year later on the same mammography unit after software upgrade and display processing parameters were set properly by the service engineer.

determined in a large part by its being able to find the line where the detector goes from being exposed to raw x-ray radiation to the area where the x-ray beam has been attenuated by tissue. If the detector is underexposed in the area exposed to raw radiation, the skin-line processing algorithm may not be able to determine where the skin line starts and may fail to process the skin line properly.

Shading artifacts

A shading artifact occurs when the display parameters of the processing are not set properly. Figure 8.18a is an RMLO image with a shading artifact. The image was taken with the correct technique factors and the breast was properly compressed. At the acquisition station, no artifacts or problems with the image were noted, and the technologist accepted the image and sent it to PACS for storage and viewing. Upon viewing the image, the radiologist noted a gray halo around the image in the area that was exposed to direct radiation. The radiologist also noted that the skin-line processing and the processing for the rest of the breast appeared to be normal and decided that the artifact would not interfere with the diagnostic interpretation of the image. The image was not repeated.

The image was sent off to technical support for review so that a solution could be found to ensure that the background around the breast would be black, as it should be. The technical support team consulted with the service engineer on site, and it was determined that some parameters in the Digital Imaging and Communications in Medicine (DICOM) header that were being sent with the image were set incorrectly. Apparently the manufacturer has a set of display parameters that are used when displaying the image at

the acquisition station and a different set of display parameters for display on the radiologists' review station. Adjusting the display parameters for the radiologists' workstation display eliminated the gray halo around all subsequent images taken on this system. Figure 8.18b is the RMLO view of the same patient taken a year later on the same mammography unit.

This artifact was not seen on acceptance testing of the mammography unit and was not seen until after the first detector replacement on this system. When the detector was replaced, some of the display parameters were not set properly. The artifact was only noticed on images that were taken using the large field size, and acceptance testing of the new detector did not pick up the artifact. It was only after patients were imaged that the artifact was noted. Ensuring that all the display parameters are set to their proper values before imaging patients will eliminate this artifact and the need for a service call.

Pixel reversal artifacts

Usually, high-density objects or highly attenuating objects are displayed white in the image. However, sometimes the processing algorithm causes these high-density objects to be displayed with their pixel values reversed or black. Figure 8.19a is an RLM spot view of the patient's breast. The compression paddle is held by a metallic arm, which is highly attenuating. The processing algorithm on this system attempts to black out the arm to prevent a large amount of white light from reaching the eye of the radiologist. In the process of blacking out the compression paddle arm, the processing algorithm also inverts

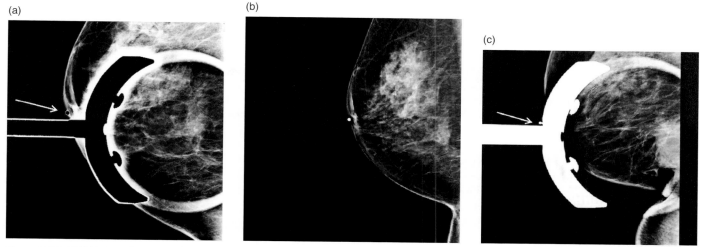

Figure 8.19 (a) RLM view of patient with nipple marker, with pixels displayed black instead of white (arrow). (b) RLM view of the breast, showing the nipple marker as it is normally displayed (white). (c) RLM image after a software upgrade that changed the image processing algorithm so that high-density objects would be displayed white instead of black.

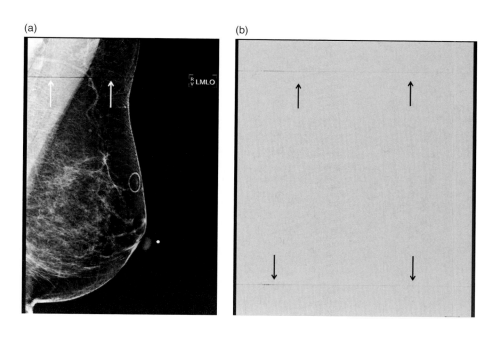

Figure 8.20 (a) Patient image showing the effect of the gain calibration artifact. This image was taken on a Hologic Selenia system using the 18 × 24 cm compression paddle with the paddle shifted to the right. The line artifact (arrow) is where the field is collimated when the 18 × 24 cm paddle is used. (b) Artifact due to improper gain calibration. The procedure for weekly gain calibration was not followed precisely, and this artifact (arrows) was created.

the pixels of the nipple marker, making it appear black (arrow). Also of note is the pixel-value reversal along the chest-wall edge of the image in the area of the pectoral muscle. Figure 8.19b is the standard RLM view that was obtained on the same day. Note that the nipple marker is white on the image and there is no pixel reversal in the pectoral muscle.

Recently, the manufacturer of this mammography machine, the Hologic Selenia, has come out with a software upgrade that has changed the way the processing algorithm reacts when there is a high-density object in the field of view. Instead of the high-density object being blacked out, the object is displayed as it would be with a film-screen system. This prevents the loss of information in other high-density areas of the image (Figure 8.19c).

Gain and offset calibration artifacts

Several manufacturers of digital mammography equipment require that the QC technologist perform a gain and offset calibration of the detector weekly. To perform this procedure, the technologist must follow a set of instructions exactly as described. If the procedure is not followed precisely, artifacts may be introduced into the image when the gain and offset calibration is applied to the patient image.

In Figure 8.20, the imaging technologist imaged a patient after the QC technologist had performed the weekly gain and offset calibration of the system. The first image taken was the RCC view of the left breast using the 18 × 24 cm field size. No artifacts were noted. The second image taken was the RMLO view of the left breast (Figure 8.20a). The imaging technologist immediately noticed the line artifact on the image and placed a service call. The imaging physicist and service engineer were called in to troubleshoot and determine the cause of the artifact. Figure 8.20b is the flat-field image taken by the imaging physicist to troubleshoot the problem. The flat-field image is taken using the entire detector (24 × 29 cm) without the compression paddle.

It was determined that the lines on the flat-field image corresponded to the position of the collimator blades when the gain and offset calibration was done for the magnification mode on the detector. The service engineer called technical support and sent the image for analysis. Technical support reported that this artifact was caused when the gain and offset procedure was not followed precisely and one of the steps had been missed or done out of sequence. A new gain and offset calibration was performed to remove the artifact.

Storage-related artifacts

Storage-related artifacts are artifacts that are created by transmission and storage of the image to PACS. These artifacts can be created by noise during transmission or problems when the image is stored to disk.

Figure 8.21 shows what can happen when the image is stored improperly. The PACS system that was used uses a wavelet coefficient scheme to store the image. When the image was viewed on the PACS review station by a radiologist, all that could be seen were white rectangles with some of the breast visible in between. The PACS vendor was asked to determine the cause of the artifact and make a repair. This required the PACS vendor to modify a script to change the coefficients used to store the images with this matrix size in order for them to be displayed properly at the review station. The image then had to be deleted from the PACS system and resent from the acquisition station to PACS for storage and review (Figure 8.21).

In this case, the radiologist discovered the artifact and the problem in the imaging chain where the artifact was created. In best practice, however, the technologist who imaged the patient should have reviewed the images once they were stored on PACS to look for artifacts and make sure that they were ready for review. The image QC process by the technologist should not be considered complete until after the images have been stored on PACS and viewed by the imaging technologist.

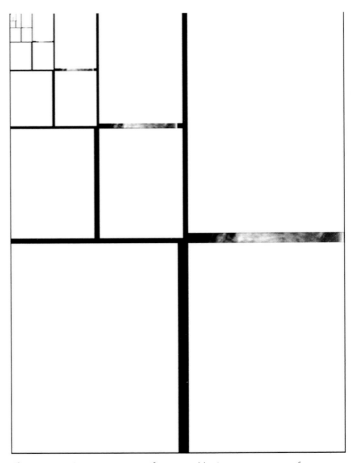

Figure 8.21 Reconstruction artifact caused by incorrect storage of frequency coefficients for image. Image could not be recovered from PACS system. This artifact would only be seen with PACS vendors that use wavelet coefficients to store images.

Conclusions

Just as in film-screen mammography, artifacts in digital mammography are inevitable. To reduce the impact that artifacts have is a team effort that requires good communication between the interpreting physician, the imaging technologist, the medical physicist, and the service engineer working on the equipment. With a proper QC program in place and due diligence by everyone on the imaging team, the number of artifacts can be minimized and their impact on the diagnostic process reduced.

References

1. Eklund GW, Cardenosa G, Parsons W. Assessing adequacy of mammographic image quality. *Radiology* 1994; **190**: 297–307.

2. Ayyala RS, Chorlton M, Behrman RH, Kornguth PJ, Slanetz PJ. Digital mammographic artifacts on full field systems: what are they and how do I fix them? *Radiographics* 2008; **28**: 1999–2008.

3. Pisano ED, Cole EB, Hemminger BM, *et al.* Image processing algorithms for digital mammography: a pictorial essay. *Radiographics* 2000; **20**: 1479–91.

4. Coscia J, Jaskulski S, Wang J. Clinically challenging mammographic artifacts: a pictorial guide. *Curr Probl Diagn Radiol* 2001; **30**: 6–18.

5. Mammography Quality Standards Act, 21 CFR 900, 1994, http://www.fda.gov/Radiation-EmittingProducts/MammographyQualityStandardsActandProgram/default.htm (accessed April 2012).

6. Rill LN, Huda W, Gkanatsios NA. View box luminance measurements and their effect on reader performance. *Acad Radiol* 1999; **6**: 521–9.

7. American College of Radiology. *Mammography Quality Control Manual.* Reston, VA: ACR, 1999.

Mobile digital mammography

Michael Ryan

Introduction

Breast cancer is currently the most common malignancy in American women. Recently, breast cancer has become the second leading cause of death in women after lung cancer. But it is a distant second. The rather remarkable difference in mortality rate comparing breast cancer to lung cancer is related to our ability to detect breast cancer at an early and more readily curable stage. Prior to the emergence of modern mammography, beginning in the early 1960s, the five-year survival rate for breast cancer was on the order of 45% [1]. Mortality reductions in breast cancer began to emerge in the late 1960s and early 1970s when the results of two major randomized controlled trials were reported. These trials were the HIP study in New York City [2] and the Swedish Two County Trial led by Dr. Laszlo Tabár [3]. The HIP study reported a 33% mortality reduction over a five-year follow-up period between women who had both screening mammography and clinical examination on a regular basis and those who did not. The Swedish study, which was started in the mid-1970s and continues today, has demonstrated a steadily increasing survival advantage, now on the order of 50%, for women who participate in regular screening mammography.

Evolution of mammographic technology

In the early days of mammography, no particular attention was given to providing specialized imaging equipment specifically designed to interrogate breast tissue. Standard overhead x-ray tubes were employed using the typical 40-inch tube-film distance commonly used for imaging the body. Breast compression was rudimentary at best, and the image receptor was nothing more than a single emulsion film in a cardboard cassette. This system was improved upon by Robert Egan, who recognized the limitations of mammography at that time. He introduced the "double film pack." This was not much more than two separate pieces of x-ray film in the same cassette with differing speeds or contrast curves. In the late 1960s, x-ray tubes were introduced which used molybdenum targets and filters [4]. This produced substantially better image contrast, particularly in women with fatty breasts.

In the 1970s, grids specifically designed for mammography began to appear, and in an attempt to improve film-screen contact, the DuPont Company developed a vacuum cassette. In this device, the x-ray screen and the film were more or less sucked together by applying vacuum to a valve on the outside of the cassette. In the 1980s, modern film-screen mammography gradually emerged through a series of improvements in x-ray tubes and in x-ray film specifically designed for mammography. The 1970s and the 1980s also ushered in an era of popularity for Xerox mammography. The Xerox process was more or less the prototype of more modern full-field digital mammography (FFDM). Xero-mammograms were quasi-digital in the sense that discrete blobs of blue dye were applied to the image in proportion to the photon absorption pattern. Xero-mammography produced an image with a number of discrete tiny blue dots and gave the reader the impression that there were sharply defined edges and calcifications.

In the 1990s, several forms of digital mammography began to emerge. These were, for the most part, at university medical centers and in research institutions. The first FFDM unit was approved for clinical use by the United States Food and Drug Administration (FDA) in 2000. To some extent, digital mammography has not grown as rapidly as other emerging technologies in the field of radiology. This is in part because mammography has always been a relatively low-cost examination, and insurers have been reluctant to pay significantly higher reimbursement for this new technology. In addition, there is a lack of data supporting substantially improved diagnostic accuracy using digital techniques. Until the Digital Mammographic Imaging Screening Trial (DMIST) [5] and Oslo II [6] studies, there had been no convincing demonstration that digital mammography was superior to film-screen mammography. The DMIST study showed that in women with dense breasts, women under age 50 years, and pre- and perimenopausal women, digital mammography was superior in accuracy compared to film-screen mammography. The Oslo II Study showed that women aged 50–69 years were more accurately examined using digital technique compared to film. Cost-effectiveness in the general population continues to be of concern.

Digital Mammography: A Practical Approach, ed. Gary J. Whitman and Tamara Miner Haygood. Published by Cambridge University Press.
© Cambridge University Press 2013.

Compliance problems

In spite of the emerging studies relating decreased mortality to regular screening, patient compliance has been, and continues to be, a problem. In the mid-1980s it was suggested that 50 million women in the United States should undergo regular mammographic screening [7]. At that time only 5–15% of women actually underwent regular mammographic screening. These numbers have improved to some degree, but patient compliance in general is poor. Numerous impediments to mammographic screening have been suggested [8]. These include cost, anticipated discomfort, inaccessibility, not having or intending to ask a healthcare provider for an order, fear of the diagnosis of cancer, and the belief that not having a family history of breast cancer renders the disease unlikely. Various studies have shown that medically underserved women have higher breast cancer mortality rates, and this is usually attributed to insufficient screening frequency and later-stage cancer at diagnosis [9]. Similarly, other studies show that access to mammography is inversely correlated with breast cancer stage at the time of diagnosis [10]. There are several demographic groups who have lower than average screening rates [11]. Low-income women and women with less than average education tend not to undergo screening mammography. Age is yet another issue. In the elderly this is the largely a result of immobility and inconvenience. Primary care physicians may further complicate compliance issues, because they anticipate that screening will have a low detection rate. They are also concerned about radiation and equivocal radiology reports that will generate additional medical studies. Problems can also occur for women who are members of health maintenance organizations (HMOs). Some HMOs restrict access to screening programs if they are not included in the HMO plan [12].

Possible solutions

Reducing costs

Lowering the cost of a medical examination is always an attractive alternative. Unfortunately, in the case of mammography, costs are already prohibitively low. Many departments operate in the red or at best break even. Many states have a variety of subsidy programs to provide screening mammography services to women. In Idaho, women are entitled to a state-subsidized mammogram when they turn 40 years old. There are additional programs for indigent women that cover the cost of diagnostic mammographic examinations, ultrasounds, and even surgery and advanced therapies. There are similar programs in most states.

Addressing convenience or accessibility

Mammography at the worksite is an excellent albeit not frequently utilized solution to the problem of patient access. Screening mammography is provided at appropriate intervals either as an employee benefit or at very low cost to the employees of the company. This solves many of the problems that women complain of when having to schedule a mammogram. It solves the problem of taking time off work and minimizes the amount of time necessary for the examination, since no travel is involved. There is frequently a lot of social support and camaraderie among the women employees of the company. This factor alone tends to improve compliance statistics. In addition, the company can sponsor educational opportunities for the women, frequently with the participation of a radiologist or a nurse [13]. This is a viable alternative for any company with a large workforce in one location. In general, women who have had screening mammography examinations performed at their worksite have reported high satisfaction ratings.

Mobile mammography

One of the major factors in achieving compliance with screening mammographic guidelines involves convenience for the patient and accessibility to the mammography site. Screening rates are correlated inversely with the distance a patient lives from the mammography unit and other factors such as the need to take time off from work. Many women who live in a rural setting are at a very inconvenient distance from the nearest fixed-site mammography facility.

Early mobile mammography
Portable mammography units

The earliest form of mobile mammography was the transport of a regular mammographic x-ray machine to a remote site on the back of a pickup truck or inside a van. The machine would arrive at the site, which was often a church, a community center, a business, or a local doctor's office. A technologist would accompany the x-ray machine. Once at the site, the technologist would work her way through the patient list and "black-box" the exposed x-ray films as the studies were completed. Once the run was finished, the technologist, mammography machine, and black-box would return to the parent radiology department, where the films would be processed. There were obvious problems in this design. The x-ray machines were heavy and were at least moderately fragile. Getting the machine on and off the truck required additional equipment and strength. Delayed processing of the images made it impossible to know if the equipment was working properly, and follow-up of improperly exposed films and abnormal examinations was a major logistical problem.

True mobile mammography

In a report written in 1996, DeBruhl et al. noted that at that time 2.4% of all mammography units were mobile [14]. As of this writing, there were 343 mobile units (Figure 9.1) out of about 8500 total certified mammography sites in the United States, or about 4% of the total. Regarding the earliest true mobile units, several decisions had to be made. The first decision involved whether screening only or screening and

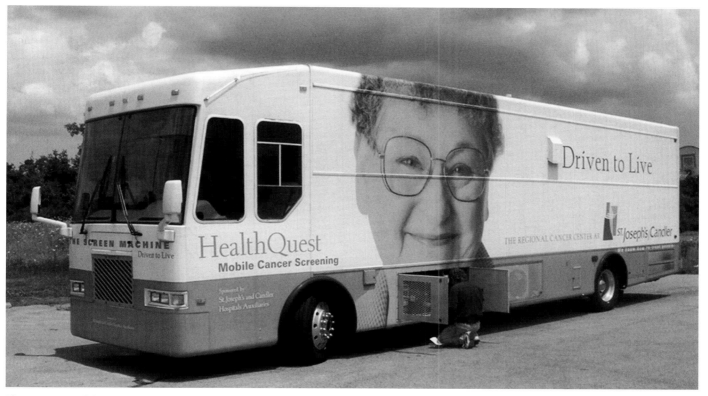

Figure 9.1 A mobile mammography van.

diagnostic mammography would be carried out by the unit. In 1996, screening-only mobile units made up 67% of the total number of mobile mammography units. Screening only was proposed as a strategy to lower costs and to increase through-put. Examination cost is one of the factors negatively influencing compliance. It was felt that by restricting the mobile mammography unit's business to screening examinations, the higher volume resulting from faster throughput would make up for lost revenue in the less expensive screening examinations. By the same token, most of the units did not perform clinical breast examinations, in order to save time and further increase patient throughput.

The second major decision concerned onboard versus batch-film processing at the parent radiology site. There are many inherent problems in attempting to process films on a mobile mammographic unit. The processor itself and the necessary plumbing add significant cost, as do the necessary chemicals and maintenance. There are frequently problems in achieving correct developer temperature and then maintaining that temperature. There is also a significant loss of time in waiting for the developer temperature to come up to operating level. Technologists have reported that 1–1.5 hours each day was devoted to starting up and shutting down the film processor. This is time that cannot be devoted to examining patients. Advantages of onboard processing include being able to develop the films and correct obvious technical errors before the patient leaves the mobile unit. In addition, there is no risk

of the "black box" having a light leak and spoiling a large number of exposed images.

The report by DeBruhl *et al.* in 1996 showed that only 47% of mobile units were either profitable or broke even [14]. This study also noted that portable units were more likely to break even or to be profitable, probably because of substantially lower equipment costs. The high cost of mobile mammography includes amortization of the mobile unit itself, additional personnel costs relating to additional staff, and costs pertaining to marketing, patient education, and promotion. A further complication of the profit–loss scenario is the imposition of government-mandated reimbursement rates for Medicare patients. Because a large proportion of mammography patients are Medicare age, the imposition of a regional reimbursement rate places significant restrictions on a mobile unit's ability to generate revenue. In a 1988 study, one mobile unit had calculated fixed and variable costs of $83 US per examination. This was in a setting where Medicare had established a global reimbursement of $55 for a screening mammogram [12]. Radiology departments operating mobile units are frequently forced to decide whether to operate in a "loss-leader" setting or to find ways to subsidize their mobile program. Many departments operate under the loss-leader scenario, realizing that the positive screening mammograms will generate additional revenue for the radiology department and hospital through diagnostic mammography, breast ultrasound, breast MRI, and referrals to surgical colleagues, radiation therapy, and medical oncology. Subsidies can appear in many forms, such as personnel provided by sponsoring institutions, processing facilities, and grants to help offset the cost of purchasing a mobile van.

Upgrading a film-screen mobile unit to full-field digital mammography

The decision to convert an existing film-screen mobile mammography unit to FFDM is not an easy one. The overwhelming factor is the much higher cost of the digital machine. It is hard to pin down the exact cost of any of the major machines on the market, because the price varies depending on whether one buys a single machine or multiple machines, whether the hospital has a corporate-rate purchase agreement with the vendor, and other factors. Suffice it to say that a digital machine costs three to four times what a new analog unit does. There are substantial benefits to be obtained with digital mammography units, not the least of which is that digital mammography is an excellent marketing tool. In spite of the various peer-reviewed studies which show, at best, a marginal improvement in diagnostic efficacy, digital mammography is perceived by the general public and by non-radiologist physicians as an inherently superior form of technology. By converting to a full-field digital unit, one eliminates the need for film processing, either onboard or back in the main radiology department. Many medical facilities in the United States have converted to computed radiography (CR) or digital radiography (DR) and eliminated the need for film processing and archiving. If the mammography department, including its mobile unit, converts entirely to digital imaging, the processing and archiving needs inherent to film go away permanently. The digital process allows for vastly improved image retrieval, copying, and transmission, as well as easier computer-aided detection (CADe) implementation. Digital imaging workstations, including those dedicated to mammography, allow application of various processing algorithms. These algorithms allow manipulation of image contrast and generally reduce the need for repeat mammograms, benefiting the patient significantly. Probably the largest single cost saving achieved by digital imaging is the elimination of the space and shelving required for film archiving. Transmission of digital mammographic images to other sites for consultation is far easier than when dealing with film, and the same can be said for sending prior mammograms to other sites.

Digital telemammography

The ability to transmit images by various methods opens up a whole new realm of possibilities in patient management on a mobile unit. If the technologist has the ability to transmit images to an expert mammographer, she can be given instructions for obtaining additional images to complete the study, eliminating the need for a later callback examination. There are inherent image transmission challenges in moving digital mammographic images from one site to another. The images require very high spatial resolution for detection of tiny calcifications and to show lesion edge detail. The file size for a single mammographic image ranges between 25 and 55 megabytes (MB). The variation in file size is related to the mammographic machine in use and the size of the patient's breast. A standard four-view mammogram would, therefore, be in the size range of 100–200 MB. Most of the available transmission technology is not fast enough to allow transmission of large file sizes in a reasonable amount of time. Telemedicine has for several years transmitted data from electrocardiography (ECG) machines, digital thermometers, and digital blood-pressure devices. These devices usually produce files on the size of 10 kilobytes (kB), which are easily transmitted over standard 56 kB telephone modems, cell phones, or T-1 lines. To put the time constraints in focus, consider a single digital chest radiograph [15]. Its file size would be on the order of 6 MB, far smaller than a mammogram. Using a 56 kB modem for transmission would require 15 minutes to move the chest x-ray from one site to another. Faster modes of landline transmission include Ethernet, T-1 and T-3 lines, and asynchronous transfer mode (ATM) at 155 MB per second. Using the ATM mode would move the chest x-ray in 325 ms. The four-view mammogram mentioned above would transmit for 240 minutes, or 4 hours, using a telephone modem, down to as little as 5.2 seconds using ATM technology. Unfortunately, ATM technology is very expensive, and there is very little of it available. In addition, many communities, particularly rural ones, have only phone lines (modems) or possibly Ethernet lines. A few have T-1 lines between certain sites.

Swedish Medical Center in Seattle has developed a fully functional satellite transmission system for at least one of its mobile mammography units [16]. This is an elaborate method of image transmission which was developed with the thought of providing almost real-time image interpretation. It was imagined that patients could wait for a few minutes after finishing a screening examination to get the results. This system uses a satellite dish on top of the mobile unit and sends a satellite signal over the Ku band to Atlanta, Georgia. The signal is then routed to Seattle over a T-1 line network. Transmission time is about 15 minutes for a four-view mammogram. Since transmission can be ongoing throughout the workday, it would be theoretically possible nearly to keep up with the patient throughput. The mobile unit also can store mammographic images on a laptop computer hard drive and download four days' worth of mammograms in about an hour when the mobile unit returns to its home base.

Mobile mammography in a medium-sized population area

It would be neither feasible nor practical to attempt to analyze all of the factors that go into putting together a digital mobile mammography unit. There are simply too many iterations and possibilities. The United States has a wide variety of patient populations to serve. Reimbursement rates vary widely, and amortization of the not inconsiderable cost of equipment varies accordingly. The list price of equipment is seldom the final bottom line in purchasing the digital mammography machine and its associated workstation. Many radiology departments have established relationships with vendors, and hospital chains can usually save considerable money in making multiple unit purchases. Acquisition of and financing for the mobile coach is usually the largest cost item. All of the major manufacturers of digital mammography equipment can provide comprehensive packets of information to prospective buyers. This information covers, among other things, mobile unit planning; cost analysis and possible revenue raising strategies; comparisons of the imaging chain from vendor to vendor across the market; projected workload changes between film-screen mammography and digital mammography; and sample operational analysis for the first and ensuing years of operation. There are independent consulting companies that deal with the details of site and mobile unit development and appropriate equipment purchases. This chapter uses the author's experience to illustrate the various decisions, problems, and solutions involved in establishing a digital mobile mammography program.

Demographics of Boise, Idaho

Boise, the capital city of Idaho, has undergone recent rapid growth, chiefly the result of the outflow of population from nearby states, particularly California. From 1959 to 1989 the population increased from approximately 50 000 to 100 000 people. Since 1989, the population of Boise has doubled again to about 200 000 people, and the surrounding environs bring the total service area population to about 400 000. In spite of the relatively small population, local citizens have enjoyed remarkably sophisticated medical care, probably because the lifestyle opportunities in Idaho have always attracted highly skilled physicians.

Since the early 1900s, there have been two major hospitals serving the Boise area. For much of this time, the hospitals engaged in duplication of service and the various forms of competitive marketing that is typical in a free-market economy. In the early 1980s, local medical politics forced the hospitals to engage in separate and well-defined areas of specialization and expertise. In a very short period of time, all of the obstetricians abandoned one of the hospitals and set up a practice in the other hospital. This rapidly resulted in loss of pediatric services as well as gynecology services for one hospital to the benefit of the other. The hospital which lost its women's services concentrated on trauma services, neurosurgery, and orthopedic surgery. The other hospital subsequently became second tier in these three service areas. The competing hospital responded by investing substantial resources in developing a cardiac surgery and coronary care service as well as a standalone tumor institute, providing medical and radiation oncology. This new status quo persisted until the early 1990s. In the early 1990s, both

hospitals began exploratory attempts to revitalize some of the services which they had abandoned in past years. The author's hospital embarked on a campaign to focus on women's medicine in early 1995. The concept was simple; execution, however, was difficult, since the hospital "across town" had long been thought of as the place where obstetrics and pediatrics were practiced. Initially, the hospital recruited, and at least partially subsidized, several new obstetricians and gynecologists. Once the obstetrics service began to put new babies into the healthcare system, pediatrics was quick to follow. Eventually, a neonatal intensive care unit became a reality. A women's center building was constructed adjacent to the main hospital. To support the obstetrical services, floor space in the new building was reserved for pregnancy and lactation counseling.

The mammography service was moved from the radiology department to the women's center and was established as a full-fledged breast care service, modeled after the comprehensive breast care schemes pioneered by Tabár and others in Europe. A weekly breast care panel meeting, or breast care tumor board, was established with the participation of a large number of surgeons. Over time, the number of surgeons who participated has decreased to include only those surgeons with a substantial interest and practice in breast care. The decision was made to move diagnostic breast ultrasound to the breast care center, which occupies about half of the first floor of the women's center. Osteoporosis screening was quickly added as a service to provide to women who are having screening mammography.

During the decades that the hospital across town was the sole provider of women's services, that hospital established primacy in providing mammography to the Boise area. The cornerstone of its marketing strategy, insofar as breast care was concerned, was to establish in the Boise area small, standalone mammography screening centers. The screening centers sent the screening mammograms and the diagnostic patients generated therefrom to the main hospital for further workup and treatment. The other hospital initially had a single mammography machine in the 1980s that was sufficient for the department's rather minimal needs. When the breast care center was established in 1996, two additional machines were put in the center. The original machine in the hospital department continued to be used for screening and diagnostic examinations as well as for wire localizations. In its first year the new breast care center did about 4000 screening mammograms. The cross-town competition, by comparison, performed approximately 14 000 screening mammograms in the same timeframe. Over the next four years, there was gradual growth in the number of screening examinations carried out by both hospitals.

In 1999, the Idaho Department of Health and Welfare estimated that only 28% of eligible women had had a single screening mammogram. (M. Inzer, personal communication). For some time, consideration had been given to instituting mobile medical services at the author's hospital. Initially a mobile health unit was conceived that could carry out multiple functions. It was planned to provide mammography, screening prostate examination, screening gynecologic examinations,

Table 9.1 Percentage of positive (BI-RADS 0, 4, and 5) examinations in Boise, Idaho, 2000 to 2009.

	2000	2001	2002	2003	2004	2005	2006	2007	2008	2009
Breast care center	15.08%	12.86%	9.58%	10.82%	12.58%	12.27%	12.12%	10.04%	9.72%	10.34%
Mobile unit	24.09%	10.31%	8.31%	11.00%	11.50%	13.59%	13.93%	11.89%	9.30%	7.60%

including Papanicolaou smears, and potentially cardiovascular screening, employing ECGs, carotid ultrasound, and even echocardiography. It became clear, however, that the complexity of equipment for several of these endeavors would overwhelm the available space in a standard recreational vehicle or even a tractor-trailer unit. Eventually, the decision was made to implement mobile medicine utilizing several different vehicles, each with specific configurations for the services provided. The mobile mammography unit was conceived as a method of increasing the percentage of women undergoing regular screening mammography as well as a means of increasing the hospital's market share in the breast care realm. It was envisioned that the treatment of breast cancer would become a major revenue stream for the hospital. This notion has been shown to be true over time.

Initiation of the film-screen mammography unit

The major task of any radiology department contemplating a mobile unit is to ensure its continuing financial success. Many radiology departments have experienced losses, sometimes substantial, in operating their mobile units. The author's hospital elected to put the cost of the x-ray machine and the onboard processor into the routine radiology equipment budget cycle. Financing of the van was eventually achieved by vigorous promotion of the outreach concept of mobile mammography to several philanthropic groups in the Boise area. A local foundation underwrote the unfunded portion of the cost of the mobile van by establishing a grant. The total outlay for the street-ready mobile mammography unit was $423 000, with an additional $200 000 earmarked for operational support for the first two years. At the same time, marketing plans were developed to promote the unit in the surrounding medical service area. Letters were sent to the offices of primary care physicians, surgeons, and gynecologists. The letters explained the concept and solicited suggestions and feedback. News coverage was arranged in the local newspaper and local television stations. The author and the lead mammography technologist undertook personal follow-up visits to many of the practices that had responded to the initial letters. Eventually, a preliminary schedule was established. In the meantime, two mammographic technologists were selected, and both of them trained for and obtained commercial driver's licenses. Some mobile units operate with a separate driver, but that adds substantially to the operating cost. Onboard processing was selected in the initial planning to permit maximum efficiency as demand for the unit grew over time. In addition, it was hoped that having onboard processing would prevent a log jam from occurring at the breast care center's processor whenever the mobile unit returned to the main base. The unit started operations in October 2000. In October 2007, the unit was taken out of service for 45 days for conversion to FFDM.

Initial quality assurance (QA)

Because the images from the mobile unit were brought back to the breast care center for CADe encoding and interpretation, it was anticipated that there would be no substantial differences in the sensitivity, specificity, and positive predictive value of the examinations, because the same breast radiologists were reading all the mammograms whether they originated on the mobile unit or on the fixed units at the breast care center. This proved to be the case over time. A positive examination was considered to be BI-RADS 4, BI-RADS 5, or BI-RADS 0. Aside from the first year of the mobile unit operation, there are no statistically significant differences between the mobile unit and the main breast care center (Table 9.1). The relatively high percentage of positive examinations for the mobile unit in the year 2000 is most likely an aberration due to the very low total number of examinations done on the mobile unit (138). It is interesting that the percentage of positive examinations decreased after the institution of the full-field digital service in both the breast care center and on the mobile unit. This is contrary to what most institutions have experienced.

Conversion to full-field digital mammographic unit

In early 2007, the breast care center made the decision to convert the entire department to FFDM, including the mobile unit. At that time, there were four vendors in the United States with FDA approval. The choice of vendor in this sort of conversion is largely driven by financial considerations. In our particular case the existing analog machines were all manufactured by Siemens. The company was able to present a significantly less expensive bid for a package deal of five digital mammographic machines. Three of these were to go to the breast care center, one to the mobile unit, and one to a new imaging center, a joint venture between the hospital and the radiology group. In addition to the economy realized in purchasing five machines at a time, the hospital also belongs to a large multi-campus hospital system that purchases medical equipment in even larger batches at significant savings. There are several advantages in having all of the mammographic machines of the same type. Among the various manufacturers, there is a range in pixel size ranging from 50 to 100 μm. As pixel size diminishes, spatial resolution increases along with noise.

In addition to using different pixel sizes, the different manufacturers use differing proprietary algorithms for image processing and display. This can lead to display problems when there is a mismatch between the acquisition device and the proprietary workstation. If two different mammograms are done on the same patient at different times on different machines, the display of the current images and the prior images can result in mismatches in size, image contrast, and gray scale. This makes accurate comparison of the image sets very difficult. If all the mammographic machines in a department are of the same type, the images will display similarly on the workstations. Some vendors' workstations have more elaborate and complicated display algorithms. Generally the window width/window level curves are either sigmoidal or linear. If an outside mammogram done on a different type of digital machine is displayed, the images will often be presented improperly. A final mismatch can occur when images from two different companies are displayed together if the image display tags are not identical. This can lead to images being displayed in a rotated or inverted orientation. This is more of a nuisance than a diagnostic problem, because the images have to be reloaded in order to display properly.

To address the various inconsistencies between the products of many vendors, the Radiological Society of North America (RSNA) and the Healthcare Information and Management Systems Society (HIMSS) formulated a set of schemes, referred to as "profiles," to allow for smooth integration of the information generated by the various systems in the marketplace. This effort is referred to as Integrating the Healthcare Enterprise (IHE) [17]. Recently, IHE profiles were developed to address pixel size issues by allowing images to be scaled to the same size. For outside images, this is referred to as import reconciliation workflow. This scheme helps in the management of importing images from compact disk (CD), hard copy, and online digital sources. It allows for reconciling identifiers to match local values, and, in a sense, updates the Digital Imaging and Communications in Medicine (DICOM) header for the image. Another component of the IHE system is the "basic image review" [18]. This defines a set of baseline features and user interfaces relating to the review of DICOM images. Although these systems have provided much more certain image display across different manufacturers' platforms, it is easier to deal with images produced and viewed on equipment manufactured by one company. Two additional advantages in buying all machines and workstations from the same manufacturer are that technologists do not have to master different architectures, and service for the equipment is easier to manage.

Advantages of computed radiography digital mammography

There are significant financial advantages in using CR digital mammography. First, with CR, it is not necessary to purchase a full-field digital machine, which is the largest cost item in digital mammography. An old analog machine can be modified for CR with the installation of a new x-ray tube and modification of the automatic exposure control. In several large studies, image quality of the CR systems was not significantly different from that of the full-field digital machines [19]. The major disadvantage of a CR mammography system is the requirement of having an "image reader" to process the images. If the radiology department already uses CR, the reader will already be on site, and there will be no additional cost. There is, however, a loss of throughput speed. Having to load plates into the reader is analogous to loading cassettes into the film processor. The author's radiology group decided to put a CR mammography unit at an outpatient imaging site that it solely owned. This decision was made because of lower equipment costs. The aforementioned problems in imaging and displaying on systems from two different manufacturers were encountered. Image sizes for the CR images sent into the picture archiving and communication system (PACS) at the breast care center were about 50% larger than the same breast imaged on one of the center's machines. In addition, image contrast was substantially different and had to be windowed and leveled for every case interpreted. There was a significant display problem caused by quantum mottle, in part introduced by a differing bit rate for the CR machine. This was eventually corrected by a bit rate increase by the machine's manufacturer and by increasing the milliampere (mA) setting during acquisition of images.

Problems inherent to digital machines on mobile units

The most crucial and delicate part of the FFDM image chain is the image sensor. In addition to CR mammography, there are two major schemes utilized by today's digital mammographic equipment. The indirect method uses cesium iodide scintillation screens to convert x-ray photons to light. The light is then detected by various methods including selenium plates, charge-coupled devices, or silicon diode arrays. The direct digital detectors utilize a silicon array that makes a direct measure of the absorbed x-ray photons. The end result is a device which is both expensive and fragile.

Environmental stability is a critical factor in ensuring proper performance and a long life for the imaging device. Ambient temperature is probably the most critical environmental concern. Once operational, the sensor device must be maintained in a temperature range of roughly 20–30 °C. The different manufacturers have slightly different temperature ranges, but they are all in this range. The rate of temperature change is also limited to less than 10 °C per hour increase or decrease. It is important to understand that temperature stability is important 24 hours a day and 7 days a week, which means that stable temperature must be maintained even when the unit is not in use, and the mobile van is parked for the weekend. This requires that the onboard heating, ventilation, and air conditioning (HVAC) system remains operational constantly. The array of necessary heating and air conditioning equipment depends largely on where the van is likely to be operated. In Idaho, summer temperatures in July and August are often in excess of 100 °F (38 °C), and, in the winter, the temperature can fall below 0 °F (−18 °C).

During operation of the van, the heating and cooling systems rely on the onboard power generator for their operation. At the home base, after operational hours, the van is attached to a docking station which provides three-phase power in a variety of configurations. All of the major manufacturers provide several options for power line connections, ranging from 208 V single-phase power to 480 V three-phase power. To mitigate damage to the sensor device if the docking station power fails, there must be a warning device capable of notifying the mobile van manager. Most mobile vans have a web-based system that monitors onboard temperature and sends out a notification if the temperature goes out of range. Some of the available systems will automatically start the onboard generator and switch over to onboard power when the docking-station power fails. The mobile van operated by the author's department has both an automatic power change-over device and a telephone notification system contacting radiology department senior management.

In addition to maintaining the ambient temperature, the relative humidity must be held in the range of 30–70% for most manufacturers, and this is usually the task of the HVAC. Other environmental concerns include vibration, which is usually mitigated by the suspension system of the van or bus where the mobile unit is installed. Some equipment manufacturers will not warrantee their installations if a lighter-weight recreational vehicle is used. Generally, vibration should be kept below 1.0 G with occasional accelerations up to a maximal level of 2.0 G.

The second enhanced requirement for digital mammographic machines is that the electric power itself needs to be "cleaned." The device that carries out this task is known as a "line conditioner" or "power conditioner." It is also referred to as an uninterruptible power supply (UPS). It is analogous to a combined surge protector and backup battery supply that many computer users employ to protect their personal computers (PCs). Its function is, first of all, to stabilize the frequency and the phase of the incoming power as required by the more sensitive digital equipment. Both shore power and the onboard power generator are connected to the input of the UPS, and the output goes to the digital x-ray machine and the technologist workstation. The unit also provides battery backup if there is a power failure, and there is sufficient stored power available to complete the current examination and do an orderly shutdown and image storage routine. UPS devices come in several sizes and can be hooked together in tandem if necessary. Cost for an individual UPS device is on the order of $10 000.

Power requirements are generally higher for digital units. Onboard generators are usually on the order of 30 kW or larger, and most manufacturers recommend purchasing a unit that meets commercial and industrial standards. Analog machines generally have onboard generator size requirements in the 20 kW range, and temperature and humidity stability are

not as stringent. Dock power or shore-station power is usually provided as 480 V three-phase at 150 A. Some vendors specify 240 V.

Finally, image download technology is different in the digital environment. With film-screen mammography, the technologist simply carried the completed images into the radiology department for hanging and interpretation. In the world of digital mammographic images, there are three broad possibilities for image transfer. The most commonly utilized mode of transfer is to put the images as they are completed onto the hard drive of a laptop computer or a portable hard drive attached to the acquisition workstation. When the mobile unit returns to the base site at the end of the day, the laptop is carried into the radiology or mammography department and attached to a digital workstation. From there the images are downloaded to the PACS gateway, where they are matched with hospital information system (HIS) and radiology information system (RIS) data. Once data-matched, the images are put online for interpretation.

A second approach is to download the images through a docking station connection or port. Depending on the configuration of the PACS, this connectivity could be an optical cable, a T-1 or T-3 line, or an Ethernet connection. From that point, the same data-matching process occurs, and the images are eventually put online for reading. The author's department uses this approach most of the time. There is also a backup pair of hard drives on the mobile unit for use when there is a problem with the docking-station download method.

The third method of downloading images is to employ a local area network or LAN, if one is available. Mobile units that operate in large cities may have access to a LAN and can utilize that for downloading some or all of the images that have been obtained. Satellite telemammography is yet another method for downloading, although this method is not in common use.

Digital mammography also imposes higher-resolution display requirements. The Mammography Quality Standards Act (MQSA) requires that soft-copy images be viewed on 5 K × 5 K monitors, instead of the 2 K × 2 K monitors more commonly deployed. As one might expect, the higher-resolution monitors are considerably more expensive. Many radiology departments are currently using a CADe system for their mammography services, whether film-screen or digital. There is a considerable time advantage in converting from analog mammography to digital mammography. Film mammograms have to be run through a digitizer before a CADe algorithm can be applied, and for a standard four-view mammogram approximately five minutes is required. In addition, the images from several studies have to be loaded separately and sequentially. In digital imaging, the CADe process is applied after the images are sent to the PACS gateway. Images in the system reside as both "for processing" or "for presentation." The "for processing" images are what is usually referred to as "raw" images. There is a separate server for the CADe process that is linked to the PACS "for processing" images. The CADe server uses these images to generate a "structured report" for each image set in the gateway. This report is available online, usually with a workstation toggle to turn the overlay images on and off as the radiologist requires. Online images are in the "for presentation" form.

Operational details

Making the schedule for a mobile unit is almost always a work in progress. It takes time to develop and implement an effective schedule. The demographics and geography of a service area have a lot to do with how a mobile schedule evolves. There are very obvious differences between the patient populations and logistics in a dense urban area and those in a rural setting such as southwest Idaho. Accordingly, no cookbook formula can be provided.

As noted earlier in this chapter, preliminary marketing was carried out by the mammographic radiologists and the breast care center staff. The initial schedule tasked the mobile unit to be on the road approximately two days a week. Ten patients per day were set as the minimum target. There was initially more business than anticipated. Over time, the number of patients seen for repeat visits to the same sites decreased. New sites were added, and gradually a schedule evolved serving some sites as often as twice weekly and other sites only on a monthly basis. In the 10 years that the mobile unit has been operating, the schedule has expanded to five and sometimes six days a week on the road. A typical schedule is now 20–24 patients per day, and on occasion the unit will perform up to 30 mammograms per day. The most distant site is on an Indian reservation in northern Nevada. This site requires 2½ hours' driving time each way. The mobile schedules two days and 60 mammograms each time it visits this site. Scheduling is carried out at the individual sites,

and prior to the mobile unit's visit, the schedule is sent by fax to the breast care center. Most of the sites are medical facilities, small clinics, schools, and a few private companies or corporations. At the breast care center, the mobile unit manager interrogates the mammography reporting system database, and, if the patient has been seen previously, uses the data to generate an outpatient registration for each scheduled patient. If the patient is new to the system, the mobile unit manager uses the contact telephone numbers supplied by the scheduling site to call the patient and complete the outpatient registration. Somewhere between 50% and 75% of patients are preregistered by this method. Some of the patients, who are added late to the schedule, fill out a "downtime registration form" when they arrive at the mobile unit. This is used retroactively to complete the registration after the fact.

The mobile unit staff is 3.1 full-time equivalents (FTEs) (Figure 9.2). Two of the staff are onboard the mobile unit, and are either two mammographic technologists or one technologist and one registered nurse. The third full-time person is a mobile unit manager who is at the breast care center. The extra 0.1 FTE is for anticipated overtime.

When a patient enters the front of the mobile unit (Figure 9.3), one staff person greets the patient, obtains a signed consent and a signed Health Insurance Portability and Accountability Act (HIPAA) form, and then takes a history. The patient then proceeds to the front examination room and gowns for the examination. The front person carries out a clinical breast examination and instructs the patient in breast self-examination (BSE) if she desires. The patient is then directed to the back person in the mammographic room. The technologist there obtains the mammogram, and when

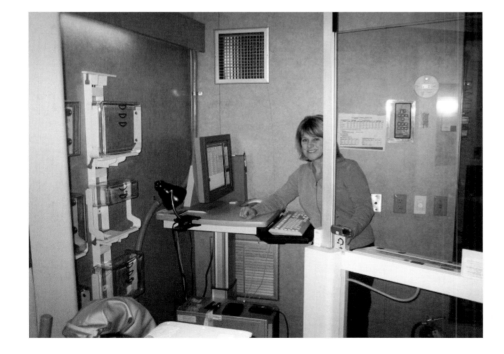

Figure 9.2 A technologist working in the mammography area on a mobile van.

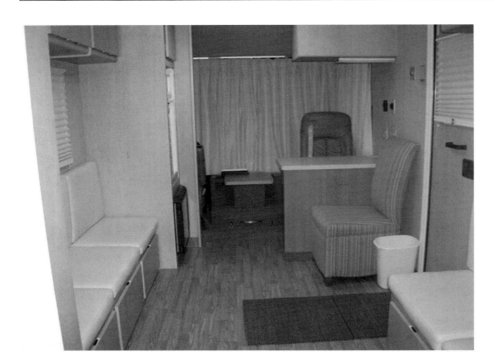

Figure 9.3 The reception area in the front part of the mobile van.

completed, gives the patient an information packet dealing with BSE and breast health in either English or Spanish. The patient dresses and exits from the rear of the unit. The mobile unit supplies the patient with disposable pads for removing and later reapplying deodorant. There is also an osteoporosis screening device consisting of a heel stiffness scanner, if the patient or the referring physician wishes the patient to be screened.

When the mobile unit returns to the base, the images are downloaded at the breast care center and are sent to the PACS gateway. The charts from the day's run are handed off to the mobile unit manager, who order-matches each patient to the appropriate DICOM headers for each image set in the gateway, and from there the images go online to be read. When the cases are read, the billing module is activated and reports are generated for the patient's physician as well as for the patient. When archived, the images are saved using lossless JPEG compression with average compression ratios of 1.5–2 : 1.

Cost analysis of digital mobile mammography

The original analog unit had a price tag of $423 000, with an additional $200 000 earmarked for operational support for its first two years. It was used from 2000 to mid-2007, at which time the digital conversion was carried out for an additional cost of $258 644. This included the cost of the new digital mammographic unit and an associated workstation, a CADe unit, all of the mammographic compression plates and devices, a UPS power conditioner, seismic protection for the equipment, and additional modifications necessary for installation of the equipment in a mobile coach. All of the other onboard facilities including the generator, HVAC, onboard water system, and front examination room remained in use from the original installation. In 2009, gross revenues of $472 800 were generated from 3080 examinations. This includes a $144 technical fee for digital screening mammography and a CADe charge of $23. Costs included $170 000 for 3.1 FTEs' productive labor and benefits; $23 000 for supplies, communications, coach repair and maintenance; $9200 for fuel; and $26 000 for imaging-equipment maintenance contracts. Most sites use a five-year straight-line depreciation schedule for the cost of equipment.

Summary

Regularly performed screening mammography has been shown to reduce breast cancer mortality substantially. For various reasons, many women do not undergo routine screening mammography at regular intervals. Among these reasons are difficult access to imaging centers and convenience issues. Mobile mammography service attempts to address these problems. The investment costs in mobile mammography are substantially higher than for a fixed site, mainly because of the van or coach needed for operations. Deciding to use digital technology adds additional costs above film-screen systems. At present, there is only a marginal improvement in performance for the extra costs, but there are marketing advantages as well as continuing savings in image storage and manipulation. Digital systems generally allow significantly greater patient throughput, increasing the revenue stream. Most hospitals derive significant spin-off revenue from an increase in mammographic throughput, by referrals for additional imaging, surgical consultations, and delivery of oncologic services.

References

1. Haagensen CD. *Diseases of the Breast*, 2nd edn. Philadelphia, PA: Saunders, 1971.

2. Strax P. Mass screening for breast cancer. *Rev Fr Gynecol Obstet* 1973; **68**: 457–66.

3. Tabár L, Fagerberg CJ, Gad A, *et al.* Reduction in mortality from breast cancer after mass screening with mammography: randomised trial from the Breast Cancer Screening Working Group of the Swedish National Board of Health and Welfare. *Lancet* 1985; **1**: 829–32.

4. Haus AG. Historical technical developments in mammography. *Technol Cancer Res Treat* 2002; **1**: 119–26.

5. Pisano ED, Hendrick RE, Yaffe MJ, *et al.* Diagnostic accuracy of digital versus film mammography: exploratory analysis of selected population subgroups in DMIST. *Radiology* 2008; **246**: 376–83.

6. Skaane P, Skjennald A. Screen-film mammography versus full-field digital mammography with soft copy reading: randomized trial in a population-based screening program: the Oslo II Study. *Radiology* 2004; **232**: 197–204.

7. Sickles EA, Weber WN, Galvin HB, Ominsky SH, Sollitto RA. Mammographic screening: how to operate successfully at low cost. *Radiology* 1986; **160**: 95–7.

8. Kessler HB, Rimer BK, Devine PJ, Gatenby RA, Engstrom PF. Corporate-sponsored breast cancer screening at the work site: results of a statewide program. *Radiology* 1991; **179**: 107–10.

9. Peek ME, Han J. Mobile mammography: assessment of self-referral in reaching medically underserved women. *J Nat Med Assn* 2007; **99**: 398–403.

10. Marchick J, Henson DE. Correlations between access to mammography and breast cancer stage at diagnosis. *Cancer* 2005; **103**: 1571–80.

11. Reuben DB, Bassett LW, Hirsch SH, Jackson CA, Bastani R. A randomized clinical trial to assess the benefit of offering on-site mobile mammography in addition to health education for older women. *AJR Am J Roentgenol* 2002; **179**: 1509–14.

12. Wolk RB. Hidden costs of mobile mammography: is subsidization necessary? *AJR Am J Roentgenol* 1992; **158**: 12434–5.

13. Reynolds HE, Larkin GN, Jackson VP, Hawes DR. Fixed-facility workplace screening mammography. *AJR Am J Roentgenol* 1997; **168**: 507–10.

14. DeBruhl ND, Bassett LW, Jessop NW, Mason AM. Mobile mammography: results of a national survey. *Radiology* 1996; **201**: 433–7.

15. Ackerman M, Craft R, Ferrante F, *et al.* Telemedicine technology. *Telemed J E Health* 2002; **8**: 71–8.

16. Kelly MM, Parikh J, Shaw KK, Hallam PS. Mobile full-field digital telemammography with satellite transmission of images. *Semin Breast Dis* 2006; **9**: 92–8.

17. IHE. IHE Technical Frameworks. IHE Radiology Technical Committee. www.ihe.net/Technical_Framework/index.cfm (accessed April 2012.)

18. Basic image review. IHE Wiki, 2010. www.wiki.ihe.net/index.php?title=Basic_Image_Review (accessed April 2012).

19. Pisano ED, Zuley M, Baum JK, Marques HS. Issues to consider in converting to digital mammography. *Radiol Clin North Am* 2007; **45**: 813–30.

Chapter 10

Procedures with digital mammography

Gary J. Whitman, Malak Itani, Callie Cheatham, and Philip M. Tchou

Introduction

The history of mammography dates back to 1913, when the German surgeon Albert Salomon published his work after doing x-rays on 30 000 specimens of breast tissue removed surgically and then studied histologically [1]. It was not till the 1980s that mammography assumed a major clinical role, with the beginning of the practice of regular mammographic screening [2]. Currently, about two-thirds of breast cancers are detected by mammography. An important recent advancement in mammography has been the introduction of digital mammography.

Mammographically guided procedures performed with digital imaging include stereotactic biopsies, needle localizations, galactography, and specimen radiography. Stereotactic guidance may be used for core biopsies and for needle localizations. Galactography involves the administration of contrast through the nipple to delineate the mammary ducts. These procedures have been markedly improved with the use of digital imaging, compared to film-screen imaging. Digital imaging results in a shorter time for image display, with less patient discomfort and anxiety. Digital imaging guidance has allowed physicians and technologists to operate more efficiently, and procedure room utilization has been improved. Specimen radiography is radiography of excisional or percutaneous biopsy specimens (including mastectomy specimens) in order to document removal of the targeted lesions. Digital mammography has made it possible for radiologists, surgeons, and pathologists to view specimen radiographs simultaneously in different parts of the hospital, improving communication between multidisciplinary team members and decreasing operating room times and procedure times.

Digital mammography has allowed for electronic image annotations, and enterprise-wide image distribution. This chapter discusses the benefits of digital imaging in stereotactic biopsies, needle localizations, galactography, and specimen radiography (Figure 10.1).

Stereotactic biopsy

Stereotactic guidance is the use of angled mammographic views to determine the three-dimensional (3D) location of a lesion. Stereotactic guidance initially started with brain biopsies, but in the early 1990s stereotactic guidance was applied in diagnostic breast procedures. Currently, stereotactic guidance is widely used for breast biopsies, especially for biopsies of microcalcifications (Figure 10.2). Most physicians prefer ultrasound guidance for biopsies of masses visible by ultrasound because ultrasound is cheaper, provides real-time imaging, and is associated with no ionizing radiation. Stereotactic guidance, however, is commonly used to sample microcalcifications [3], which are usually difficult to visualize by ultrasound, and sometimes for small masses and areas of architectural distortion. A small percentage of nonpalpable breast masses seen on mammography are not seen on ultrasound, and these masses may be biopsied with stereotactic guidance.

Stereotactic biopsy is especially helpful in diagnosing ductal carcinoma in situ (DCIS) and atypical ductal hyperplasia (ADH). Following biopsies resulting in DCIS, the targeted lesion is then surgically excised in order to attain clear margins. At surgery, approximately 28% of DCIS cases will be upgraded to invasive ductal carcinoma [4]. Likewise, about 20% of cases yielding ADH on stereotactic biopsy are upgraded to DCIS or invasive ductal carcinoma on excision [5]. Thus, nearly all patients with ADH diagnosed by stereotactic biopsy subsequently undergo surgical excision.

Stereotactic biopsies are performed with specialized mammography units called stereotactic breast biopsy systems, designed to image the breast with angled views and identify the biopsy site in the x, y, and z planes. The major components of stereotactic biopsy systems are a patient table, a digital mammographic imager (with compression capability), and a biopsy device. The biopsy table is designed for the patient to lie in the prone position, with an opening for the pendant breast. The mammography unit is located underneath the table. The mammography unit applies compression to the breast and the x-ray tube can be rotated around the breast. Most prone stereotactic biopsy systems use charge-coupled device (CCD)-based cameras coupled to x-ray phosphor screens to provide digital imaging. The biopsy device is mounted securely to a supporting device.

During a stereotactic biopsy procedure, mammographic images are taken, usually in sets of three: one is taken as a

Digital Mammography: A Practical Approach, ed. Gary J. Whitman and Tamara Miner Haygood. Published by Cambridge University Press. © Cambridge University Press 2013.

(a)

(b)

(c)

(d)

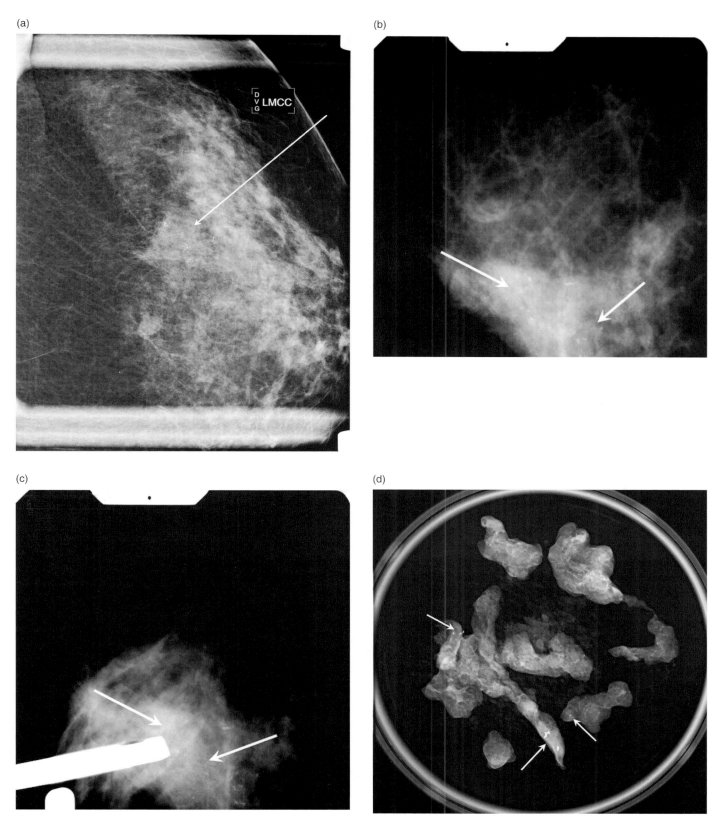

Figure 10.1 (*cont.*)

(e)

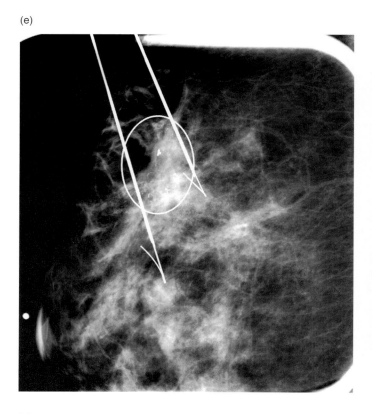

(f)

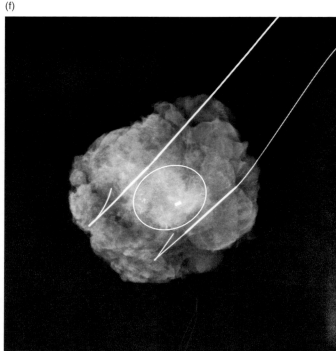

(g)

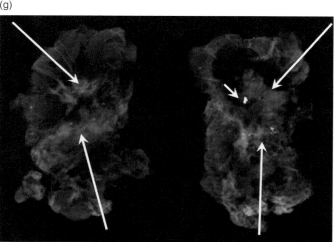

Figure 10.1 (a) Left craniocaudal magnification mammography in a 55-year-old woman shows pleomorphic calcifications (arrow). (b) Straight-on craniocaudal image shows the targeted calcifications (arrows). (c) Stereotactic angled view following needle insertion shows the biopsy needle and the targeted calcifications (arrows). (d) Specimen radiography shows the targeted calcifications (arrows). Pathology revealed high-grade ductal carcinoma in situ (DCIS) with comedonecrosis. (e) Left breast lateromedial mammogram at the time of the needle localization shows the targeted calcifications (circle) and a clip marker, bracketed by a Kopans needle wire device and a Hawkins needle wire device. (f) Specimen radiography revealed the excised calcifications (circle) in the center of the specimen, along with the clip marker. (g) Sliced specimen radiography shows the targeted calcifications (long arrows) and the clip marker (short arrow).

straight-on image, and two angled views are acquired (typically ± 15 degrees from the straight-on position). Lesions noted on the mammograms will shift in the opposite direction of the tube's rotation. The degree of shift will depend on the distance of the lesion relative to the tube. Lesions located closer to the tube will produce a greater shift in the offset images, while more distant ones will only shift slightly. The distance that the lesion shifts in these images is used to calculate its position relative to the detector using trigonometric relationships. This information is then used to calculate a trajectory and a depth for the biopsy needle, controlled by the computer. The radiologist then positions the needle device to sample tissue from the designated region of the breast. Tissue samples are extracted using either a core needle or a vacuum-assisted device (VAD), which can collect multiple samples with one needle insertion [3]. In general, stereotactic biopsies, especially those targeting microcalcifications, are performed with VADs. Additional insertions at different depths or positions may be performed as deemed necessary by the radiologist. Verification of removal of the appropriate targeted lesion is then done using specimen radiography.

Currently, most stereotactic core biopsies in North America are performed with VADs. Previously, fine needle

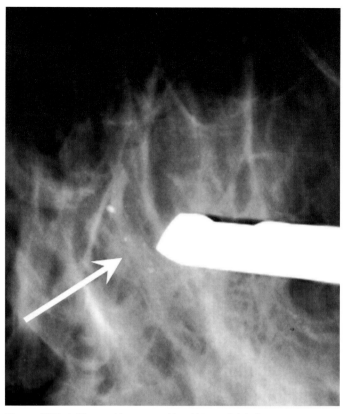

Figure 10.2 A 59-year-old woman with a history of right breast cancer underwent mammography which showed indeterminate calcifications in the left breast. Stereotactic biopsy was performed, targeting the calcifications (arrow). Pathology revealed no evidence of malignancy.

aspirations and 11–16 gauge core biopsies were performed. If a core biopsy is performed, the number of cores obtained is controversial. The number of cores should be greater than three [4], and probably close to 12. Lomoschitz *et al.* noted no increase in diagnostic yield when more than 12 cores where obtained with an 11 gauge needle [5]. A clip marker is usually placed at the biopsy site. Clip markers are helpful for demonstrating the biopsy site, especially when all or most of the lesion was removed. The immediate post-clip image may be obtained as a stereotactic image. Thereafter, a two-view mammogram should be obtained to document the position of the clip. The two-view mammograms are helpful for noting evidence of clip migration as well as hematoma formation. If there is evidence of clip migration, the biopsy site should be annotated on the post-biopsy images, and the radiology report should describe the direction of the clip migration and indicate the distance between the clip and the biopsy site.

Needle localization

Needle localization, also known as wire localization, involves placement of a guide wire and/or a needle leading from the outside of the breast to the site of a targeted nonpalpable abnormality within the breast. Needle localizations are performed prior to excisional biopsies and lumpectomies to ensure accurate localization of the targeted lesion.

Needle localizations are typically performed using a standard mammography system or a stereotactic biopsy system. Ultrasound-guided (and MRI-guided) localizations may also be performed for mass lesions. Local anesthesia (1% lidocaine buffered with sodium bicarbonate) is usually administered [6] prior to mammographically guided needle localization procedures. Initially, the breast is compressed, and images are taken to localize the targeted lesion and to determine the best path for the needle. During the procedure, images are taken as necessary to determine the position of the needle relative to the targeted lesion. When the needle is in the correct place, images are taken for verification and the hookwire is deployed. The outer needle may remain in place or it can be removed, with the lesion localized by the hookwire. The needle and/or the hookwire serve to direct the surgeon to the nonpalpable abnormality identified on mammography. Bracketing with two or more needles may be performed (Figure 10.3).

In general, mammographically guided needle localizations are well tolerated by patients. Bleeding and/or pain, especially at a prior biopsy site, may occur, but these complications are usually minimal. Also, vasovagal episodes may occur, and nearly all of these episodes resolve with conservative measures. At the conclusion of the procedure, the needle is taped to the patient's skin, and the patient is escorted to the surgical holding area. Following surgery, the resected lesion is then submitted for pathologic analysis, and specimen radiography is performed.

Galactography

Galactography (or ductography) is a mammographic procedure that uses contrast material to obtain images of the patient's ductal system. Galactography is commonly used to evaluate patients with abnormal nipple discharge. Galactography helps to define the cause of pathologic nipple discharge, identify abnormal ducts, and provide guidance for surgical excisions. Discharge may be sanguineous (bloody), serosanguineous, clear, milky, yellow, blue, green, or black. Clear, sanguineous, and serosanguineous are the most worrisome types of discharge, and spontaneous discharge is considered more worrisome than non-spontaneous discharge [7]. Suspicious areas usually appear as filling defects, which may be caused by fibrocystic changes, papillomas, and carcinomas. These defects often occur in dilated ducts.

Galactography is performed with a standard mammography unit. Pressure is placed on the breast until the trigger area is found that produces the discharge. A blunt-tipped needle, or cannula, is guided into the correct duct towards the location of the discharge. It is necessary that the breast be stabilized during this procedure. Occasionally, it will be necessary to dilate the duct, or a warm towel may be placed over the breast to facilitate duct dilation. This is especially necessary when abnormalities exist such as nipple retraction, dried secretions along the duct, or deep crevices in the duct. When the cannula is in the correct

(a)

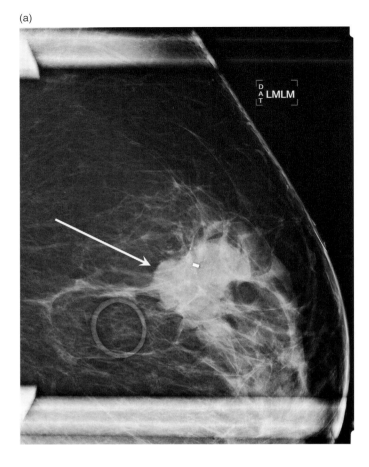

(b)

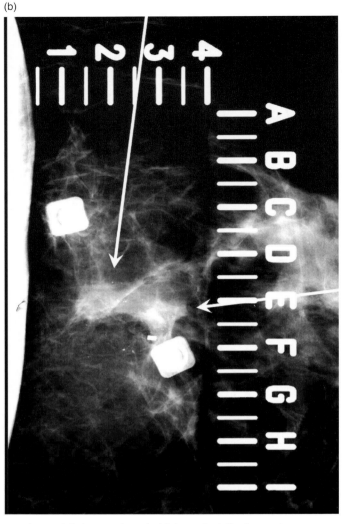

Figure 10.3 (a) Magnified lateromedial view of the left breast in a 64-year-old woman shows a lobular mass (arrow) with internal calcifications and a clip marker. Ultrasound-guided biopsy revealed mixed invasive ductal and lobular carcinoma. The patient was then treated with neoadjuvant paclitaxel and trastuzumab. (b) Left craniocaudal mammogram obtained during the needle localization shows two Kopans needles bracketing the targeted calcifications (arrows) and the clip marker. (c) Left mediolateral mammogram obtained during the needle localization shows the two localizing needles and hookwires bracketing the targeted calcifications (circle) and the clip marker. (d) Sliced specimen radiography shows the targeted calcifications (arrows) and the clip marker. Pathology revealed fat necrosis and associated calcifications, with no residual malignancy identified.

location, a syringe is used to insert 0.2–0.3 mL of low-osmolar, non-ionic contrast material into the duct. The cannula and the syringe are taped in place during the procedure. The patient is positioned in the mammography unit under mild compression. Images are obtained using standard mammographic techniques. The contrast material may affect the phototiming, but usually not by much since only a small amount of contrast material is used. Magnification imaging is often used for better visualization of the ducts and to identify small filling defects. If duct filling is incomplete, more contrast may be injected. Backflow may occur if the ducts are obstructed. At the conclusion of the procedure, the catheter is removed, and a final mammographic image may be taken.

It is possible that extravasation, leakage of contrast material into the surrounding tissues, may occur immediately or after

some time. Excessive pressure due to too much contrast injected or puncture of the duct while placing the needle can cause extravasation. Patients undergoing galactography may experience minimal pain. Patients may experience vasovagal syncope (or fainting). In rare cases, the patient may have a mild to severe allergic-type reaction to the contrast material. Prior history of contrast reactions should be noted. In some cases, patients may require premedication [7]. In patients with prior severe contrast reactions, galactography may be cancelled, and another procedure, such as ultrasound or magnetic resonance imaging (MRI), may be performed.

Care should be taken by the operator to avoid injecting air bubbles, which may simulate filling defects. When filling defects are noted on galactography, it can be difficult to determine whether an abnormality is benign or malignant, which

(c)

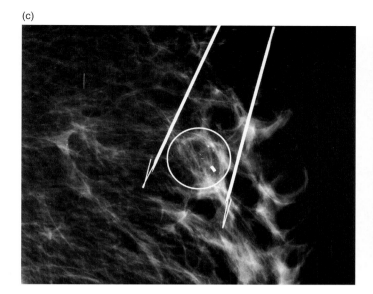

(d)

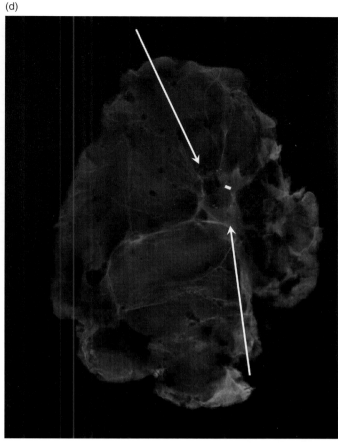

Figure 10.3 (*cont.*)

gives galactography a somewhat high false-positive rate. Studies are ongoing, comparing galactography, sonography, and MRI.

Preoperative galactography can be performed to facilitate surgical removal of a known intraductal lesion. During preoperative galactography procedures, the contrast material is mixed with methylene blue, allowing the surgeon to excise a blue-stained duct. In addition, preoperative galactography may be combined with preoperative needle localization in order to facilitate excision of lesions noted distant from the nipple (Figure 10.4).

Specimen radiography

Specimen radiography is used for immediate assessment of tissue samples following biopsies or surgical excisions, including mastectomies. Specimen radiography involves x-ray imaging of the excised tissue using a standard mammography system or a dedicated specimen radiography system. Specimen radiography is used to verify that calcifications were removed following stereotactic biopsies. Specimen radiography also plays a major role following surgical excisions, demonstrating that the lesion, with appropriate margins, was removed.

Specimen radiography of surgical specimens allows for less breast tissue to be removed, often an important consideration in breast-conserving surgery. When a known malignancy is being surgically excised, one needs to make certain that the margins of excision are sufficiently clear of any malignant tissue (Figure 10.5). Positive margins increase the chance of recurrence. After excision, the removed tissue is sent to pathology for examination. The excised tissue may be inked, examined, and imaged. At many centers, specimen radiography is performed while the patient is under anesthesia in the operating room. Specimen radiography images may be obtained with a standard mammography unit or with a dedicated specimen radiography unit. There are various techniques, including obtaining one view and obtaining two orthogonal views. Another approach involves radiography of the entire specimen, followed by slicing the specimen, and then radiography of the sliced tissue sections. The specimen radiographs are compared with the preoperative mammograms to verify that the targeted abnormalities were removed at surgery (Figure 10.6).

The speed of the process is critical because the patient is usually in surgery, under anesthesia, during the time of specimen radiography. At The University of Texas MD Anderson Cancer Center (UTMDACC), a specialist in breast imaging

(a)

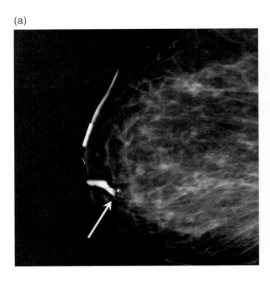

(b)

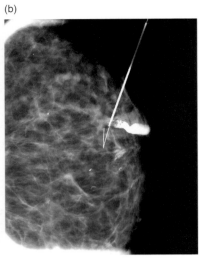

Figure 10.4 An 86-year-old woman presented with spontaneous bloody left nipple discharge. (a) Ductography revealed a dilated duct on the left lateromedial view with an abrupt cut-off (arrow), secondary to an intraluminal lesion. Preoperative needle localization was performed for surgical guidance. (b) Left craniocaudal mammogram shows the filling defect localized with a Kopans needle wire device. Pathology revealed an intraductal papilloma.

carefully analyzes the specimen radiographs, obtained using computed radiography, and annotates the images to indicate the location of the targeted abnormalities and any close or involved margins. The annotated images are then sent on the picture archiving and communication system (PACS) and viewed by the pathologist and the surgeon. If the margins are appropriate and the malignancy has been removed, the surgical site will be closed, and the patient will be sent to the recovery room. However, if the margins are positive or close, additional tissue will usually be excised, as determined by the findings on specimen radiography. Specimen radiography reduces the number of patients needing a second surgery, and also reduces the likelihood that the patient will have a recurrence in the area of the resection [8].

Following stereotactic biopsies, specimen radiography is utilized to determine if the targeted calcifications were removed (Figure 10.7). The findings on specimen radiography determine whether or not it is necessary to obtain additional tissue. At UTMDACC, specimen radiography is used as a guide, and the cores containing calcifications are marked with India ink. Thereafter, all of the cores are placed in formalin and sent for pathologic analysis. At UTMDACC, the radiologists report the number of cores removed and the number of cores with calcifications. In addition, the radiology report includes an assessment of the percentage of the targeted calcifications that were removed during the biopsy.

Digital mammography improvements

The multiple steps that were necessary for image formation with film-screen mammography have been replaced by one or two steps in digital mammography (depending on whether it is a direct or an indirect capture device), and digital imaging has provided important improvements, including speed and reproducibility. Having the mammogram in the form of a printed film is a major limitation because it is the sole medium

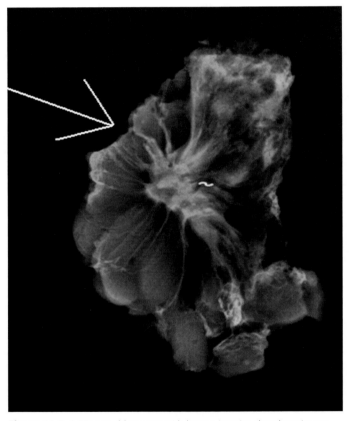

Figure 10.5 A 77-year-old woman with known invasive ductal carcinoma underwent breast conservation surgery. Sliced specimen radiography shows an irregular spiculated mass, representing the known malignancy, with a clip marker. The malignancy extended close to the anterior margin (arrow).

for acquisition, display, and storage [9,10]. The optimization of these three processes in digital mammography has resulted in flexibility in post-processing, electronic measurements and annotations, and simultaneous and quick accessibility by multiple users.

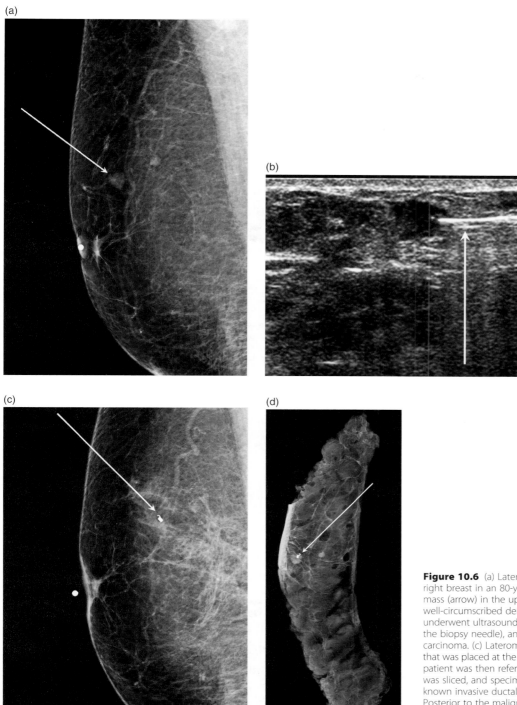

Figure 10.6 (a) Lateromedial mammographic view of the right breast in an 80-year-old man demonstrates a small mass (arrow) in the upper breast, along with a smaller well-circumscribed density posterior to it. (b) The patient underwent ultrasound-guided core biopsy (arrow points to the biopsy needle), and pathology revealed invasive ductal carcinoma. (c) Lateromedial mammogram shows a clip (arrow) that was placed at the biopsy site with ultrasound guidance. The patient was then referred for surgery. (d) The surgical specimen was sliced, and specimen radiographs were taken, showing the known invasive ductal carcinoma with the clip marker (arrow). Posterior to the malignancy, a small mass was noted, representing a benign intramammary lymph node on pathology.

Speed

Digital mammography has improved many of the procedures used in the diagnosis and treatment of breast cancer. One of the key changes is the amount of time the entire imaging process takes. During a procedure with film-screen mammographic guidance, the physician must wait for the images to be completed, then, several minutes later, the physician can resume the procedure based on analysis of the images. This waiting time is extremely critical, as the patient's breast is in compression. Studies have shown that a digital image is received in approximately 15 seconds, while

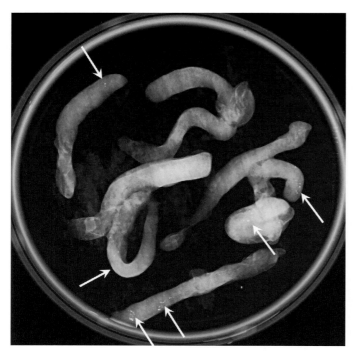

Figure 10.7 Specimen radiography following a stereotactic biopsy shows several microcalcifications (arrows). Pathology revealed benign tissue associated with microcalcifications; an incidental focus of atypical lobular hyperplasia was noted.

it may take up to 3 minutes for a film to be processed [11,12]. Digital imaging has decreased procedure times by up to 50% in some cases, particularly in needle localizations [13]. The procedure time decreases when digital imaging is used, primarily due to faster image acquisition and not decreased reading times [14].

Practical improvements

Faster imaging allows more time for physicians to see more patients, minimizes patient fear and anxiety during procedures, and allows the physician to quickly identify and act upon any complications that may arise during a procedure (e.g., extravasation in galactography or the needle in an inappropriate position in needle localizations). Digital mammographic guidance allows patients to have a more comfortable experience. The ability to perform more procedures in the same room during the same period of time, with the same staff, allows for improved efficiency.

Enterprise-wide distribution

Digital storage of mammographic images can be a huge asset to a hospital or a radiology department. A digital network allows enterprise-wide image display within the hospital or the hospital system [15]. Enterprise-wide image distribution decreases the time a clinician must wait to view imaging studies and facilitates consultations between various specialists. At UTMDACC, enterprise-wide image distribution has been particularly helpful in assessing specimen radiographs

following segmental resections and mastectomies. PACS has allowed the radiologist to view the specimen radiographs, annotate them, and then send the annotated images via PACS to the pathologist in the pathology laboratory across the street.

Computer enhancements and post-processing

The ability of digital imaging to enhance and manipulate imaging data has been a major improvement compared to film-screen systems. One study showed that digital mammography provides advantages over film-screen mammography by eliminating film-related inefficiencies, reducing technical repeats, and allowing for magnification at the workstation [16]. With digital systems, the image can be manipulated easily to improve visualization of the breast tissue. The contrast of the image can be enhanced, the gray scale can be modified, the image can be magnified, edge enhancement can be applied, and the modified image can be annotated, displayed, and stored digitally. The ability to modify the contrast of the image can be especially helpful when the breast tissue is dense [17].

With film-screen mammography, the data available on the film is what the radiologist has to work with. The only enhancements available are to view the image with a hot light and to use a magnifying glass as the film is examined. Digital imaging data can be modified to help improve image analysis [18]. By modifying the digital data on the workstation, subtle changes or abnormalities can more clearly be seen and are less likely to be missed by the radiologist. These improvements are particularly important in planning needle localization procedures, because of the need to visualize subtle microcalcifications. In addition, digital mammography clearly delineates the skin, which may be poorly visualized on film-screen mammography. Clear visualization of the skin is a key issue in needle localization procedures, as the skin-to-lesion distance dictates the length of the needle used. In addition, at UTMDACC, the skin-to-needle tip distance is communicated to the surgeon by the radiologist following needle localization procedures.

Specific digital mammography improvements related to procedures

Mammographically guided procedures have been improved by digital mammography, mostly due to improved speed of image acquisition and display, enterprise-wide distribution, and the ability to save image modifications and annotations.

Regarding stereotactic biopsies, procedure planning has become easier with digital systems, as post-processing and image enhancement allow better visualization of microcalcifications and the skin line. Planning the procedure is also easier because of the ability to draw needle trajectories and make accurate measurements. In addition, PACS allows quick and easy comparison of current images with previous ones. Becker *et al.* reported that in stereotactic core biopsy, digital

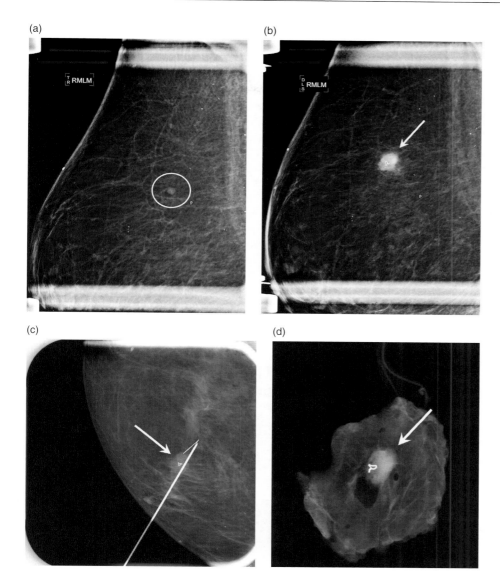

Figure 10.8 (a) Right magnified lateromedial mammogram in a 72-year-old woman reveals a 4 mm mass (circle). Stereotactic biopsy demonstrated mucinous carcinoma. (b) Right magnified lateromedial post-biopsy mammogram shows the post-biopsy clip and an associated hematoma (arrow). (c) Craniocaudal image from the needle localization shows the clip and the hematoma (arrow), localized with a Kopans needle wire device. (d) Sliced specimen radiography shows the clip and the hematoma (arrow). Pathology revealed focal residual mucinous carcinoma.

mammography decreased missed lesions from about 7.4% to 3.6% and missed microcalcifications from 13% to 4.5% [19].

A significant improvement in stereotactic biopsies with digital imaging is the marked reduction in the procedure time, compared to film-screen systems. The time previously needed for processing films has been markedly reduced due to the fact that mammographic images taken before, during, and after the procedure, as well as specimen radiographs, are now all processed using digital imaging. Reduced time for processing images obtained during the procedure and specimen radiography is important, as the patient is in an uncomfortable position, lying prone, with the breast compressed, and the needle in the breast.

The advantages of digital mammography for procedure planning also apply for needle localizations. Artifacts due to patient motion have been reduced significantly after shifting to digital mammography because the time for image display has decreased, thereby decreasing the time in compression, patient discomfort, and anxiety. These factors result in quicker, more accurate needle localizations (Figure 10.8).

For galactography, the time it takes for the images to be processed is of concern because of patient discomfort and the need to quickly identify complications such as extravasation. The speed gained with digital mammography reduces the time during which a patient has the galactography catheter in her breast (Figure 10.9).

After surgical excision of breast lesions, a specimen radiograph is usually obtained to ensure clear margins (Figure 10.10). In general, specimen radiography has similar accuracy and image quality to conventional digital mammography [20]. Specimen radiography with digital systems has several advantages, including speed, enterprise-wide availability of images, and the ability to add annotations. As for speed, the time needed to assess specimen radiographs is critical because the patient remains under anesthesia in the operating room while the surgeon awaits feedback on the specimen radiograph in the operating room. Digital mammography decreases the time required for specimen radiography [21].

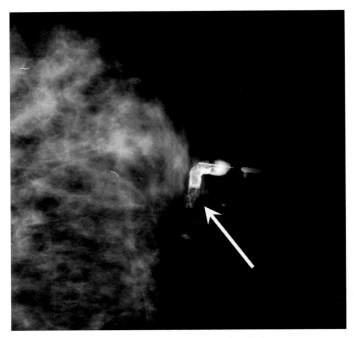

Figure 10.9 A 58-year-old woman presented with right breast spontaneous clear-to-white nipple discharge. Galactography demonstrates a tubular filling defect (arrow) near the base of the nipple on the right lateromedial view. Surgical excision revealed an intraductal papilloma.

Simultaneous access to digital specimen radiographs by the surgeons, pathologists, and radiologists improves communication regarding close and/or positive surgical margins. The radiologist assesses the specimen radiographs and then communicates with the pathologist and/or the surgeon. With digital mammography, the radiologist can annotate the areas of concern on the specimen radiograph (Figure 10.11), and provide the pathologist and the surgeon with a visual map of where margins may be close or involved by tumor.

Specimen radiography is usually performed following stereotactic biopsies. The speed of digital mammography has allowed for quick image processing, minimizing patient discomfort and compression time, and decreasing overall procedure time. The biopsy needle remains in the breast at the site of the suspicious lesion until the radiologist has analyzed the specimen radiographs and made sure that the biopsied sample is representative of the targeted lesion. With digital imaging, the radiologist can annotate the targeted findings (usually microcalcifications) on specimen radiography, and the annotated images are available for the pathologist to view during histopathologic evaluation of the biopsy samples.

The future of procedures performed with digital mammography

The introduction of digital mammography has directly influenced mammographically guided procedures and specimen radiography, mainly by facilitating procedure planning, decreasing procedure times, simplifying communication between

(a)   (b)

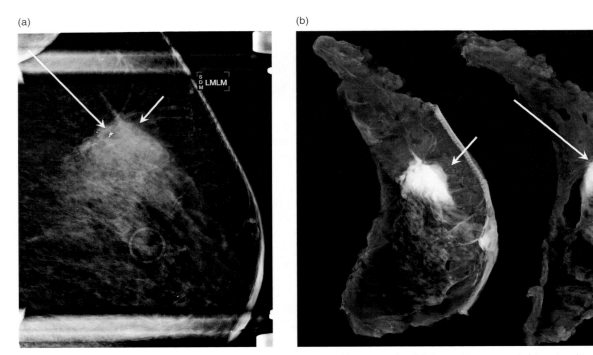

Figure 10.10 Diagnostic mammography was performed on a 67-year-old woman after left breast biopsy revealed invasive ductal carcinoma. (a) Magnified left lateromedial mammogram shows an irregular mass (short arrow) representing the malignancy, with an associated clip marker (long arrow). (b) Specimen radiography after a left mastectomy shows the malignancy (short arrows) with clear margins. The clip marker is noted (long arrow).

(a)

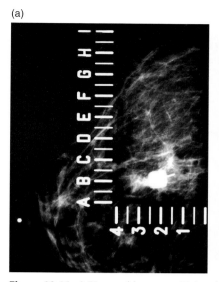

(b)

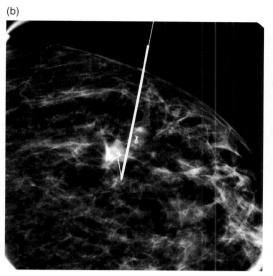

(c)

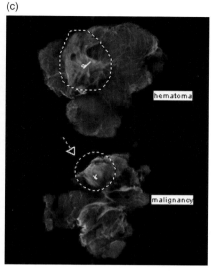

Figure 10.11 A 73-year-old woman with invasive ductal carcinoma underwent breast conservation surgery. Needle localization was performed using a lateral-to-medial approach. Shown are (a) lateromedial and (b) craniocaudal views from the needle localization procedure, localizing two clip markers. (c) Specimen radiography shows the targeted malignancy (circle), with an internal clip, extending to the posterior margin (arrow). On the adjacent slice, a hematoma (oval) was noted with an internal clip.

radiologists and other physicians (mainly surgeons and pathologists), and minimizing patient discomfort and time in compression. Although digital imaging is associated with increased costs [17], the benefits outweigh the costs over time. Digital imaging is evolving, with recent improvements in image quality and workstation functionality. In the future, there will be further advancements in digital imaging and procedures with digital imaging guidance. These advancements should lead to improved accuracy and further decreases in procedure times.

Acknowledgments

We thank Barbara Almarez Mahinda for assistance with manuscript preparation.

References

1. Picard JD. [History of mammography]. *Bull Acad Natl Med* 1998; **182**: 1613–20.

2. Van Steen A, Van Tiggelen R. Short history of mammography: a Belgian perspective. *JBR-BTR*. 2007; **90**: 151–3.

3. O'Flynn EA, Wilson AR, Michell MJ. Image-guided breast biopsy: state-of-the-art. *Clin Radiol* 2010; **65**: 259–70.

4. Koskela AK, Sudah M, Berg MH, *et al.* Add-on device for stereotactic core-needle breast biopsy: how many biopsy specimens are needed for a reliable diagnosis? *Radiology* 2005; **236**: 801–9.

5. Lomoschitz FM, Helbich TH, Rudas M, *et al.* Stereotactic 11-gauge vacuum-assisted breast biopsy: influence of number of specimens on diagnostic accuracy. *Radiology* 2004; **232**: 897–903.

6. Kopans DB, Swann CA. Preoperative imaging-guided needle placement and localization of clinically occult breast lesions. *AJR Am J Roentgenol* 1989; **152**: 1–9.

7. Slawson SH, Johnson BA. Ductography: how to and what if? *Radiographics* 2001; **21**: 133–50.

8. Ciccarelli G, Di Virgilio MR, Menna S, *et al.* Radiography of the surgical specimen in early stage breast lesions: diagnostic reliability in the analysis of the resection margins. *Radiol Med* 2007; **112**: 366–76.

9. Mahesh M. AAPM/RSNA physics tutorial for residents: digital mammography: an overview. *Radiographics* 2004; **24**: 1747–60.

10. Pisano ED. Current status of full-field digital mammography. *Radiology*. 2000; **214**: 26–8.

11. Irwin MR, Downey DB, Gardi L, Fenster A. Registered 3-D ultrasound and digital stereotactic mammography for breast biopsy guidance. *IEEE Trans Med Imaging* 2008; **27**: 391–401.

12. Yang WT, Whitman GJ, Johnson MM, *et al.* Needle localization for excisional biopsy of breast lesions: comparison of effect of use of full-field digital versus screen-film mammographic guidance on procedure time. *Radiology* 2004; **231**: 277–81.

13. Dershaw DD, Fleischman RC, Liberman L, *et al.* Use of digital mammography in needle localization procedures. *AJR Am J Roentgenol* 1993; **161**: 559–62.

14. Haygood TM, Wang J, Atkinson EN, *et al.* Timed efficiency of interpretation of digital and film-screen screening mammograms. *AJR Am J Roentgenol* 2009; **192**: 216–20.

15. Carrino JA. Digital imaging overview. *Semin Roentgenol* 2003; **38**: 200–15.

16. Houssami N, Ciatto S. The evolving role of new imaging methods in breast screening. *Prev Med* 2011; **53**: 123–6.

17. Pisano ED, Gatsonis C, Hendrick E, *et al.* Diagnostic performance of digital versus film mammography for breast-cancer screening. *N Engl J Med* 2005; **353**: 1773–83.

18. Van Ongeval C, Bosmans H, Van Steen A. Current status of

digital mammography for screening and diagnosis of breast cancer. *Curr Opin Oncol* 2006; **18**: 547–54.

19. Becker L, Taves D, McCurdy L, *et al.* Stereotactic core biopsy of breast microcalcifications: comparison of film versus digital mammography, both using an add-on unit. *AJR Am J Roentgenol* 2001; **177**: 1451–7.

20. Kuzmiak CM, Millnamow GA, Qaqish B, *et al.* Comparison of full-field digital mammography to screen-film mammography with respect to diagnostic accuracy of lesion characterization in breast tissue biopsy specimens. *Acad Radiol* 2002; **9**: 1378–82.

21. Kaufman CS, Bachman BA, Jacobson L, *et al.* Intraoperative digital specimen mammography: prompt image review speeds surgery. *Am J Surg* 2006; **192**: 513–15.

Digital breast tomosynthesis

Alexis V. Nees

Introduction

Digital breast tomosynthesis is a breast imaging technology that provides three-dimensional-like information. Tomosynthesis has been developed to improve the characterization of breast lesions and cancer detection, particularly in dense breasts. However, an understanding of mammography and its limitations is necessary to fully appreciate tomosynthesis and its potential uses and advantages. The purpose of mammography is the early detection of breast cancer. Mammography is the only imaging method scientifically proven with the ability to detect clinically occult breast cancer and result in a decreased mortality rate from breast cancer. Several large controlled trials have demonstrated the efficacy of screening mammography, reducing breast cancer mortality rates by 18–30% [1,2]. However, screening mammography does not detect all breast cancers. Film-screen mammography does not detect 10–20% of palpable breast cancers, particularly in dense breasts, as there may not be a sufficient difference in contrast between the normal breast tissue and the cancer [3,4].

Film-screen mammography is an analog detection system, in which x-ray photons pass through the breast and are converted to light by a fluorescing screen. A reaction on the film emulsion is triggered by the light. The film is developed by a chemical process, thus producing a gray-scale image of the photon distribution. Digital mammography differs from film-screen mammography in that the x-ray photons strike a digital detector, which converts the absorbed energy into an electronic signal. This signal is received, processed, and stored as a matrix. The signal is linearly proportional to the intensity of the transmitted x-ray. This results in a wider dynamic range than for film-screen mammography [5]. Digital mammography provides a broader dynamic range of densities and greater contrast resolution. However, the spatial resolution of film-screen mammography is better than that of digital mammography. Spatial resolution is measured in terms of the smallest high-contrast object that can be distinguished as distinct. Film-screen mammography resolves 12 and 15 line-pairs/mm, which is equivalent to 42–30 μm pixels. For digital mammography, spatial resolution ranges from 100 to about

50 μm pixels in whole-breast mode or 5–10 line-pairs/mm [6]. Because of reduction in quantum mottle and elimination of granular artifacts from film emulsion, digital images have lower noise than film-screen images [5,7]. The radiation dose of film-screen and digital mammography is comparable, with average mean glandular doses of 4.7 and 3.7 mGy for film-screen and digital mammography, respectively [8,9].

Digital mammography addresses some of the limitations of film-screen mammography. Digital mammography decouples or separates the processes of image acquisition, processing, and display. Therefore, each process can be optimized. Decoupling of acquisition and processing enables post-acquisition processing of the image, which can optimize image quality. The degree of image contrast can be manipulated for optimization. This is advantageous compared to film-screen mammography, as digital mammography can provide additional diagnostic information without requiring additional imaging and exposing the patient to additional radiation. Processing tools may change the contrast and brightness of an image (i.e., window and level) or enlarge part of or the entire breast. Since different parts of the breast may be viewed with different brightness and contrast settings, an optimal analysis of the fatty and the dense components of the breast is made possible. Post-acquisition processing may compensate for underexposure or overexposure, which can reduce the need for repeat images and consequently expose the patient to less radiation. Manufacturers have developed different algorithms, specific to their systems, to optimize the images. These algorithms can change the window width and the level automatically, depending on the range of the intensity values present. Algorithms can enhance the sharpness of the borders of a lesion. Peripheral equalization algorithms can enhance the visualization of structures in the periphery of the breast. Other processing techniques include image inversion and noise suppression.

However, the primary limitation of mammography is geometry, where two views of a complex object result in the superimposition of normal structures over or around abnormal masses, in effect hiding them. This limitation exists for both film-screen and digital mammography. Differences in the conspicuity of a

Digital Mammography: A Practical Approach, ed. Gary J. Whitman and Tamara Miner Haygood. Published by Cambridge University Press.
© Cambridge University Press 2013.

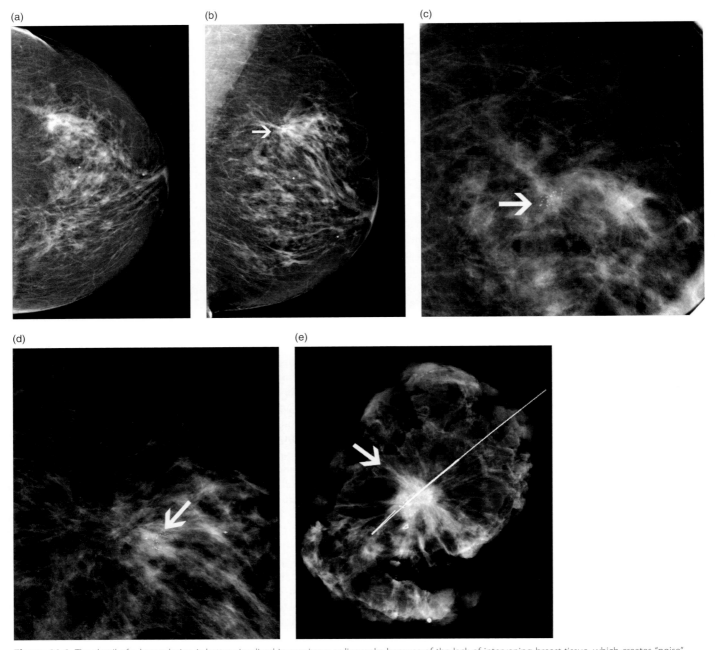

Figure 11.1 The detail of a breast lesion is better visualized in specimen radiographs because of the lack of intervening breast tissue, which creates "noise" that may obscure a lesion. (a, b) Craniocaudal (CC) and mediolateral oblique (MLO) views in a 63-year-old woman demonstrate architectural distortion (arrow) and asymmetry. (c, d) Spot compression CC and lateromedial (LM) views show persistent asymmetry and pleomorphic calcifications (arrow). (e) The spiculated margins (arrow) of this invasive ductal carcinoma are clearly visible in the specimen radiograph because of the lack of structural "noise" of normal breast tissue. A clip marker is noted at the periphery of the malignant mass.

lesion on specimen radiography compared with the standard mammographic views demonstrates this problem. Specimen radiography has better geometry, as the object/specimen is immediately adjacent to the detector, rendering a superior image of the lesion/mass. Thus, the lesion is more clearly identified on specimen radiography (Figure 11.1). However, the detail of the lesion is also better seen because of the lack of

intervening breast tissue, which creates "noise" that may obscure the lesion. This noise from the surrounding breast tissue decreases the ability of mammography to detect breast cancers.

In an effort to resolve the problem of noise from overlapping structures, Miller *et al.* developed a technique in which several radiographs were taken with the tube at various angles

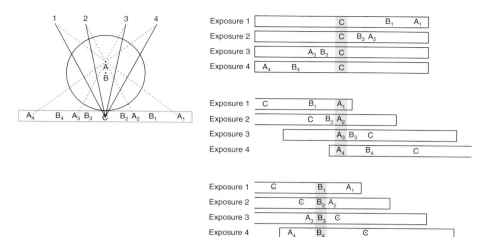

Figure 11.2 Parallax shift. Multiple exposures are obtained from different angles (points 1–4) with the central beam centered on the radiograph (B) in constant relationship to the object (A). The projections of structures onto the detector shift less between images obtained at different angles if the object is closer to the detector. Note that the shift is greater from image to image if the distance of the object from the detector is greater. Radiographs are photographed serially on a single film with only one plane in register. Top right schematic shows initial composite exposure. Middle right schematic shows A in register in all exposures, creating a sharp image of A (and all other points in plane of A); B and C are not in register. The lower right schematic shows B (and all other points in plane of B) in register.

and the central beam centered on the radiographs in a constant relationship to the object [10]. The radiographs were photographed serially on a single film with only one plane registered. The separation of objects in the image depends on the object size and its distance from the plane and the total travel of the tube (Figure 11.2). Smaller objects will appear separate on the final image, even if close to the plane. Larger objects appear separate only if located further from the plane, those closer to the plane will overlap. The projections of structures onto the detector shift less between the images obtained at different angles if the object is closer to the detector. The shift is greater from image to image if the distance of the object from the detector is greater. This is known as parallax shift. Miller *et al.* demonstrated that structures in the same plane could be aligned with objects in other planes not in register or alignment. The structures in alignment were more visible and those not in alignment or register were more difficult to see. Thus, the structures that were not in alignment were eliminated. If images are shifted and added, each plane through the imaged structure can be viewed in registration. This technique, referred to as "shift and add," creates a series of images, with each image displaying one plane in registration or sharp focus [11].

Tomosynthesis differs from conventional linear tomography. Tomography requires the x-ray source and detector to be moved for each slice with a full exposure. With tomosynthesis, all the planes of the imaged object are "synthesized" from fewer projections. The registration process is complex. It requires an electronic detector to allow the images to be "shifted and added" with a computer. Images in the same plane are aligned and reinforced, which makes them more visible. Structures out of alignment are more difficult to see and eliminated. With "shifting and adding" the images in a programmed manner, each plane through a structure can be "synthesized" in sharp registration; the structures in this plane are well seen. Structures out of plane are not well seen, because of misregistration [12] (Figure 11.3). Tomosynthesis has been investigated in parts of the body other than the breast [13,14]. The reduction of streak artifacts by use of one-dimensional filtering of linear tomosynthesis images resulted in image quality superior to that of conventional tomograms [14–17]. However, imaging of the breast requires high resolution, which initially delayed the clinical application of tomosynthesis. The development of full-field digital mammography (FFDM) provided a full-field, flat, digital detector suitable for tomosynthesis of the breast. Complex computer reconstruction algorithms are used to reconstruct the image datasets into thin slices or thick slices (slabs) for viewing and interpretation.

Image acquisition

Prototype tomosynthesis systems have been developed by several vendors. There are several ways of acquiring the images. For all methods, the breast is held in standard compression and the x-ray tube is moved in an arc about the stationary breast. One method of acquisition is the "step-and-shoot" method. With "step-and-shoot," the detector is uncoupled from the x-ray tube. Therefore, the x-ray tube can move independently of the stationary detector.

Alternatively, the x-ray tube and detector can move simultaneously about the stationary breast. However, the patient's shoulder can obstruct the moving detector in the mediolateral oblique (MLO) projection, which may limit the angle through which the images can be acquired. Also, the detector must be located further from the breast to allow for its movement. A potential benefit of moving the detector is the ease of incorporation of a scatter rejection grid into the system. This is the method of continuous acquisition.

The acquired images are not truly three-dimensional, because of the limited angle of scanning. Images would need to be acquired over an arc of 180 degrees or more (similar to computed tomography [CT]) to produce accurate cubic voxels (volumetric information). With tomosynthesis, a series of

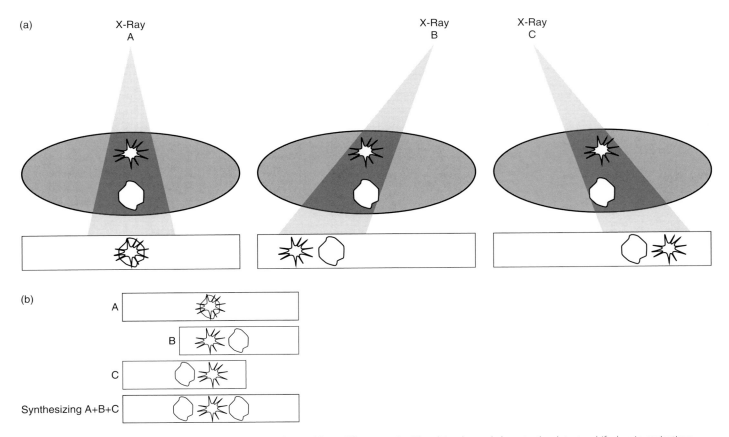

Figure 11.3 Parallax shift in tomosynthesis. (a) Images are obtained from different angles. The object located closer to the detector shifts less in projections obtained at different angles. The shift is greater for the object located a further distance from the detector. (b) The individual images are arranged and reinforced with a single object in alignment, which allows the object to be seen more clearly. The structures out of alignment are more difficult to identify. "Shifting and adding" the images in a programmed manner allows each plane to be synthesized in sharp registration.

low-dose exposures is obtained throughout the angular range. The x–y plane is perpendicular to the x-ray beam and has the highest resolution. The z-axis (thickness or depth) is parallel to the beam, with less resolution. Therefore, tissue located behind a structure in the breast is not as well seen from a lesser angle. Increasing the number of images or projections over a larger (wider) angular range will improve the z resolution of the system. It will also improve the signal-to-noise ratio. This is similar to CT. However, as the angle increases, the amount of breast tissue to be traversed is greater, resulting in increased scatter and increased dose.

Images are acquired with the breast in compression similar to conventional mammography. Imaging can be performed with the breast in the craniocaudal, mediolateral oblique, or true lateral positions. The compression force is similar to that used in conventional mammography. The time required to obtain the images must be short to avoid patient motion. Acquisition time is dependent upon the manufacturer's system, approximately 4.3–15 seconds. Approximately 11–49 projections are obtained from different angles over a 15–60-degree angular range. Each projection/exposure is a fraction of the total dose of conventional mammography (approximately 5–10% of a single-view mammogram). Since each exposure is

low in dose, an image receptor with high quantum efficiency and low noise is required.

Breast compression is necessary during mammography to reduce overlap of structures and reduce the radiation dose and scatter, thus improving the image quality. In addition, compression stabilizes the breast and decreases artifacts secondary to patient motion. However, some patients complain of pain or discomfort due to breast compression during mammography. Applying less compression may result in less patient discomfort. Some studies indicate that it may be possible to perform tomosynthesis with less compression, while maintaining image quality.

Saunders and colleagues investigated the effect of reduced conspicuity of masses and calcifications in a voxelized anthropomorphic breast phantom with reduced compression in tomosynthesis [18]. The Monte Carlo program was used to simulate tomosynthesis projections, which were reconstructed and analyzed for conspicuity of masses and calcifications at two compression levels (standard and 12.5% reduced compression). The glandular radiation dose was kept constant. The conspicuity of masses and calcifications was constant with decreased compression, suggesting that reduced compression in tomosynthesis would have minimal effects on diagnostic performance. Förnvik and colleagues investigated the use of reduced compression in an observer study of symptomatic women undergoing tomosynthesis with standard full compression and half compression force [19]. Three readers with tomosynthesis experience scored one of the paired structure volumes as superior. No difference in image quality was found between full and half compression. The patients felt that half-compression tomosynthesis was more comfortable (83%) or of equal comfort (17%) to tomosynthesis with standard compression.

Reconstruction

With tomosynthesis, the digital data are acquired in multiple two-dimensional projections and then reconstructed into three-dimensional-like information for display. Since imaging is not performed in a complete 180-degree arc, a true volume is not obtained. Thus, images cannot be reconstructed in sagittal or coronal projections. Images are reconstructed at 1 mm slice thickness parallel to the plane of the detector. This results in a series of images, each displaying one plane in sharp focus. Objects at different depths are separated horizontally in the projections. There is increased visibility of objects by "blurring" out objects from different heights (Figure 11.4). Thus, tomosynthesis provides the opportunity to view mammographic slices throughout the breast, analogous to CT. Several reconstruction algorithms exist, including shift and add, tuned aperture CT, matrix inversion, filtered back projection, maximum likelihood reconstruction, and simultaneous algebraic reconstruction techniques. The specific reconstruction algorithm used is manufacturer-dependent. Different algorithms have their own strengths and weaknesses. While source images are typically reconstructed to 1 mm slice thickness, this can be varied without the need to acquire additional images. Maximum-intensity projections can be used to reconstruct to 10 mm thick slices or slabs.

Dose

The dose of tomosynthesis will depend upon the specific manufacturer's system and method of image acquisition. Single-view tomosynthesis has a mean glandular dose comparable with a two-view mammogram [20]. The total dose of single-view tomosynthesis is approximately 1.5 times the dose of a single conventional MLO view. The total radiation dose delivered by tomosynthesis will depend on the image acquisition strategy, i.e., single-view tomosynthesis, two-view tomosynthesis, or a combination of tomosynthesis and conventional mammography (single-view tomosynthesis in combination with craniocaudal mammography, or two-view mammography versus two-view tomosynthesis in combination with conventional mammography in one or two views). All systems result in doses less than the US Food and Drug Administration (FDA) limit (300 mrad/exposure). The slight increased dose of tomosynthesis compared with standard mammography is thought to be acceptable if it leads to a decreased recall rate or an increased cancer detection rate.

For a better perspective on dose due to breast imaging, one should consider the dose from background radiation. The average effective dose from natural background radiation in the United States, excluding man-made and medical sources, is about 3 mSv per year [21,22]. The average effective dose from two-view mammography is 0.56 mSv for film-screen and 0.44 mSv for digital mammography, equivalent to about two months of natural background radiation.

Image interpretation

Digital tomosynthesis is interpreted in soft-copy format on a high-resolution monitor. Reconstructed images are viewed with 1 mm slice separation. This slice separation can be reduced without requiring additional imaging. It is similar to cross-sectional imaging with the spatial resolution of digital mammography. The detail in the slices is superior to a

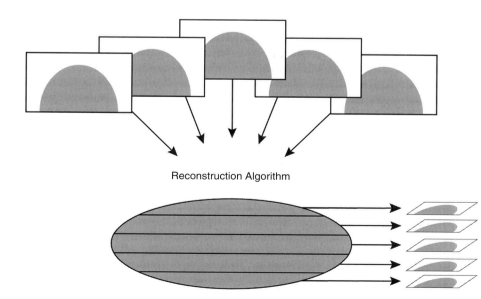

Reconstruction Algorithm

Figure 11.4 Reconstruction. Multiple low-dose projection images are obtained through the breast at differing angles. Images are reconstructed in a plane parallel to the detector, resulting in a series of thin-slice images. Each image displays one plane in sharp focus. Objects at different depths in the breast are separated horizontally in the projections.

conventional two-dimensional mammogram, as the "noise" due to overlapping structures and breast tissue has been removed. The three-dimensional reconstruction allows the depth (z-axis) of a lesion in the breast to be calculated.

The image series can be reviewed slice by slice (with manual or automated image advancement tools) or in a continuous fashion, such as a ciné loop. The radiologist can scroll back and forth through the breast in a matter of seconds. The slice thickness can be adjusted to view thin slices or thicker slices (slabs). Reconstruction at 0.5 mm thickness provides a thinner slice, which may be advantageous for the evaluation of some lesions, such as the morphology of calcifications or masses. Thinner-slice reconstruction will produce more images for review by the radiologist. Images may also be constructed at 10 mm thickness using maximum-intensity projections to produce slabs for viewing. Slabs may be helpful to view the distribution of calcifications in a volume of tissue. The raw projection image datasets initially obtained for reconstruction are available for review, but not typically interpreted.

The advantages of the decoupling of the processes of image acquisition, processing, and display, as with digital mammography, are also true with tomosynthesis. Decoupling enables post-acquisition processing of the images, which can help to optimize image quality. The degree of image contrast can be manipulated as needed. Soft-copy display and interpretation allow the use of processing tools to change the contrast and the brightness of the images. Parts of the breast or the entire breast may be enlarged for optimal analysis. The gray scale can be inverted. A moving magnified square can be used, which is analogous to using a magnifying glass when interpreting film-screen images. Annotation and measurement tools are also available.

Time for interpretation in tomosynthesis depends on multiple variables. The number of images for the radiologist to review depends on the breast thickness, reconstruction thickness (i.e., 0.5–1 mm thickness), and the number of raw images acquired. For example, a 6 cm thick breast with 10 image projections reconstructed at 1 mm slice thickness will result in 60 images to review in one projection (e.g., craniocaudal, mediolateral oblique, or true lateral). Thinner reconstruction at 0.5 mm thickness will provide twice the number of images, while thicker (slab) reconstruction will give fewer images for review. The image acquisition strategy also affects the number of images for review. If tomosynthesis is performed in two projections (e.g., craniocaudal and mediolateral oblique) or interpreted in conjunction with one-view or two-view mammography, there will be more images for interpretation. More images will likely take more time to interpret. An initial learning curve may exist for those new to interpreting tomosynthesis. Finally, reading with comparison images may also affect interpretation time. To date, none of the published studies has evaluated reading with comparison images.

Interpretation time in tomosynthesis has been evaluated in several performance studies. Gur and colleagues conducted a reader study to compare the diagnostic performance of FFDM and tomosynthesis [23]. Eight readers independently reviewed full-field digital mammograms alone, the 11 low-dose tomosynthesis projections (acquired for reconstruction), the reconstructed tomosynthesis, and FFDM in combination with tomosynthesis. The readers were asked to detect and rate masses and clusters of calcifications independently in each imaging mode. The readers marked the detected abnormalities and indicated the type of abnormality (mass versus calcifications). The likelihood of presence of an abnormality and the likelihood of malignancy were rated on a "semicontinuous" scale. If no abnormality was detected, the reader clicked a "done" button. The reader then provided a screening Breast Imaging Reporting and Data System (BI-RADS) assessment (0, 1, or 2). The total time each mode was displayed was automatically recorded to serve as an estimate of time of viewing, interpretation, and rating. The mean times in minutes were 1.22 ± 1.15 for digital mammography, 1.38 ± 0.99 for source images, 2.05 ± 1.46 for tomosynthesis, and 2.39 ± 1.65 for combined digital mammography and tomosynthesis. The mean time was longest for the combined mode of FFDM in combination with tomosynthesis, which is expected. The shortest time was for viewing FFDM alone. However, the interpretation times in this study reflect an experimental setting, asking the reader to identify, mark, and independently report each abnormality. The experimental process is likely more complex and likely more time-consuming than clinical interpretation and assessment. The authors also indicated that the review and reporting times would likely not be a large limitation in the incorporation of tomosynthesis into clinical practice, as some false positives will be eliminated with tomosynthesis. False-positive examinations result in increased time, cost, and potential inconvenience for the patient. If some of these false-positive studies are obviated, time will be saved, possibly equivalent to the additional time spent viewing tomosynthesis.

In another paper, Zuley and colleagues reported a retrospective reader study comparing the diagnostic performances of digital mammography and tomosynthesis [24]. Three radiologists independently reviewed digital mammography alone and then reviewed the reconstructed tomosynthesis in combination with digital mammography. The readers were asked to identify, mark, and rate each abnormality. All examinations were reviewed and rated twice with each mode following a specified delay of 60 days following the first reading. Results demonstrated that the use of tomosynthesis did require a longer time for interpretation than digital mammography alone. On average, the time required to interpret and rate examinations did not decrease regardless of changes in recall performance. The interpretation time also did not decrease during the repeat readings; however, there was a shift in the total interpretation time (digital mammography alone and combination of digital mammography and tomosynthesis) to rely more on combined display, while the time spent on interpretation of digital mammography alone decreased.

Equipment

Tomosynthesis is performed with a two-dimensional (2D) system for digital mammography with capability of moving the x-ray tube about the stationary breast. The detector remains stationary for the "step-and-shoot" method of acquisition and moves below the stationary breast for the "continuous" method of image acquisition. Imaging can be performed in the craniocaudal, mediolateral oblique, and true lateral projections. A specific workstation is needed for image reconstruction and viewing. The datasets are very large and require much memory for storage. A picture archiving and communication system (PACS) is necessary for data storage.

FDA approval

Tomosynthesis is a relatively new technology. In the USA, to date a single manufacturer has received approval from the FDA to market a 2D FFDM and tomosynthesis system. Two other manufacturers have systems under development and investigation. On February 11, 2011, Hologic, Inc. received FDA approval to market its Selenia Dimensions 2D Full Field digital mammography and tomosynthesis system. The 2D modality was approved two years earlier [25]. Facilities with this system have been using the 2D system with the tomosynthesis mode locked. Facilities with accredited units must apply for and obtain FDA approval to extend the certificate to include the tomosynthesis modality. These facilities must meet Mammography Quality Standards Act (MQSA) requirements. Personnel (interpreting physicians, technologists performing examinations, and medical physicists performing equipment evaluation and/or surveys) must obtain at least 8 hours of tomosynthesis training, the unit must undergo mammography equipment evaluation prior to use, and the facility must follow the manufacturer's recommended quality control procedures. FDA approval is for tomosynthesis to be used/performed in conjunction with FFDM, not *instead of* FFDM. No information with regard to reimbursement is available at the time of writing this chapter.

Digital breast tomosynthesis: potential advantages

Tomosynthesis has several potential clinical benefits or advantages, including improved mass detection (sensitivity), better mass characterization, decreased recall rates, and improved lesion localization. These advantages may be realized in the screening or diagnostic settings. However, there are no published clinical randomized controlled trials to date.

Improved detection of lesions with tomosynthesis may be due to several factors. Tomosynthesis allows viewing of slices throughout the breast and eliminates some of the noise due to overlapping structures. Thus, some lesions obscured by overlapping breast tissue may be better seen with tomosynthesis than conventional mammography (Figure 11.5). This may be particularly true in dense breasts. Reduction of overlap can lead to increased lesion conspicuity and thus increased detection rates. Improved lesion detection will lead to improved sensitivity and an increased cancer detection rate. Tomosynthesis is advantageous not only in dense breasts. Smaller lesions, which may not have been identified on conventional mammography, may be detected in patients with non-dense breasts. This results in increased sensitivity and potentially improved clinical outcomes.

The reduction in obscuration of lesions by overlapping structures provided by tomosynthesis can improve the characterization of masses, asymmetries, or architectural distortions (Figure 11.6). Lesion margins are better seen, which allows for better characterization. Thus, it may be easier to characterize lesions as benign or malignant from their morphologic appearance (Figure 11.7). This could mean improved specificity. In addition, characterization of more lesions as benign on imaging could lead to a decrease in biopsy rates. It is unlikely that tomosynthesis will provide improved characterization of calcifications.

The need for additional imaging following screening evaluation may be decreased with tomosynthesis. Some false-positive examinations, such as those due to "pseudo-lesions" caused by superimposed structures, will be eliminated with tomosynthesis. In addition, the improved characterization of the morphology of masses with tomosynthesis may decrease the need for additional diagnostic mammographic images. These developments may result in a decrease in the recall rate from screening.

Another potential advantage of tomosynthesis is improved localization of lesions in the breast. Similar to conventional mammography, a lesion can be identified in the x–y plane. However, tomosynthesis provides three-dimensional reconstructed information and z-axis or depth information. When viewing reconstructed images, the slice location in which the lesion is viewed provides information with regard to the depth of the lesion in the breast. The slice number, slice thickness, and total number of slices define the depth of the lesion in the breast.

At this point, it remains unclear what the accepted image acquisition strategy will be for the clinical utility of tomosynthesis. Currently, the only FDA-approved manufacturer advocates using tomosynthesis in conjunction with two-view digital mammography. However, there are currently no published randomized clinical trials of tomosynthesis. Therefore, a true standard of care has yet to be established. Since the MLO mammographic projection includes virtually all of the breast tissue, some would suggest that a single MLO tomosynthesis image set as opposed to two-projection tomosynthesis image sets may provide adequate information, alone or in combination with conventional mammography. Rafferty and colleagues evaluated how often mammographically detected cancers were not imaged in the MLO projection during two-view (CC and MLO) conventional mammography [26]. In a review of over 380 malignant cases, only three (0.8%) cancers were not seen on the MLO view. All three cancers were not imaged because of suboptimal positioning and located in the posterior inferior breast. Michell and colleagues compared two-view digital mammography with single (mediolateral)-view tomosynthesis in patients with abnormal screening mammograms. Receiver operating characteristic (ROC) analysis for two-view digital mammography was 0.915, and 0.960 for single-view tomosynthesis (difference 0.045; $p = 0.009$). In this series, single-view (MLO) tomosynthesis had superior sensitivity compared with two-view digital mammography [27]. If tomosynthesis is performed in only the mediolateral projection with

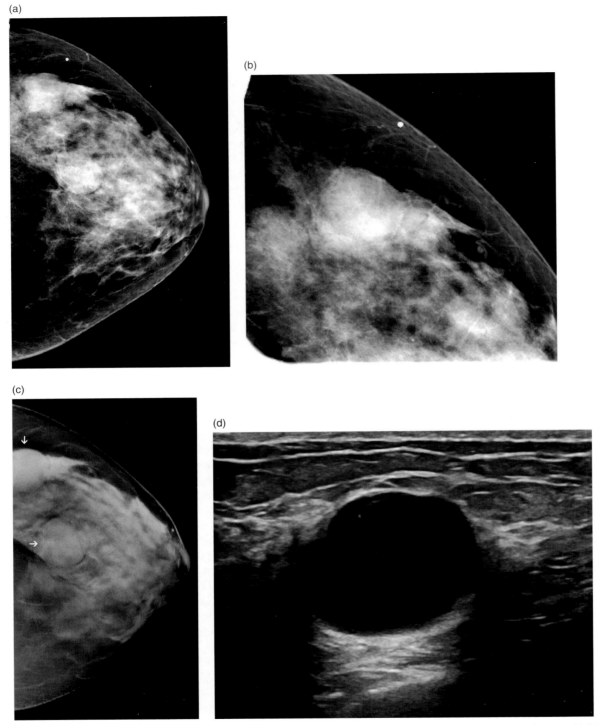

Figure 11.5 The reduction of overlapping breast tissue on digital breast tomosynthesis leads to increased conspicuity of lesions. (a) CC view from a diagnostic mammogram in a 49-year-old woman with a palpable abnormality demonstrates asymmetry in the lateral breast; a mass is incidentally noted in the central breast. (b) Spot compression CC view did not improve characterization of the mass margins. (c) Tomosynthesis slice demonstrates two masses with circumscribed margins (arrows). (d) Ultrasound demonstrates that one of the masses is a simple cyst.

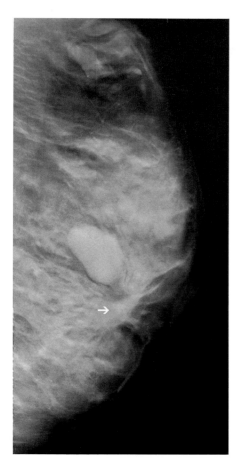

Figure 11.6 Reduction of overlapping structures improves visibility of mass margins, asymmetries, and architectural distortions. Tomosynthesis demonstrates a circumscribed oval mass, which corresponds to simple cyst on ultrasound. The architectural distortion in the retroareolar region (arrow) is due to a prior surgical biopsy for atypical ductal hyperplasia.

optimal positioning, this approach may provide adequate information and require less time for review, with a potential increase in patient compliance as less imaging and less compression (because of fewer views) may be required.

Digital breast tomosynthesis: potential disadvantages

No breast imaging technology is perfect. Tomosynthesis may have some potential disadvantages. Disadvantages include increased interpretation time, the need for additional training, and increased cost. There is non-uniformity among manufacturers. In addition, not all breasts may fit the detector. There is currently no approved method for biopsy or wire localization of lesions requiring surgical removal.

Tomosynthesis provides a greater number of images for review and interpretation by the reader. This could result in a longer time for interpretation. Zuley and colleagues found that the time to review and rate examinations increased by an average of 33% between the initial reading of digital mammography alone and the second reading of combined digital mammography and tomosynthesis [24]. Gur *et al.* found the mean time of interpretation and rating of abnormalities was longest for FFDM in combination with tomosynthesis; the shortest time was for viewing FFDM alone [23]. However, both of these studies measured interpretation times in an experimental setting, requiring the readers to identify, mark, and independently report each abnormality. In addition, the studies were performed on an enriched patient population with more abnormalities seen on imaging than would be expected in a typical screening population. Finally, clinical decisions were not made on the basis of these examinations. All of these factors may affect the interpretations and the interpretation times. If tomosynthesis does require longer interpretation times, the increased times for tomosynthesis interpretation may be offset by increased sensitivity and decreased recall rates.

Additional training and education for the interpreting radiologists, technologists, and medical physicists is only a relative disadvantage. If personnel are already trained for digital mammography, the requirement is only an additional eight hours of training. Although it has not yet been stated, one would assume there will be a requirement to complete continuing medical education category 1 credits specifically for tomosynthesis. These requirements should have minimal to no impact on the clinical implementation of tomosynthesis.

Increased cost is another potential drawback for tomosynthesis. There will be costs associated with the purchase of equipment for those facilities that do not currently own a system with tomosynthesis capability. It is likely that manufacturers will produce systems which perform digital mammography with a tomosynthesis mode. Tomosynthesis is viewed on a high-resolution workstation similar to that used for interpretation of digital mammography. Typically two monitors are used. The current FDA-approved system uses the same workstation for the interpretation of digital mammography with a software upgrade for tomosynthesis. No additional hardware is required for the workstation. It is likely that other manufacturers will utilize a similar arrangement. The datasets for tomosynthesis are very large and will require additional storage space in PACS. This may add to the cost. Tomosynthesis is interpreted in soft-copy mode with no printed hard-copy images, which may result in decreased cost with no requirement for film or a printer. However, it is unlikely these savings will offset the cost of equipment and storage. Finally, there may be costs incurred from the need to redesign the workspace to accommodate digital units performing tomosynthesis examinations and/or to provide ample space for workstations in the reading room. These modifications will be dependent upon the current setup of individual facilities, including the space allocation and the associated workflow.

Unfortunately, there is a lack of uniformity among different manufacturers. Different methods of image acquisition and reconstruction are utilized. A manufacturer may use "step-and-shoot" or continuous methods of image acquisition. Other parameters that may vary include the angular degree of movement of the x-ray tube, the number of projection images acquired, the exposure settings, the x-ray source/filter source, the effective size of the pixels, patient positioning, and the total dose of the examination. While each technique has its own advantages and disadvantages, the lack of uniformity makes direct comparison in clinical trials difficult.

(a)

(b)

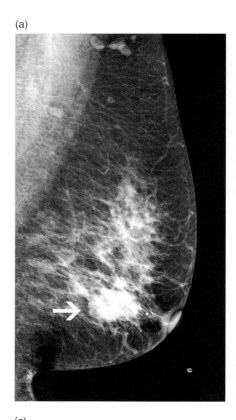

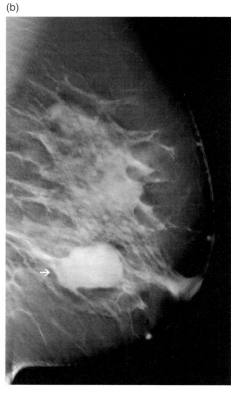

Figure 11.7 Tomosynthesis can improve margin visibility, resulting in improved characterization of masses as benign or malignant. (a) MLO view demonstrates a mass (arrow) corresponding to a palpable abnormality in a 46-year-old woman. (b) Tomosynthesis 1 mm thick slice shows improved visibility of the margins (arrow) of this invasive ductal carcinoma. (c) Ultrasound shows that the invasive ductal carcinoma is a microlobulated hypoechoic mass.

(c)

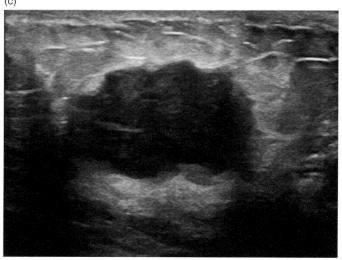

Another relative disadvantage is that all breasts may not fit the detector. One size does not fit all in tomosynthesis units. Some breasts may be too large for the detector size. Other breasts may be too thick to obtain optimal imaging. These are issues that will need to be addressed as more clinical experience is gained with tomosynthesis.

At the time of writing this chapter, there is no reimbursement for tomosynthesis. It is likely that reimbursement issues will be addressed in the near future, as tomosynthesis is incorporated into clinical practice.

Review of the current literature

Review of the current literature shows the early experience with tomosynthesis in an experimental setting. Most studies utilized patient populations enriched with cancer cases. Cases were often interpreted without clinical history. No published studies have been performed with comparison mammograms. No decisions with regard to direct patient care were made in these studies. Published studies have evaluated reader preference of tomosynthesis versus conventional mammography, characterization of masses and asymmetries, time of interpretation, recall rates, sensitivity, specificity, and detection and characterization of calcifications. To date, there are no published large randomized clinical trials.

Reader preference

Several studies have assessed reader preference for tomosynthesis images versus conventional mammography. Poplack *et al.* assessed the quality of tomosynthesis compared with diagnostic film-screen mammography [20]. Ninety-nine cases recalled from digital screening mammography were evaluated with diagnostic film-screen mammography in 98 women. The women also underwent tomosynthesis of the affected breast in the same projections obtained with diagnostic mammography. Following clinical interpretation of the diagnostic mammograms, one of two readers evaluated the tomosynthesis and diagnostic film-screen mammography images in direct comparison. The readers subjectively rated the quality of the tomosynthesis images compared with conventional mammography, based on lesion conspicuity and feature analysis specific to the type of finding (mass, asymmetry, focal asymmetry, architectural distortion, or calcifications). Image quality for tomosynthesis was rated better than, equivalent to, or worse than conventional mammography. In 52% (51/99) of the cases, the image quality of tomosynthesis was rated equivalent to that of mammography. Tomosynthesis image quality was rated superior to mammography in 37% (37/99) of cases. For masses, tomosynthesis was rated equivalent in 26% (5/19) of cases and superior in 68% (13/19) of cases. The benefit of tomosynthesis was attributed to improved lesion conspicuity, better margin-feature analysis, detection of additional findings (such as multiple circumscribed masses, suggesting benignity), and the increased ability to detect fat in a mass. However, the image quality of tomosynthesis was rated inferior in 57% (8/14) of cases with calcifications as the finding. The comparison diagnostic film-screen mammography did include focal magnification views. Based on this subjective analysis, tomosynthesis demonstrated superior image quality compared with diagnostic film-screen mammography for all types of findings, but was less effective for the evaluation of calcifications. It should be noted that this study was performed with a research prototype tomosynthesis unit (Genesis, Hologic) with image acquisition requiring 19 seconds. Subsequent prototype units have lower acquisition times, which may decrease potential motion-related blur affecting the detection and characterization of calcifications. This study utilized a 1 mm equivalent slice thickness without slabs, which may have affected the ability to evaluate the distribution of clustered calcifications in a volume of breast tissue.

In an observer performance study, Good and colleagues assessed ergonomic and performance-related issues of tomosynthesis interpretation [28]. Nine readers interpreted 30 cases (from an enriched study population containing only five negative examinations) in three different modes (FFDM alone, 11 low-dose tomosynthesis projection images, and reconstructed tomosynthesis). Readers were asked to identify and mark the finding on the examination and indicate the type of abnormality (masses versus calcifications). The likelihood of the presence (or the absence) of an abnormality and the likelihood of malignancy were rated on a "semicontinuous" scale. If no abnormality was detected the reader clicked a "done" button. The reader then provided a screening BI-RADS assessment (0, 1 or 2). For the low-dose tomosynthesis projection images and the reconstructed tomosynthesis mode, the reader was asked to rate the image quality in comparison to FFDM on a five-category Likert scale (significantly better, somewhat better, comparable, somewhat worse, and significantly worse). Subjective analysis found that none of the readers rated the reconstructed tomosynthesis significantly worse than FFDM. Tomosynthesis was rated comparable in 31.1%, somewhat better in 44.1%, and significantly better in 23% of the cases. In 1.9% of the cases, reconstructed tomosynthesis rated as somewhat worse than digital mammography.

Andersson *et al.* compared cancer visibility in single-view tomosynthesis with one- or two-view digital mammography in 36 patients with 40 cancers known to be subtle or occult on conventional mammography [29]. Tomosynthesis was performed in the same projection as the conventional mammogram in which the finding was least visible or the MLO view if the lesion was mammographically occult. Cancer visibility was ranked higher for tomosynthesis in 55% (22/40) of the cases and equal to digital mammography in 32.5% (13/40) of cases. In one case (2.5%), tomosynthesis was considered inferior to conventional mammography. In this case, the cancer was in a juxtathoracic location and not included in the field of view on tomosynthesis. Four of the 40 cancers (10%) were occult on conventional mammography and tomosynthesis. These cancers were visible with sonography only. The difference in cancer visibility when tomosynthesis was compared to digital mammography was statistically significant ($p < 0.01$).

Hakim and colleagues compared additional mammographic views with tomosynthesis in the characterization of known masses, architectural distortions, or asymmetries in 25 cases [30]. Four readers subjectively assessed preference for combination FFDM and tomosynthesis or FFDM with additional views to evaluate the index lesion. A Likert scale was used to assess image quality. Combination digital mammography and tomosynthesis was ranked better for diagnosis in 50% of the cases, at least equivalent in 31%, and worse in 19%. In 3 of 13 cases in which digital mammography and tomosynthesis was rated worse than digital mammography with additional views, the rating was attributed to the posterior location of the lesion, which was not included in the tomosynthesis field of view.

Diagnostic performance

Multiple studies have evaluated diagnostic performance of tomosynthesis. It should be noted that none of these studies was performed with comparison examinations or with both breasts viewed as one case. The lack of comparison examinations, clinical information, and the ability to view both breasts simultaneously may impact recall rates and does not reflect most breast imaging scenarios in which clinical decisions are made. Since most studies contained enriched patient populations, recall rates higher than those seen in clinical practice may not be unusual.

Poplack and colleagues also evaluated the diagnostic potential of tomosynthesis by estimating its recall rate when used in conjunction with digital screening mammography [20]. One of two readers assessed whether the tomosynthesis findings would have prompted recall. They found that tomosynthesis used as an adjunct to screening mammography led to a decrease in the recall rate by 52% (52/99). It should be noted that due to a difference in the recall threshold between the clinical radiologist and a study reader, seven cases would not have been recalled based on the screening mammograms. Tomosynthesis resulted in eight additional recalls at a site different than the index lesion. (These findings were evaluated with additional imaging if the finding was identified retrospectively on conventional mammography and deemed necessary for evaluation.) With adjustment for fewer recalls due to reader threshold differences and additional tomosynthesis findings, the final recall rate reduction was 40% (37/92). In this study, screening-detected asymmetries, focal asymmetries, and architectural distortions were less likely than masses or calcifications to be recalled with the addition of tomosynthesis.

Teertstra and colleagues compared diagnostic digital mammography with tomosynthesis in 513 women with abnormal screening mammograms, clinical symptoms, or referrals for a second opinion [31]. One of seven breast imagers interpreted the clinical examination. Further evaluation was performed for BI-RADS category 0, 3, 4, or 5 cases. All tomosynthesis was interpreted by one reader blinded to the clinical history, mammography, and pathology reports. In contrast to previously reported studies, both breasts were viewed, one after the other. Clinical decision making did not utilize information from tomosynthesis. Histologic proof was available for 344 cases, including 112 newly detected cancers. Eight of these cancers (7%) were not identified with tomosynthesis. Three of the eight cancers not visualized with tomosynthesis were invasive lobular carcinomas. However, conventional mammography also had eight false-negative examinations, which were detected with ultrasound ($n = 4$ palpable cancers), MRI ($n = 2$ contralateral breast cancers), tomosynthesis ($n = 1$), and following prophylactic bilateral mastectomy ($n = 1$). Five of the eight false-negative mammograms were classified as BI-RADS 4 on tomosynthesis. The sensitivity of both mammography and tomosynthesis was 92.9% using a positive threshold of BI-RADS 0, 3, 4, or 5. The specificity was 86.1% for mammography and 84.4% for tomosynthesis. However, if a positive threshold of BI-RADS 0, 4, or 5 was used, the sensitivity of mammography decreased to 73% and the sensitivity of tomosynthesis decreased to 80%; the specificities were 97% and 96% for mammography and tomosynthesis, respectively. The change in numbers can be attributed to cancers assigned BI-RADS category 3 (21% with mammography and 12% with tomosynthesis). The authors also suggested that a number of benign lesions assigned BI-RADS 4 with tomosynthesis might

have been due to the lack of comparison examinations, which were available for interpretation of conventional mammography. Several cases demonstrated calcifications that were mammographically stable for several years and thus deemed benign.

When comparing single-view digital mammography to single-view tomosynthesis in patients with subtle or occult cancer on conventional mammography, Andersson et al. found a significant upgrade in the BI-RADS classification of 21 patients ($p < 0.01$) [29]. The BI-RADS classification was significantly upgraded for another 12 patients from two-view digital mammography compared with single-view tomosynthesis ($p < 0.01$).

In their observer performance study, Good and colleagues assessed the detection of abnormalities for each mode (FFDM alone, 11 low-dose tomosynthesis projection images, and reconstructed tomosynthesis) and the overall proportion of nonmalignant examinations recalled for each mode [28]. The proportions of malignant examinations recalled (i.e., detection rate) varied for different readers for the different modes. However, the results were not statistically significant as to the effect of the mode on the proportion of examinations recalled.

Gennaro et al. [32] compared the performance of tomosynthesis with FFDM in the diagnostic setting. Patients with a screening-detected mammographic abnormality and/or sonographic abnormality underwent single-view (MLO) tomosynthesis of each breast. Six readers reviewed the cases (CC and MLO digital mammography and single MLO tomosynthesis), rated lesion conspicuity, and provided a BI-RADS assessment for slabs and slices. The BI-RADS score associated with the highest conspicuity value was used for ROC analysis. Lesion conspicuity with tomosynthesis was at least as good as lesion conspicuity with digital mammography in 79.4% of cases. The results were similar for the conspicuity of benign and malignant lesions separately. The overall clinical performance of tomosynthesis and digital mammography for malignant cases versus all other cases was not statistically significant.

Calcifications

There is less published information on the detection and characterization of calcifications with tomosynthesis. The results vary in different studies. Many of the results suggest that digital mammography is more sensitive than tomosynthesis for the detection of calcifications. There are several reasons for this. Breast imagers have long-standing experience with the evaluation of digital mammography for calcifications, whereas search patterns on tomosynthesis have not yet been established. In addition, calcification conspicuity is dependent upon slice thickness. Increasing slice thickness (slabs) may increase the ability to detect a cluster of calcifications. Some of the earlier studies did not include evaluation with slabs. However, slabs compromise the spatial resolution of the individual calcifications. Therefore, viewing at multiple slice thicknesses is necessary for optimal interpretation of tomosynthesis and assessment of calcifications. Since tomosynthesis contains more images and should be viewed at multiple slice thicknesses, reader fatigue may be a factor in interpretation. A few technical factors may also contribute to the difference in sensitivity. Longer acquisition time of tomosynthesis may result in motion artifact, which can render the calcifications less distinct on the images. This may have been more of an issue in earlier research. New-generation tomosynthesis machines typically have shorter acquisition times. Tomosynthesis exposure parameters, processing algorithms, reconstruction algorithms, dynamic range display, and workstation tools can be modified to address some of the issues related to decreased sensitivity.

Poplack *et al.* found that calcifications typically had superior image quality on diagnostic film-screen mammography compared to tomosynthesis [20]. Seventy-three percent (8/11) of cases in which tomosynthesis was rated inferior to film-screen mammography had calcifications as the finding. The difference in performance for evaluation of calcifications was attributed to improved conspicuity of calcifications and better assessment of particle number and morphology on diagnostic mammography, which included focal magnification views. The tomosynthesis system used for this research study had limitations of lengthy exposure time and lack of slab (thick-slice) reconstruction. These limitations have been addressed with the development of subsequent systems.

Helvie and colleagues evaluated the visibility and characterization of calcifications with tomosynthesis [33]. Readers independently reviewed 1 mm thin slices and slabs. The visibility of calcifications and the probability of malignancy were rated. Readers also provided descriptors of the calcifications and a final BI-RADS assessment. Calcifications were visible in 100% of cases on either the CC or the MLO view. One malignant case was occult in one view. This case was a 2 mm low-grade ductal carcinoma in situ (DCIS). Good *et al.* found that all clusters of malignant calcifications detected with conventional mammography were also seen on tomosynthesis [28].

Spangler and colleagues compared the ability of tomosynthesis and FFDM to detect and characterize calcifications [34]. In this multi-reader, multimodality observer performance study, each reader separately reviewed FFDM without comparisons or additional views and tomosynthesis in separate sessions. Tomosynthesis images could be reviewed at any slice thickness (including slabs). Readers indicated if calcification clusters were detected and provided a forced BI-RADS assessment (1–5). The calcification detection sensitivity was higher for digital mammography (84%) than for tomosynthesis (75%). The specificity was higher for digital mammography (71%) than for tomosynthesis (64%). However, the diagnostic performance as measured by the area under the ROC curve using BI-RADS was not statistically significantly different between digital mammography and tomosynthesis.

Masses and asymmetries

The potential for improved characterization of masses and asymmetries, described as an advantage of tomosynthesis, has

been assessed in several studies. Poplack and colleagues compared the image quality of tomosynthesis with conventional mammography [20]. Readers subjectively rated the equivalence of image quality of tomosynthesis compared with diagnostic mammography based on lesion conspicuity and feature analysis of the findings. The readers indicated that the primary reasons for improved image quality of tomosynthesis were lesion conspicuity, more accurate margin-feature analysis, and the ability of tomosynthesis to detect additional findings. The readers also found that tomosynthesis demonstrated normal tissue and lack of significant findings in some false-positive screening mammograms.

In their comparison of single-view tomosynthesis with one- or two-view digital mammography in cases of known mammographically subtle or occult cancers, Andersson and colleagues found that cancer visibility on tomosynthesis was superior to digital mammography [29]. For 55% (22/40), cancer visibility was ranked higher for tomosynthesis than for one-view mammography. Of the remaining 18 cancers, 13 (32.5% of the original 40) were equally visible on tomosynthesis and one-view mammography. When compared with two-view mammography, cancer visibility was ranked higher with tomosynthesis for 27.5% (11/40) of the cases. These differences in cancer visibility were statistically significant ($p < 0.01$). When tomosynthesis was compared with one-view mammography, 21 cases were upgraded in BI-RADS category (11 cases upgraded from category 1, 2, or 3 to category 4 or 5, and 10 cases upgraded from category 3 to category 4 or 5). When tomosynthesis was compared to two-view mammography, 12 cases were upgraded (four from category 1 or 2 to category 4 or 5, and eight from category 3 to category 4 or 5).

Helvie and colleagues compared the characterization of biopsy-proven benign and malignant masses by tomosynthesis [35]. Readers rated the likelihood of a mass being present, mass visibility, and the probability of malignancy, and the readers provided BI-RADS descriptors for mass margins and shapes. The readers found that circumscribed margins were present in 70% of benign masses and only 4.9% of malignant masses. Spiculated or indistinct margins were seen in only 11% of benign masses and in 81% of the malignant masses. Eighty-four percent of benign masses were lobular or oval in shape, compared with 15% of malignant masses. Irregular shape was seen in 9% of benign masses and 81% of malignant masses. More benign masses had circumscribed margins and lobular or oval shape. In this study, if a threshold of cancer probability of 2% for BI-RADS category 3 was used, it was estimated that 39% of the masses recommended for biopsy might have been classified as BI-RADS category 1, 2, or 3 with tomosynthesis [36].

In their comparison of tomosynthesis with additional mammographic views in the characterization of known masses, architectural distortions, and asymmetries, Hakim *et al.* asked the readers to provide a BI-RADS assessment for each index lesion [30]. For the benign cases, 69% were rated BI-RADS category 1, 2, or 3. Ninety-two percent of the malignant cases were rated as BI-RADS 4 or 5. In 32% of cases, at least one reader indicated that tomosynthesis eliminated the need for diagnostic ultrasound because of the visibility of the mass margins on the optimal tomosynthesis slices; all of these cases were benign.

Clinical implementation: how do we do this?

Facilities wanting to incorporate tomosynthesis into clinical practice must first acquire the equipment. The Hologic Selenia Dimensions 2D Full-Field digital mammography and tomosynthesis system is the only system with FDA approval at the time of writing. Currently the accreditation bodies do not have the capability to review the tomosynthesis images and cannot accredit the tomosynthesis modality portion of the system. So facilities with an accredited Selenia Dimensions 2D unit will need to apply to the FDA to extend certification to include tomosynthesis. The certification extension program requires the 2D modality of the unit to be accredited by one of the current accreditation bodies and submission of additional tomosynthesis testing results with other documentation directly to the FDA for review and approval per specifications of the certificate extension application. This program will continue until the FDA has approved the accreditation bodies to accredit the tomosynthesis modality of the units. Facilities applying to obtain FDA approval to extend the certificate of approval must meet MQSA requirements, which include: eight hours of tomosynthesis training for breast imagers, technologists, and medical physicists; the unit must undergo mammography equipment evaluation prior to use; and the facility must follow the manufacturer's recommended quality control procedures. Sites that are not currently MQSA-certified in digital mammography will need to apply to the American College of Radiology or the state for FFDM certification. Physicians not currently trained in FFDM will need eight hours of digital mammography training. It will take approximately 14 days for the FDA to process and approve or deny the application request. At this time, only the FDA needs to approve the system at a specific site. To date, neither the state nor the American College of Radiology is involved in the approval process.

Tomosynthesis is interpreted in soft-copy mode on a high-resolution workstation. Facilities not currently interpreting digital mammography will need to acquire the appropriate workstation. Workspace may need to be reconfigured or redesigned to accommodate digital units to perform tomosynthesis in facilities not currently performing digital mammography. In addition, reading rooms may need to be reconfigured to accommodate workstations. Since tomosynthesis will be performed in addition to digital mammography, more than one monitor per workstation will likely be used. Interpretation of tomosynthesis in conjunction with comparison mammograms has not been evaluated in the current literature. If comparing with prior film-screen mammography examinations or printed digital mammography images, space must be allotted for alternators. The datasets for tomosynthesis are very large and require much memory. An adequate PACS is needed. In addition, ancillary personnel will need to be trained to assist in image storage and data retrieval.

Workflow issues are important. Tomosynthesis has received FDA approval to be performed in conjunction with digital mammography, not instead of mammography. The strategy for image acquisition needs to be established. Will one-view or two-view tomosynthesis be obtained? Clinical trials may assist with establishment of the standard of care. Although the time for image acquisition of tomosynthesis is short, the number of views obtained should be considered in the scheduling of patients. In addition, the number of views obtained will affect the time of interpretation. Finally, not all breasts will fit the detector size. When this occurs with mammography, multiple similar projections are taken to include all of the breast tissue. In addition, some breasts may be too thick for acquisition of optimal tomosynthesis images. It remains unclear how these issues will be addressed with tomosynthesis. At the current time, there are no approved methods for biopsy or wire localization of lesions requiring surgical excision using tomosynthesis. This limitation could hinder the evaluation of lesions seen only on tomosynthesis and not on FFDM. However, it is likely that such methods of biopsy and localization will be developed and approved as tomosynthesis is incorporated into clinical practice. These new procedural methods will require additional training for physicians and technologists.

Future applications: what does the future hold for digital breast tomosynthesis?

Tomosynthesis provides the opportunity for multimodality imaging. The imaging may be coregistered with other technologies to produce fused images. Tomosynthesis can be performed with ultrasound, optical imaging, or functional imaging. Prototype machines have been developed that allow tomosynthesis, digital mammography, and automated breast ultrasound to be performed during the same examination. Following mammography and tomosynthesis, breast ultrasound is performed mechanically while the breast remains in compression. The different modalities may be reviewed independently or as a three-dimensional registered examination. An advantage of registration is the ability to correlate lesions found in the different modalities. A simple cyst seen on the automated ultrasound can be correlated with a circumscribed mammographic or tomosynthesis mass. A clinical prototype tomosynthesis unit has been used in combination with optical imaging for noninvasive acquisition of coregistered functional optical and structural images of the breast. Normalized hemoglobin concentration (HbT) can be used to differentiate benign solid masses from malignant masses.

Significant differences in oxygen saturation (SO_2) help differentiate cystic from solid masses. Increased ability to differentiate benign from malignant lesions has the potential to result in a decreased number of unnecessary biopsies in the clinical setting [37]. Coregistration of the images allows the reader to correlate suspicious mammographic findings to the corresponding optical images. Other modalities for use in multimodality imaging include positron emission tomography (PET), magnetic resonance imaging (MRI), and technetium-99m sestamibi imaging.

Computer-aided detection (CADe) is another potential future application of tomosynthesis. Chan and colleagues have developed a computer-aided detection system for tomosynthesis for the purpose of mass detection [38]. In a preliminary study, the system achieved a sensitivity of 85% with 2.2 false positives per case. As tomosynthesis may detect mammographically occult lesions, biopsy and wire localization capability will be necessary in future applications. Another potential future application is telemedicine or teletomosynthesis/telemammography. This would require the rapid transmission of source images and reconstruction from one site to another in digital/electronic form. The information could be transmitted via a variety of methods, including high-speed internet, satellite, or wireless links. However, patient information must be vigilantly protected during transmission. The transmission of digital information allows the images to be acquired at one location/site and interpreted at another. Therefore, a breast imager with tomosynthesis expertise can either perform primary interpretation or consultation. Teletomosynthesis/telemammography could potentially allow more patients to have access to this new technology.

Contrast-enhanced tomosynthesis is another potential future application. As breast cancers grow, new and abnormal blood vessels develop, a process called angiogenesis. MRI has detected breast cancers by the identification of leaked gadolinium-based contrast material from these abnormal vessels. Tomosynthesis could be performed after administering intravenous iodinated contrast material with the hope to identify abnormalities based on angiogenesis, which may be obscured by overlapping breast tissue. Two methods have been used for contrast-enhanced digital mammography: temporal subtraction and dual-energy subtraction. Both are currently under investigation and not yet approved for widespread clinical use.

Summary

Digital breast tomosynthesis is a new technology that acquires a series of low-dose projection images about the stationary compressed breast over an angular arc, providing three-dimensional-like information. Data from these source images is reconstructed using a variety of methods to provide slices of the breast for viewing, analogous to computerized tomography (CT) scans. Tomosynthesis has been developed with the hope of improving lesion detection and characterization by eliminating the "noise" of overlapping breast tissue. The current literature is favorable with regard to reader preference, lesion detection, and the characterization of masses. The limited research relating to calcifications has produced mixed results, although some earlier studies did not include the use of slabs for evaluation of calcifications. Larger clinical trials are needed. To date, one manufacturer has obtained FDA approval to market a two-dimensional FFDM and tomosynthesis system and two other manufacturers have systems under development and investigation. Future applications include multimodality imaging with coregistration and computer-aided detection. Tomosynthesis has the potential to improve cancer detection, lower recall rates, and reduce the number of false-positive biopsies.

Acknowledgments

Thank you to Sarah Abate for assistance in manuscript preparation. Thank you to the University of Michigan Breast Imaging team and the patient volunteers for their participation and dedication to breast imaging research.

References

1. Hendrick RE, Smith RA, Rutledge JH, Smart CR. Benefit of screening mammography in women aged 40–49: a new meta-analysis of randomized controlled trials. *J Natl Cancer Inst Monogr* 1997; **22**: 87–92.

2. Nystrom L, Rutqvist L, Wall S, *et al.* Breast cancer screening with mammography: overview of Swedish randomized trials. *Lancet* 1993; **342**: 973–8.

3. Burrell HC, Sibbering DM, Wilson AR, *et al.* Screening interval breast cancers: mammographic features and prognosis factors. *Radiology* 1996; **199**: 811–17.

4. Hollingsworth AB, Taylor LD, Rhodes DC. Establishing a histologic basis for false-negative mammograms. *Am J Surg* 1993; **166**: 643–7.

5. Feig SA, Yaffe MJ. Current status of digital mammography. *Semin Ultrasound CT MR* 1996; **17**: 424–43.

6. Lewin JM, D'Orsi CJ, Hendrick RE. Digital mammography. *Radiol Clin North Am* 2004; **42**: 871–84

7. Pisano E, Yaffe M. Digital mammography. *Breast Dis* 1998; **10**: 127–36.

8. Berns EA, Hendrick RE, Cutter GR. Performance comparison of full-field digital mammography to screen: film mammography in clinical practice. *Med Phys* 2002; **29**: 830–4.

9. Hendrick RE. Radiation doses and cancer risks from breast imaging studies. *Radiology* 2010; **257**: 246–53.

10. Miller ER, McCurry EM, Hruska B. An infinite number of laminagrams from a finite number of radiographs. *Radiology* 1971; **98**: 249–55

11. Niklason LT, Christian BT, Nikalson LE, *et al*. Digital tomosynthesis in breast imaging. *Radiology* 1997; **205**: 399–406.

12. Kopans DB. *Breast Imaging*, 3rd edn. Philadelphia, PA: Lippincott Williams & Wilkins, 2007.

13. Sone S, Kasuga T, Sakai F, *et al*. Development of a high-resolution digital tomosynthesis system and its clinical application. *Radiographics* 1991; **11**: 807–22.

14. Chakraborty DP, Yester MV, Barnes GT, Lakshminarayanan AV. Self-masking subtraction tomosynthesis. *Radiology* 1984; **150**: 225–9.

15. Sone S, Kasuga T, Sakai F, *et al*. Chest imaging with dual-energy subtraction digital tomosynthesis. *Acta Radiol* 1993; **34**: 346–9.

16. Edholm PR, Quiding L. Reduction of linear blurring in tomography. *Radiology* 1969; **92**: 1115–18.

17. Edholm P, Quiding L. Elimination of blur in linear tomography. *Acta Radiol* 1970; **10**: 441–7.

18. Saunders RS, Samei E, Lo JY, Baker JA. Can compression be reduced for breast tomosynthesis? Monte Carlo study on mass and microcalcification conspicuity in tomosynthesis. *Radiology* 2009; **251**: 673–82.

19. Förnvik D, Andersson I, Svahn T, *et al.* The effect of reduced breast compression in breast tomosynthesis: human observer study using clinical cases. *Radiat Prot Dosimetry* 2010; **139**: 118–23.

20. Poplack SP, Tosteson TD, Kogel CA, Nagy HM. Digital breast tomosynthesis: initial experience in 98 women with abnormal digital screening mammography. *AJR Am J Roentgenol* 2007; **189**: 616–23.

21. Mettler FA, Bhargavan M, Faulkner K, *et al.* Radiologic and nuclear medicine studies in the United States and worldwide: frequency, radiation dose, and comparison with other radiation sources-1950–2007. *Radiology* 2009; **253**: 520–31.

22. National Council on Radiation Protection and Measurements. *Ionizing Radiation Exposure of the Population of the United States.* NCRP Report 160. Bethesda, MD: National Council on Radiation Protection and Measurements, 2009.

23. Gur D, Abrams GS, Chough DM, *et al.* Digital breast tomosynthesis: observer performance study. *AJR Am J Roentgenol* 2009; **193**: 586–91.

24. Zuley ML, Bandos AI, Abrams GS, *et al.* Time to diagnosis and performance levels during repeat interpretations of digital breast tomosynthesis: preliminary observations. *Acad Radiol* 2010; **17**: 450–5.

25. US Food and Drug Administration. Radiation-emitting products. Mammography Quality Standards Act and Program. Facility certification and inspection (MQSA). www.fda.gov/Radiation-EmittingProducts/MammographyQualityStandardsActandProgram/FacilityCertificationandInspection (accessed April 2012).

26. Rafferty E, Kopans DB, Wu T, *et al.* Breast tomosynthesis: will a single view do? Radiologic Society of North America 90th Scientific Assembly and Annual Meeting Chicago (IL), December 2004.

27. Michell MJ, Wasan RK, Iqbal A, *et al.* Two-view 2D digital mammography versus one-view digital breast tomosynthesis. *Breast Cancer Res* 2010; **12**: 3.

28. Good WF, Abrams GS, Catullo VJ, *et al.* Digital breast tomosynthesis: a pilot observer study. *AJR Am J Roentgenol* 2008; **190**: 865–9.

29. Andersson I, Ikeda DM, Zackrisson S, *et al.* Breast tomosynthesis and digital mammography: a comparison of breast cancer visibility and BIRADS classification in a population of cancers with subtle mammographic findings. *Eur Radiol* 2008; **18**: 2817–25.

30. Hakim CM, Chough DM, Ganott MA, *et al.* Digital breast tomosynthesis in the diagnostic environment: a subjective side-by-side review. *AJR Am J Roentgenol* 2010; **195**: W172–6.

31. Teertstra HJ, Loo CE, van den Bosch MA, *et al.* Breast tomosynthesis in clinical practice: initial results. *Eur Radiol* 2010; **20**: 16–24.

32. Gennaro G, Toledano A, di Maggio C, *et al.* Digital breast tomosynthesis versus digital mammography: a clinical performance study. *Eur Radiol* 2010; **20**: 1545–53.

33. Helvie MA, Chan H, Hadjiiski LM, *et al.* Digital breast tomosynthesis mammography: successful assessment of benign and malignant microcalcifications. Radiologic Society of North America 95th Scientific Assembly and Annual Meeting Program, 2009; p. 389.

34. Spangler ML, Zuley ML, Sumkin JH, *et al.* Detection and characterization of calcifications on digital breast tomosynthesis and 2D digital mammography: a comparison. *AJR Am J Roentgenol* 2011; **196**: 320–4.

35. Helvie MA, Hadjiiski L, Goodsitt M, *et al.* Characterization of benign and malignant masses by digital breast tomosynthesis mammography. Radiologic Society of North America 94th Scientific Assembly and Annual Meeting Chicago (IL), December 2008.

36. Helvie MA. Digital mammography imaging: breast tomosynthesis and advanced applications. *Radiol Clin North Am* 2010; **48**: 917–29.

37. Qianqian F, Selb J, Carp SA, *et al.* Combined optical and x-ray tomosynthesis breast imaging. *Radiology* 2011; **258**: 89–97.

38. Chan HP, Wei J, Sahiner B, *et al.* Computer-aided detection system for breast masses on digital tomosynthesis mammograms: preliminary experience. *Radiology* 2005; **237**: 1075–80.

Chapter 12

Breast computed tomography

Gary J. Whitman, Chao-Jen Lai, Xinming Liu, Malak Itani, Raunak Khisty, and Chris C. Shaw

Technical aspects

Background

The idea of breast computed tomography (breast CT) was conceived and explored not long after computed tomography (CT) was developed and commercialized. First attempts to image breasts with CT involved the use of a specially designed CT system (CT/M) [1–5] as well as a conventional body scanner [6,7]. The CT/M system suffered from poor image quality and long scanning times and did not prove to be practical. The use of a body scanner for breast imaging requires the entire chest to be exposed and included in image reconstruction. This causes two problems: first, the chest is unnecessarily exposed, increasing radiation dose to the patient; second, since the breasts are only a small part of the chest, only a small number of voxels can be used to represent the breasts, leading to poor resolution. These problems led to attempts to develop dedicated CT units in which one of the breasts was scanned with dedicated scanning hardware, sparing the rest of the chest from radiation and allowing all available voxels to be used to represent the breast in the reconstructed images, leading to much improved resolution. This new imaging technique involved a different imaging geometry, often referred to as pendant geometry, with the patient positioned prone with one breast protruding downward through an opening and scanned by a specially designed scanner underneath the table. Because of technological limitations, this concept was not pursued until the early 2000s.

In the 1990s, flat-panel detectors were developed and used to construct digital x-ray systems for general radiography as well as mammography applications. The availability of these detectors facilitated research and development of various cone-beam CT techniques in academic institutions. With these techniques, a cone-shaped beam is used to rotate around and scan the patient. Efforts were made to use the cone-beam CT technique to implement dedicated breast CT using pendant geometry, which was explored in the 1970s with fan-beam-based CT techniques. The use of cone-beam CT techniques for dedicated breast CT was first proposed by Boone *et al.* at the University of California, Davis and Ning *et al.* at the University of Rochester [8–13]. Boone *et al.*

constructed the first patient imager for clinical evaluation. Ning *et al.* initiated the first effort to commercialize the breast CT technology. Patient studies conducted to date have shown that breast CT images are superior to mammography in detecting and visualizing breast anatomy and soft tissue masses but are more limited in imaging small microcalcifications. A third group at Duke University has recently constructed a patient imager with a specially designed quasi-monoenergetic x-ray source to improve the image quality [14,15]. Two other groups, one at the University of Massachusetts and the other at the University of Texas MD Anderson Cancer Center (UTMDACC), have constructed bench-top experimental systems (Figure 12.1) to image mastectomy breast specimens in an effort to investigate the imaging properties of breast CT [16–19]. The researchers at UTMDACC have also proposed and investigated the use of a collimated x-ray beam to scan a preselected volume-of-interest to allow smaller microcalcifications or other details to be seen without increasing the breast dose [20–22]. To enhance the visibility of cancers, breast CT with contrast injection has been explored and investigated [23]. Research groups in Europe have also begun to develop and investigate improved breast CT techniques in an effort to bring breast CT (Figure 12.2) into practical use [24–27].

Two major issues may hamper the use of breast CT to replace mammography in the screening, diagnosis, and assessment of breast cancers. The first is breast CT's inability to image small microcalcifications. This is due to the limited spatial resolution of the current breast CT systems, owing not to the detector technology but to the limited alignment accuracy for CT scans, motion in relation to the heart beating during the long scanning period (10 seconds or longer), and the high photon flux required with high-resolution detectors imaging small objects. The second issue is related to the breast dose in breast CT scans. This is closely linked to the first issue because higher exposures, and hence higher doses, are required to image small microcalcifications.

General design

Like a regular CT system, a dedicated breast CT system consists of an x-ray tube and a detector assembly mounted on a

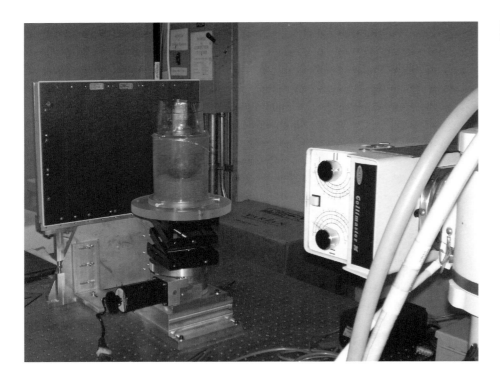

Figure 12.1 Bench-top CT system used for specimen imaging.

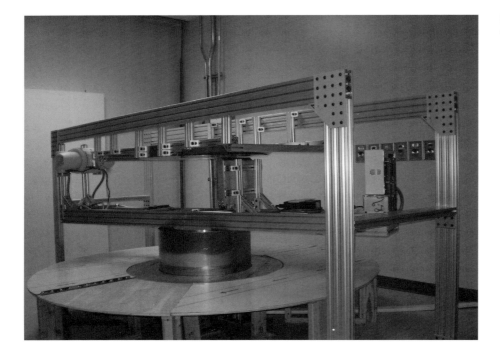

Figure 12.2 Cone-beam CT system under construction.

gantry which rotates around the breast during the scan. However, a dedicated breast CT system scans the breast only and does not image the remainder of the chest. This design has two advantages: first, the rest of the chest is spared from radiation exposure, thus reducing the patient dose; second, since the breast occupies a smaller volume, the field of view can be substantially reduced in acquiring the projection images

and the detector can be used to cover a much smaller region, which helps improve the pixel density and results in better resolution in the reconstructed images.

Breast CT units have been designed to scan the breast without exposing the rest of the body or the chest. In mammography, exposure of only the breast is achieved by collimating and orienting the x-ray field away from the chest so that one side of the x-ray field is pointing straight down along the chest wall while the breast is drawn outward, compressed, and held between the table/detector and a compression plate. The orientation can be altered by rotating the x-ray tube and the table/detector around the breast and then compressing the breast again to allow a second mammogram to be taken at a different angle. This configuration can be applied to the design of a dedicated breast CT scanner by having the gantry rotate around the breast continuously over 360 degrees. It is unnecessary and even disadvantageous to compress the breast for breast CT. Actually, the quality of the reconstructed images would be better optimized if the breast was molded into the shape of a long, skinny half-ellipsoid. The best way to achieve this shape, as it turns out, is to use pendant geometry. With pendant geometry, the patient lies prone on a table with one breast protruding through a circular opening in the middle of the table, naturally hanging downward. It may also be possible to use a bowl-shaped holder to lightly compress the breast into the shape of a half-ellipsoid. Either way, the discomfort from compression in mammography is eliminated. The x-ray tube and the detector are mounted on a gantry and rotate around the breast underneath the table. While other configurations may be possible, this is how all current dedicated breast CT systems are designed.

Gantry and table

The gantry and table configuration is very similar to that of a stereotactic biopsy system except that the gantry holding the x-ray tube and the detector need to be rotated around the breast at a reasonably fast speed over one full revolution, or 360 degrees. Because of the combined large weight of the detector and the x-ray tube, a robust heavy-duty gantry and motor-drive system must be used. One design issue is how to route the power, interface, and data cables from the x-ray tube to the generator and from the detector to the controller/acquisition computer while allowing the x-ray tube and the detector to rotate around the breast over 360 degrees. Commercial flexible cable holders are available to coil the cables during the scan and to uncoil afterwards [10]. A more elegant but more complex and expensive approach is to use a slip ring which allows the power, interface signals, and data to be connected between the rotating gantry and the stationary sources without using cables [28]. This eliminates the need to coil and uncoil cables and, furthermore, allows the gantry to be rotated continuously for multiple revolutions. However, since there is a limit on the voltage of the power that can be transmitted through a slip ring, a high-frequency switching generator must be used, with the low-voltage alternating current (AC) power first converted to direct current (DC) power and then connected to a high-frequency switching step-up transformer and high-voltage rectifiers mounted on the gantry through the slip ring.

The patient table needs to be designed for patient comfort and the ability to allow the entire breast and even part of the axillary tissue to protrude downward for the breast CT scan. The area around the opening may be specially shaped for these purposes. The position of the opening needs to accommodate either the left or the right breast. Instead of having two openings, the table may be designed with one opening, with the patient positioned prone in two opposite orientations. This design enables the use of only one opening to accommodate either breast. Due to the presence of the rotating gantry in the middle of the table, the patient needs to climb up from either end of the table.

X-ray source

While low-energy x-rays have been successfully used in mammography, it is impractical to use them for breast CT because they cannot penetrate an uncompressed breast and they would require an excessively high breast dose. Typically, 49–80 kVp x-rays generated with a tungsten target are used in breast CT [8,9,29,30]. They penetrate the breast well but produce lower contrast in the projection images. However, the low contrast of tissue structures and small calcifications are easily restored after image reconstruction. The x-ray source used in breast CT has two functional requirements. First, the focal spot needs be as close as possible to one end of the tube housing. This allows the x-ray cone-beam to be generated and used to scan at a short distance beneath the table. With some tubes used for breast CT, the focal spot is located at 4–5 cm below one end of the housing, allowing the cone-beam to be placed slightly lower than 4 cm below the table, maximizing the coverage of the breast on the chest-wall side. Secondly, the focal spot size must be small enough to allow a reasonably small pixel size to be used for image acquisition. The typical focal spot size used for breast CT is 0.3–0.4 mm. With these requirements, the power of the x-ray tube is generally on the lower side. Fortunately, the source-to-detector distance can be made short to increase the x-ray flux, and the breast, generally small compared to other parts of the body and containing no bony structures, is less attenuating. Like x-ray sources for other imaging techniques, the x-ray beam for breast CT needs to be collimated for radiation protection purposes. Furthermore, the x-ray beam should be collimated in such a way as to generate a cone-beam with its upper edge moving in a horizontal plane as close beneath the table as possible. A bow-tie filter, which varies in thickness from the edges toward the central axis of the breast, may be used to compensate for the variation of x-ray attenuation from the center of the breast to the periphery and to equalize the transmitted x-ray intensity at the detector input. This helps avoid signal saturation near the borders of the breast.

Detector

For breast CT, an image detector with efficient x-ray absorption, a smaller pixel size, a low noise level, and a fast framing rate are required. For this reason, amorphous silicon/cesium iodide (a-Si/CsI) and, more recently, complementary metal-oxide semiconductor (CMOS)/CsI flat-panel detectors have been widely used for breast CT and other cone-beam CT applications. With both types of detectors, the transmitted x-rays are converted into visible light in the CsI scintillator layer. The light propagates through the needle structures of CsI crystals, created to minimize light spread, and reaches a two-dimensional (2D) array of image elements where the built-in photodiodes convert the light into charges and store them until the signal readout process. Flat-panel detectors have been developed for various applications, ranging from digital radiography, digital mammography, small animal imaging, to cone-beam CT for use in radiation treatment procedures [31–35]. For breast CT, a large field of view is required to accommodate a magnified (by a factor of as much as 2) large breast. A fast acquisition rate (7.5–30 frames per second) is required to minimize scanning times and motion artifacts. A detector with minimal dead space on one edge, like those designed for digital mammography, is very desirable as it may allow for more coverage of the breast on the chest-wall side.

The quality of a flat-panel detector is largely determined by its pixel size, data depth, and efficiency of x-ray absorption. The pixel size reflects the spatial resolution capability of the detector. The data depth and efficiency of x-ray absorption are directly linked to the contrast sensitivity or the ability to image low-contrast objects. For breast CT, a flat-panel detector designed for fluoroscopy is more suitable than the high-resolution detectors designed for mammography applications. A detector widely used for breast CT as well as other cone-beam CT applications is the Paxscan 4030CB by Varian Medical Systems (Salt Lake City, UT). It has a native pixel size of 194 μm, which, with a magnification factor of 1.33, would provide a voxel size of 146 μm for three-dimensional (3D) breast imaging. This is considerably larger than the minimum pixel size of 100 μm for digital mammography. However, the use of higher-resolution detectors is simply impractical due to considerations regarding breast dose, system alignment, and pulsatile motion. In fact, with many breast CT systems, the detectors have to be operated in binning mode to minimize the noise level at a reasonable exposure level and to reduce the data size for speedier image acquisition, reconstruction, and manipulation. However, binning results in a larger effective pixel size (398 μm or larger), which degrades the resolution.

With the dose level commonly limited to the mean glandular dose limit for two-view mammograms, the spatial resolution becomes less important. However, the use of smaller pixel sizes is essential for imaging smaller calcifications, although higher exposure levels are required as well. Similarly, larger data depth may be important in imaging bony structures or large objects. The data depth of a flat-panel detector could be 12, 14, or 16 bits, corresponding to a maximum gray-scale value of 4095, 16 383, or 65 535. It is usually determined from the ratio of maximum signal to the root mean square dark current noise, which occurs as the result of current leakage in the photodiodes and electronic noise in the preamplifiers. Since the breast is relatively small compared to the chest or the head and does not contain bony structures, 14-bit data depth is thought to be sufficient. The

readout gains are usually variable in order to boost the signal size for low exposures. However, the visibility of low-contrast objects is still limited by the dark current noise level, which is reflected by the data depth.

Image quality

Image contrast

Image contrast in breast CT images, as in regular CT images, is linked to the difference of CT numbers between the object and background materials. Thus, microcalcifications have much higher contrast than soft tissues. However, small microcalcifications may be subjected to partial pixel effects during image acquisition and produce lower contrast in the projection images. This contrast reduction could reduce the CT numbers of small microcalcifications to a level that is no longer visible in contrast to the surrounding tissues. Since the CT numbers are proportional to the ratio of the difference in linear attenuation coefficient between the object and water to that of water, both the CT numbers and image contrast are subjected to only small variations with the x-ray kVp. The variations become even less if a filtered x-ray beam is used. For the same reason, image contrast is less affected by radiation scattering and beam hardening, although the CT numbers themselves are subjected to significant negative biases, causing the so-called "cupping artifacts" that are described in more detail below.

Spatial resolution

Spatial resolution is essential to x-ray breast imaging, in particular to imaging small microcalcifications. Spatial resolution characterizes the ability of an imaging system to resolve small details of an object. In x-ray breast imaging, such details could be the morphology of small microcalcifications or the margins of a soft tissue mass. The spatial resolution of a breast CT system correlates highly with the spatial resolution quality of the projection images. The spatial resolution of a projection image depends on the spatial resolution capability of the detector, the focal spot size, and the imaging geometry (where the x-ray source, object, and detector are placed in relation to each other).

The spatial resolution capability of a flat-panel detector may be characterized by its native pixel size. Theoretically, the spatial resolution of a flat-panel detector is also determined by image blurring in the CsI layer. Thicker CsI layers, commonly used in digital radiography systems, tend to result in greater blurring, leading to lower spatial resolution; while thinner CsI layers, commonly used in digital mammography systems, tend to result in less blurring, leading to higher spatial resolution. However, to contain the cost of the detector and subsequent image processing, storage, transmission, and display, the pixel size of the detector is usually chosen to match the resolution of the light image prior to conversion into charge signals in the image pixels. Thus, the pixel size serves as a good indicator for characterizing the spatial resolution capability of the detector. For imaging tissue structures and large microcalcifications in breast CT, a detector with a pixel size of 200 μm provides more than adequate spatial resolution. For imaging small microcalcifications, a detector with a smaller pixel size is necessary to allow the microcalcifications to be seen individually and to allow larger microcalcifications to be imaged with their true dimensions and shapes visible.

As in projection imaging, the relative positions of the x-ray source (focal spot in the x-ray tube) and the detector affect the spatial resolution capability of the breast CT system. When an object is projected onto the detector, it is magnified with a factor equal to the ratio of the source-to-detector distance to the source-to-object distance. This magnification is referred to as geometric magnification, which helps increase the apparent size of the object, thus improving the spatial resolution capability of a projection imaging system. However, there is a limit on how much the magnification can be increased. The x-ray focal spot is projected through each point of the object onto the detector and creates a shadow in the image. The image of the object is then blurred, with this shadow acting as the kernel or point spread function for the blurring process. This is referred to as the focal spot blurring effect, which increases with the magnification factor, though not proportionally. Thus the optimal geometric factor is the one at which the size of the focal spot shadows equals the pixel size and the spatial resolution performance peaks. In CT, an off-center object is magnified by different factors in different projection views. However, the magnification for an object at the center of rotation (isocenter) is usually used to estimate the average effect of magnification and the overall spatial resolution quality in the reconstructed images. In fact, the native (in non-binning mode) or effective (in binning mode) pixel size of the detector is usually projected back to the plane at the isocenter and the pixel size divided by the geometric magnification factor to select the optimal voxel size for image reconstruction. This voxel size is usually used to indicate the spatial resolution quality of the reconstructed images.

Different geometries have been used in designing the breast CT systems. With some of the breast CT systems, the detector array and the x-ray focal spot are placed at about the same distance from the isocenter, resulting in a geometric factor of close to 2 and a focal spot shadow with similar size as the focal spot itself. For instance, a 0.4 mm wide focal spot would be projected onto the detector with a 0.4 mm wide shadow in the projection image. This sets a resolution limit, which makes it unnecessary to use a high-resolution detector with a pixel size smaller than 400 μm. Thus, when a high-resolution detector (e.g., Paxscan 4030CB with a 194 μm pixel size) is used, it is usually operated in the binning mode to achieve a larger effective pixel size (388 μm with 2 × 2 binning) for speedier image acquisition and reconstruction.

The imaging geometry can also be configured with smaller geometric magnification to take full advantage of the resolution capability of the detector. This involves moving the detector closer to the isocenter, to which the object is centered, thus producing a focal spot shadow similar in size to the native pixel size of the detector. For instance, with a source-to-isocenter distance of 76 cm and a source-to-detector distance of 114 cm, the geometric magnification factor is reduced to 1.5 and a 0.4 mm focal spot would produce a 0.2 mm wide shadow, which is similar in size to the native pixel size of the aforementioned detector. This would help improve the spatial resolution of the reconstructed images and allow smaller calcifications to be detected or visualized.

Noise level

In projection imaging, the ability to image low-contrast objects is directly linked to the contrast signal-to-noise ratio, defined as the ratio of the contrast signal to the noise level, which, for small, low-contrast objects, should be similar inside the object or the background regions. However, signals in CT images are CT numbers computed as the difference of linear attenuation coefficient between the object and water divided by the coefficient for the water. Thus, contrast signals in breast CT do not vary significantly with the x-ray technique. The ability to image small, low-contrast objects is dictated more by the noise level in the reconstructed images.

Noise in breast CT images originates from noise in the projection images. During image reconstruction, noise in the projection images is propagated to the reconstructed images. Due to normalization and logarithmic mapping performed prior to reconstruction, the noise level in the reconstructed images reflects the signal-to-noise ratios in the projection images. Thus, as we increase the x-ray exposures for image acquisition, both the signal size and noise level increase in the projection images. In the reconstructed images, on the other hand, the signal size remains the same while the noise level decreases.

Noise in the projection images consists of a quantum noise component and a system noise component. The former is associated with the process of x-ray absorption while the latter is associated with the process of image signal readout. The level of the quantum noise component is affected by many factors, including the x-ray kVp, mAs, the imaging geometry, the breast size and composition, and the detector used. The x-ray kVp and mAs determine the x-ray output from the x-ray source. The x-ray kVp, the breast size, breast composition, and the source-to-detector distance determine the fluence of x-rays transmitting through the breast and reaching the detector. The quantum detection efficiency of the detector determines the percentage of the x-ray fluence absorbed and used to produce signals in the projection images. Random fluctuations occur during absorption of x-ray photons in the detector and result in quantum noise in the image with the level of noise proportional to the square root of the number of x-ray photons absorbed in each pixel. The system noise, originating from the readout electronics, is added during the image readout process. An image quality metric, referred to as the detective quantum efficiency (DQE), combines the effect of the system noise with the ability of the detector to absorb x-rays. DQE is often used to quantify the efficiency of the detector to preserve the x-ray statistics, as quantified by the signal-to-noise ratio, during the x-ray detection and image formation process.

(a)

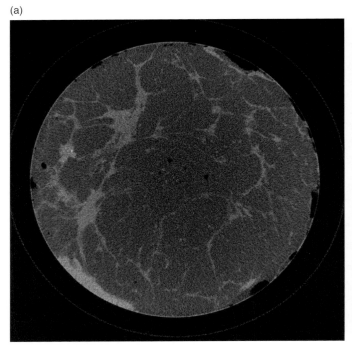

(b)

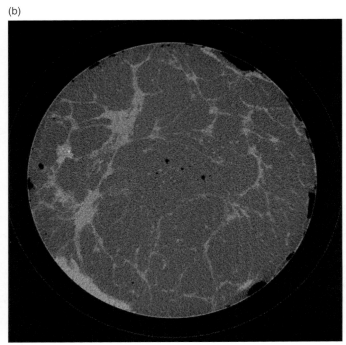

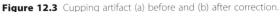

Figure 12.3 Cupping artifact (a) before and (b) after correction.

Signal accuracy and artifacts

Breast CT images differ from mammograms in that the images can be easily separated into dense tissue, adipose tissue, calcifications, and skin. Theoretically, each region should have similar CT numbers whose levels characterize the tissue types. In reality, these numbers are non-uniform, and they tend to decrease from the periphery towards the center of the breast. This non-uniformity is the result of beam hardening and the presence of scatter components in image signals. This effect is referred to as the cupping artifact (Figure 12.3). Accurate CT numbers are not essential to reading breast CT images, but they are essential to quantitative image analysis of the breast CT images (e.g., image segmentation and computer-aided diagnosis). Thus, the breast CT image data need to be corrected for biases of the CT numbers if they are to be used for quantitative analysis.

Intrinsic to 3D image reconstruction is the generation of artifacts in the reconstructed images. Artifacts may be generated in several ways. Some are more visible than others and may obscure the lesions or anatomy to be detected or examined. The first type of artifacts is associated with excessive attenuation by certain objects, which could be metal clips or large calcifications (Figure 12.4). Image reconstruction in x-ray CT relies on accurate measurement of x-ray attenuation with the projection images. Excessive attenuation by a metal clip or a large calcification could result in so much attenuation that the transmitted x-ray intensity is too low to be measurable. This means that the signals for x-rays passing through these objects become zero or hide in the noise fluctuations. This phenomenon not only makes it impossible to directly reconstruct CT signals for the objects themselves, it also affects the reconstruction of objects or structures around them.

As the result, so-called metal clip artifacts are generated. They may appear as saturated images of the objects with incorrect dimensions or shapes, star-shaped streaks around the objects, or moiré patterns in the images (Figure 12.5). Fortunately, the streaking artifacts and moiré patterns can be easily removed by replacing the projection data in the object regions with data corresponding to less attenuation. These data, while being artificially created and incorrectly reflecting the true attenuation, help reduce the streaking artifacts and moiré patterns. In addition, they can help restore, although only partially, the apparent dimension and shapes of these heavily attenuating objects and the accuracy of the CT signals in and around them.

Other types of artifacts could result from misalignment, defects of the detector pixels or improper bias offsetting or gain correction of the projection image data. These types of artifacts may sometimes appear with images generated with earlier experimental prototype imagers. However, as the alignment and signal normalization problems are ironed out, these types of artifacts tend to be reduced to an unnoticeable level.

Tissue structures

Based on the patient studies and specimen imaging studies to date, tissue structures are well resolved with an isocenter glandular dose at the same level as the mean glandular dose limit for two-view mammograms for an average-size breast. Dense tissue is visually well separated from the adipose tissue. Due to the coarseness of the structures, the spatial resolution of current breast CT systems used in patient studies is adequate even though the detector is operated in the binning mode with an effective pixel size of 388 µm. However, it is also clear that soft tissue

(a)

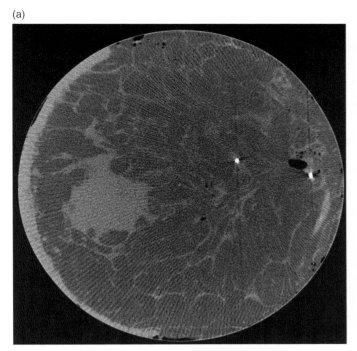

(b)

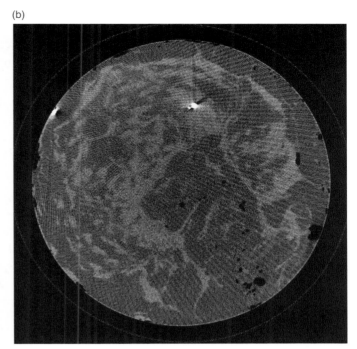

Figure 12.4 (a, b) Metal artifacts secondary to clips.

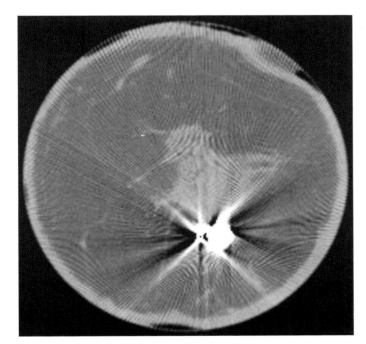

Figure 12.5 Metal clip artifact causing streaks in the image, consistent with a moiré pattern.

masses or tumors cannot be distinguished from the dense tissue solely based on the differences of their signal levels or the CT numbers. Thus, if the soft tissue masses or tumors are totally embedded in the dense tissue, they cannot be distinguished from the dense tissue. As with mammograms, only when the mass or tumors grow out of the dense tissue and spread into the adipose tissue can they be visualized and identified based on the difference of their morphology from that of the normal tissue structures (Figure 12.6). This may be expected, as the breast CT images intrinsically have higher noise levels, due to the lower exposures used and the additional noise introduced by scattered radiation, which is present in abundance. However, even with regular clinical CT, which has better scatter control and superior contrast sensitivity, masses and tumors may not be seen consistently. The real problem is that the CT numbers of masses or tumors are simply too close to those of normal dense tissue. This is where breast CT has an advantage over conventional mammography. Because mammography provides a summation shadow, the edges of a mass can be obscured by dense tissue located in a different plane, perhaps several centimeters away from the mass. Breast CT provides consecutive slice images, allowing masses or tumors to appear surrounded only by the tissue that is actually in the same plane with them (Figures 12.7, 12.8). If this tissue is dense, the mass may still be obscured (Figure 12.9), but at least it will not be obscured by dense tissue on the other side of the breast. Direct detection and visualization of abnormal masses inside dense tissue may also be achieved by breast CT with contrast injection [23]. This may result in images similar to and comparable to contrast-enhanced magnetic resonance imaging (MRI). This is a new area being explored and investigated.

Microcalcifications

Although breast CT provides true 3D images of the breast and therefore is actually a new modality, it has often been used in the same way as or compared to mammography. Thus, it must

(a)

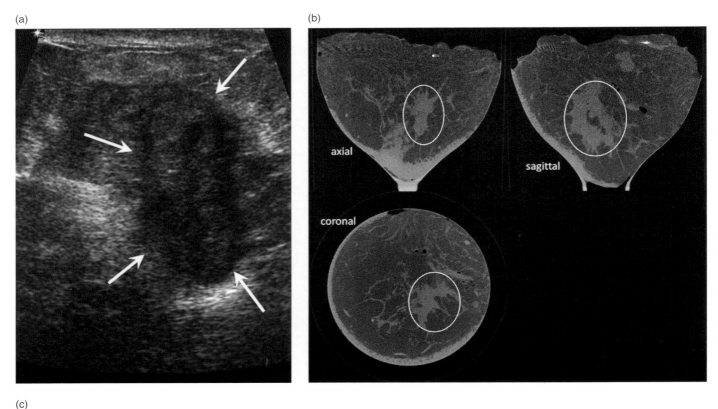

(b)

(c)

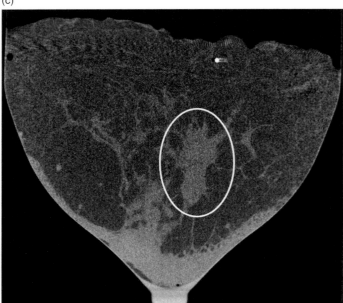

Figure 12.6 A 63-year-old-woman complained of fullness in her right breast. (a) Ultrasound showed a large right breast mass (arrows). Ultrasound-guided core biopsy revealed invasive carcinoma, and fine needle aspiration of an axillary lymph node was positive for metastatic disease. The patient underwent right mastectomy. (b) CT of the surgical specimen shows the right breast mass (circles) in the axial, sagittal, and coronal planes, with (c) a magnified view of the axial image.

demonstrate the ability to image small microcalcifications if it is to be used to replace mammography in screening or in the diagnosis or assessment of breast cancers containing microcalcifications (Figure 12.10). Early reports on patient studies suggested that breast CT has ample resolution for imaging tissue structures or soft tissue masses. However, only larger microcalcifications are visible on breast CT images

(Figure 12.11). There are several factors to prevent current breast CT systems from effectively imaging small microcalcifications. First of all, to contain the breast dose, the flat-panel detectors are often operated in the binning mode, resulting in a large effective pixel size (e.g., 388 μm for 2 × 2 binning with the Paxscan 4030CB detector). A second limiting factor is the partial pixel effect during image acquisition. Thus, although

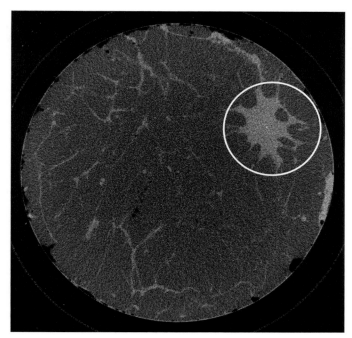

Figure 12.7 A 46-year-old woman palpated a left breast mass. Ultrasound showed an irregular hypoechoic mass in the left breast at 2 o'clock. Ultrasound-guided core biopsy was performed, and pathology revealed invasive ductal carcinoma. The patient underwent left mastectomy. CT of the surgical specimen demonstrates the malignancy (circle) as an irregular spiculated mass in the coronal view.

microcalcifications, with their high linear attenuation coefficient, should have superior contrast against a background of adipose or dense tissues, the contrast may be substantially degraded through the partial pixel effect. The degradation may be so severe that these small microcalcifications would be masked by the image noise. This problem may be resolved by increasing the x-ray technique and reducing the noise level in the reconstructed images, thus allowing the small microcalcifications to become visible. However, the higher exposures would also increase the radiation dose and the risk of cancer induction to the breast. Another solution is to use higher-resolution detectors to reduce the partial pixel effect. However, since the image pixels are smaller in size, they would absorb a smaller number of photons, thus lowering the signal size and allowing the system noise to become a limiting factor. In summary, it seems unlikely that the visibility of small microcalcifications can be improved without increasing the breast dose.

X-ray techniques and doses

The x-ray kVp used with current breast CT systems ranges from 49 to 100. Experiments have not demonstrated an advantage to using kVps in the lower end of this range. On the contrary, higher kVps are necessary to allow the x-rays to penetrate large breasts and result in projection images of reasonable quality for reconstruction. In general, 80 kVp is a practical choice for small and medium breasts

(14 cm or smaller in diameter) while use of higher kVps may be necessary for imaging larger breasts (14 cm or greater in diameter). The mean glandular dose for a breast CT scan can be estimated by measuring the open field exposure (air kerma) at the isocenter. Monte Carlo simulation may be used to determine the factor to convert the isocenter exposure to the average breast dose or mean glandular dose for the breast [36,37]. Although no legal limit on the breast dose in breast CT has been set, it is a general practice to keep the mean glandular dose the same as or below the mean glandular dose limit for two-view mammograms for a 50% adipose, 50% dense breast with a compressed thickness of 5 cm (6 mGys). As mentioned in the previous section, higher exposure levels may be necessary for imaging small microcalcifications. However, to date, there has not been consensus on whether there is a need to image small microcalcifications and whether there is sufficient justification for increasing the x-ray exposure level to achieve this goal at the expense of a higher breast dose.

There have been many efforts to use iterative algorithms to obtain reconstructed images of reasonable quality from projection images acquired at reduced exposure levels [38]. These algorithms may provide a promising approach to obtaining high-quality breast CT images with acceptable breast doses in order to image small microcalcifications. This should be a priority in breast CT research in the future.

Clinical applications and correlation with other modalities

Breast CT and mammography

Current standard guidelines in the United States follow the recommendation of the American Cancer Society that all women age 40 years and older should have a screening mammogram every year and should continue to do so for as long as they are in good health. Worldwide, nearly 516 000 deaths due to breast cancer were reported in women in 2004 [39]. Mammography has been reported to reduce the mortality due to breast cancer by 20–30% in women over 50 years old [40].

Advances introduced into mammography since 1990 have increased its accuracy. Despite its usefulness, mammography still has several limitations. With routine mammography, it is difficult to differentiate small structures of soft tissue density from parenchymal tissue [13]. The sensitivity of mammography is reduced to as low as 30% in dense breasts [41–43], and because mammography is a 2D projection of a 3D object there is resultant structure and tissue overlap [13]. In a study by Berg *et al.*, the sensitivity of mammography in detecting diagnosed breast lesions was reported to be 67.8%, while its specificity was 75% [44].

Lindfors and colleagues published the first clinical breast CT paper, and breast CT was compared to film-screen mammography (Figure 12.12). The breast CT images were compared to the conventional craniocaudal and mediolateral

(a)

(b)

(c)

(d)

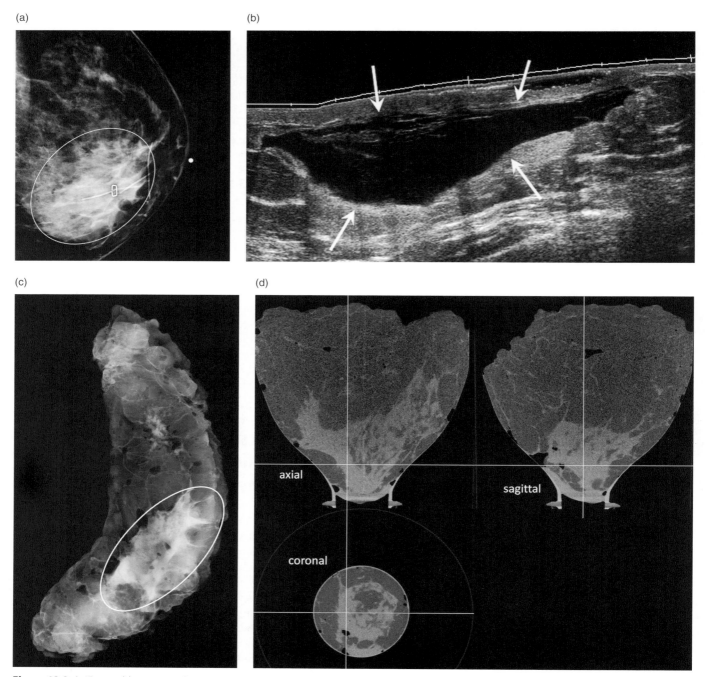

Figure 12.8 A 45-year-old woman underwent screening mammography which showed clustered calcifications in the left breast. The patient underwent left breast excisional biopsy, which revealed ductal carcinoma in situ (DCIS). (a) Left breast craniocaudal mammogram after the surgical biopsy showed post-surgical changes, a surgical clip, and residual calcifications (circle). (b) Ultrasound revealed a seroma (arrows) that was subsequently drained under ultrasound guidance. The patient then underwent left mastectomy, which demonstrated no evidence of residual tumor. (c) Sliced surgical specimen x-ray shows post-surgical changes (circle). (d) Specimen CT shows the corresponding post-surgical changes in the axial, sagittal, and coronal planes, with the crossbars for localization.

oblique views; no additional diagnostic views were used for comparison. In the study, 10 healthy volunteers were imaged with breast CT, and breast CT was performed on 69 women with Breast Imaging Reporting and Data System (BI-RADS) category 4 and 5 lesions. Lindfors *et al.* showed that breast CT was significantly better than film-screen mammography

for visualization of masses ($p = 0.002$). Film-screen mammography outperformed breast CT for visualization of microcalcifications ($p = 0.006$) [12].

Lindfors *et al.* used a prototype breast CT scanner designed at the University of California, Davis with a flat-panel detector (Paxscan 4030CB; Varian Imaging Systems, Palo Alto, CA).

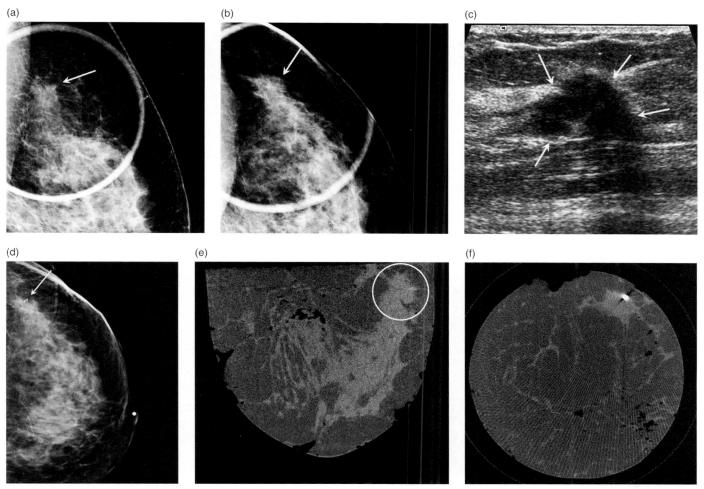

Figure 12.9 A 61-year-old woman with a left breast mass seen on screening mammography. (a) Left lateromedial and (b) exaggerated craniocaudal mammograms and (c) ultrasound demonstrate the mass (arrows). Ultrasound-guided biopsy revealed invasive metaplastic carcinoma. (d) An exaggerated craniocaudal view of the left breast shows the marker clip after the biopsy (arrow). Left mastectomy was performed. (e) Sagittal view of the specimen CT demonstrates the lesion (circle). (f) On the coronal view of the specimen CT, metallic artifacts are noted, secondary to the marker clip.

The unit used a 30-frames-per-second acquisition at a pixel matrix of 1024 × 768, resulting in 0.388 mm pixel dimensions at the detector. In the study, 500 cone-beam projection images were acquired 360 degrees around the patient's breast in 16.6 seconds. The breast CT techniques were designed to deliver the same mean glandular radiation dose as a two-view mammogram, based on Monte Carlo analyses [12].

In the study by Lindfors *et al.*, the projection images were used to reconstruct 300–500 512 × 512 images. The native reconstructed images were produced in the coronal plane, and the data could be used to produce tomographic images in any orientation. In the study, the images were viewed sequentially in a stack mode at a flat-panel liquid crystal display monitor in the coronal, sagittal, and transverse planes, using software developed specifically for breast CT. In the study, contrast and brightness could be adjusted, and a zoom function was available. Also, the section width thickness could be adjusted [12].

Lindfors *et al.* first performed breast CT on 10 healthy volunteers, followed by breast CT on 69 women with BI-RADS category 4 or 5 lesions (Figure 12.13). Motion blurring was noted in one of the first 10 scans, and all 10 volunteers were able to sustain the 16.6 second breath hold required for the scan [12]. Of the 69 women with BI-RADS category 4 or 5 lesions, four women were excluded from the study analysis. Two women were excluded because of movement during breast CT (possibly secondary to the 16.6-second breath hold). Two women were excluded because the mammographically visible lesions were not in the breast CT field of view: one lesion was situated in the axillary tail region, and the other lesion was in the anterior aspect of the breast of a large-breasted woman. Two women had bilateral breast lesions. For the study, the breast CT images were compared to film-screen mammography in 67 breasts in 65 women [12].

Fifty-eight (87%) of 67 lesions were identified on breast CT. Two lesions not seen on breast CT were proven to represent

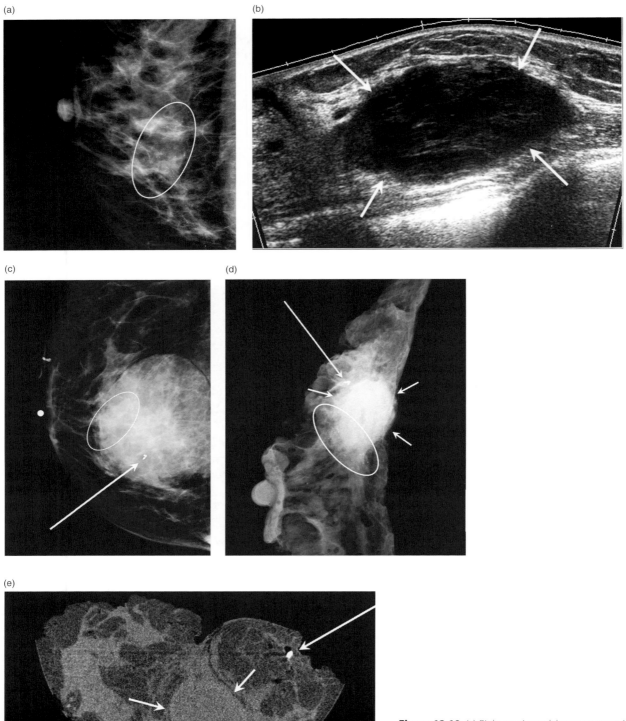

(a)

(b)

(c)

(d)

(e)

Figure 12.10 (a) Right craniocaudal mammogram in a 68-year-old woman showed suspicious calcifications (circle). The patient underwent biopsy that revealed DCIS. (b) Ultrasound and (c) right craniocaudal mammogram after the biopsy demonstrate a hematoma (short arrows), a marker clip (long arrow), and residual calcifications (circle). The patient then underwent right mastectomy. (d) Sliced specimen x-ray shows the hematoma (short arrows), the clip (long arrow), and residual calcifications (circle). (e) Sagittal view of the surgical specimen CT shows the hematoma (short arrows), the clip (long arrow), and residual calcifications (circle).

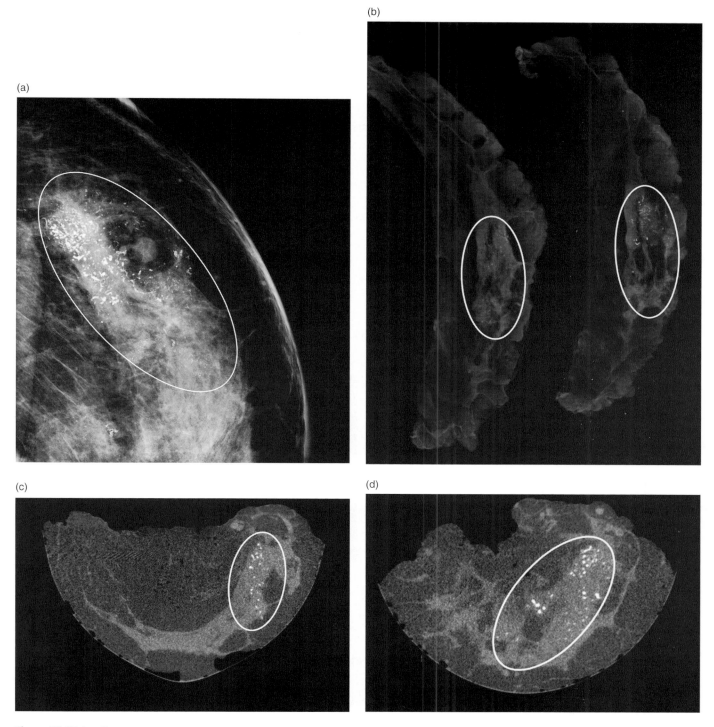

Figure 12.11 *(cont.)*

summation artifacts and biopsy was not performed. Thus, 58 (89%) of 65 true lesions on film-screen mammography were identified on breast CT. Out of seven true lesions not identified on breast CT, three were malignant. The malignancies not identified on breast CT included a 5 mm cluster of microcalcifications (proven to represent ductal carcinoma in situ [DCIS]), an area of

diffuse microcalcifications in dense tissue (proven to be DCIS), and a 15 mm mass that was subtle on mammography and best seen with sonography (representing invasive ductal carcinoma). There were four benign lesions not identified with breast CT, including palpable diabetic mastopathy (poorly visualized with film-screen mammography); lobular carcinoma in situ

(e)

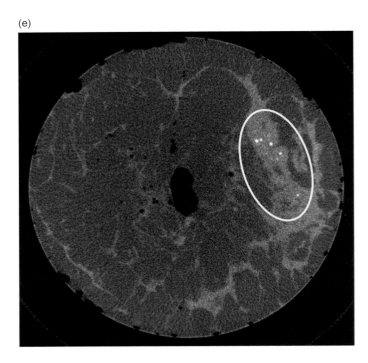

Figure 12.11 A 58-year-old woman presented with pleomorphic calcifications noted in the left breast (circle) as seen on (a) the left breast magnified exaggerated craniocaudal mammogram. Core biopsies showed multicentric left breast DCIS. The patient underwent left mastectomy. Sliced specimen (b) x-ray and (c) axial, (d) sagittal, and (e) coronal CT images showed the pleomorphic calcifications (circles).

(b)

(a)

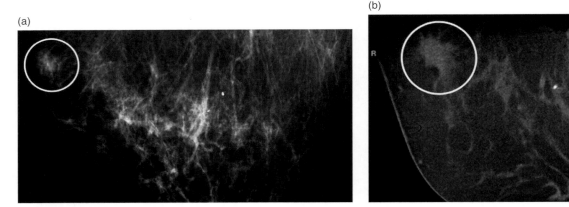

Figure 12.12 (a) Right craniocaudal mammogram shows a round mass (circle). (b) CT was performed, demonstrating a spiculated mass (circle). Pathology revealed infiltrating ductal carcinoma. Courtesy of Dr. Karen Lindfors, University of California, Davis, Sacramento, CA.

(LCIS), seen as a 2 mm microcalcification cluster on film-screen mammography; fibrocystic changes, noted as a 3 cm area of microcalcifications on film-screen mammography; and a 4 mm cyst. In one patient, a small satellite cancer was identified with breast CT adjacent to the index lesion (proven to be invasive ductal carcinoma). The satellite lesion was not visualized on screening or diagnostic film-screen mammography [12].

Lindfors *et al.* undertook a patient comfort survey on 82 women who underwent breast CT (10 healthy volunteers, 69 women with BI-RADS category 4 or 5 lesions, and three women with BI-RADS category 5 masses who underwent contrast-enhanced breast CT). The survey indicated that many women found it difficult to arch forward into the breast CT unit, had neck pain while arching forward, or found the table-top to be too firm. When asked to compare comfort with

breast CT compared to comfort with film-screen mammography, two-thirds of the women indicated a very pronounced preference for breast CT ($p < 0.001$) [12].

In the study by Lindfors *et al.*, the pectoralis musculature was visualized on breast CT in only 18% of the patients. Visualization of the axillary tail region was also limited. Efforts have been directed towards redesigning the table in an effort to image more of the chest wall and the axillary tail regions [12].

O'Connell *et al.* evaluated 40 breasts in 23 women with breast CT. The breast CT images were compared to mammography (digital mammography was performed in 20 women and film-screen mammography was performed in three women). All of the mammograms were assessed as BI-RADS category 1 or 2. O'Connell *et al.* used a flat-panel detector (PaxScan 4030CB, Varian Medical Systems) mounted on a gantry, with an

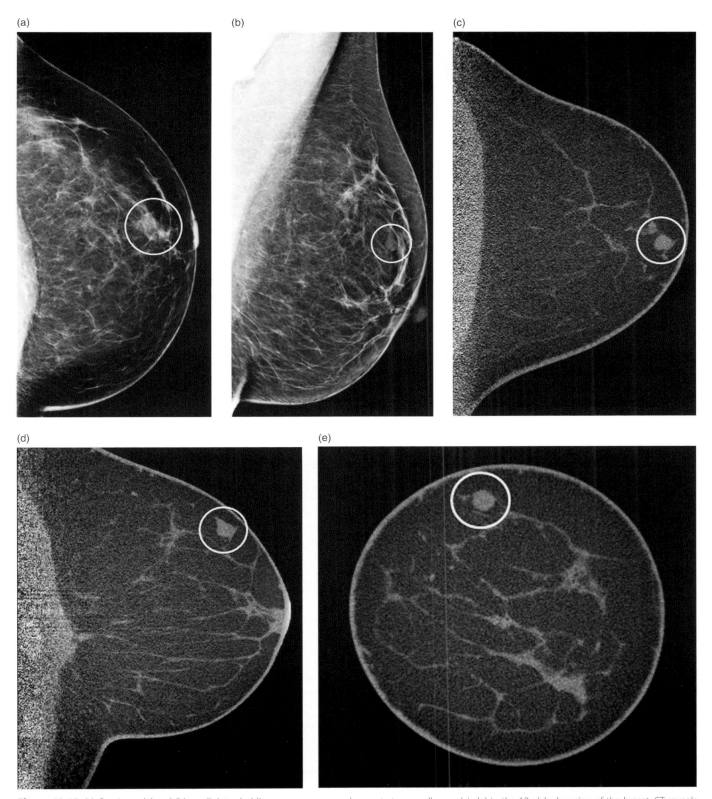

Figure 12.13 (a) Craniocaudal and (b) mediolateral oblique mammograms demonstrate a small mass (circle) in the 12 o'clock region of the breast. CT reveals a small mass in the anterior aspect of the breast. (c) Axial, (d) sagittal, and (e) coronal CT views are shown. Pathology revealed pseudoangiomatous stromal hyperplasia. Courtesy of Dr. Karen Lindfors, University of California, Davis, Sacramento, CA.

ergonomically designed patient table. The x-ray tube had a 0.3 mm focal spot size, and images were acquired at 49 kVP and 50–200 mA. Thirty frames were acquired per second over a scan time of 10 seconds. The imaging volume was 28 × 28 × 16 cm. The reconstructed images were loaded into 3D visualization software (Visage CS Thin Client/Server, Visage Imaging) for 3D rendering, visualization, and display. The reconstructed images were visualized in three orthogonal planes (transverse, sagittal, and coronal) and with 3D rendering. The average time to scroll through the images was approximately five minutes [13].

In the report by O'Connell and colleagues, the average glandular dose for breast CT (4–16 mGy) was within the range of the dose for mammography. Breast tissue coverage was statistically significantly better with breast CT than with mammography in the lateral ($p < 0.0001$), medial ($p < 0.0001$), and posterior ($p = 0.0002$) aspects of the breast. Mammography had statistically significantly better coverage than breast CT in the axilla and the axillary tail ($p < 0.0001$). Most calcifications and all masses detected on mammography were visualized with breast CT. In this study, 85% of the calcifications less than 1 mm and all of the calcifications greater than 1 mm were identified with breast CT. Overall, 60 (89.6%) of the mammographic findings were visualized with breast CT [13].

O'Connell et al. noted that 20 women (86.9%) found breast CT to be as comfortable as, or more comfortable than, mammography. For women who reported discomfort during breast CT, the predominant areas of discomfort or pressure points included the neck, the shoulders, and the ribs. Efforts are under way to redesign the table with the goal of improving patient comfort [13].

In their study of the feasibility of breast CT, Chen et al. emphasized the advantage of breast CT over mammography in two main aspects: significantly better low-contrast detectability of breast tumors, and more accurate 3D localization of breast lesions [9]. Breast CT can potentially reduce examination times with comparable radiation doses. Breast CT may also eliminate the need for compression and additional workup views [18].

In summary, breast CT has been shown to be better than mammography for detection of small masses, especially in dense breasts. Mammography has been shown to be better than breast CT for visualizing the axilla and for detecting microcalcifications.

Breast CT and conventional tomosynthesis

Breast CT and breast tomosynthesis both have potential because of their abilities to visualize the 3D structure of the breast tissue and to decrease obscuration of masses by overlapping normal tissue. As compared with breast CT, digital breast tomosynthesis uses lower kVps (in the same range as mammography) and this gives tomosynthesis better differentiation among low-contrast objects. The use of mammography equipment also gives tomosynthesis better spatial resolution than breast CT, but the disadvantage is that tomosynthesis measures only a limited angular range of projection data. Observer performance, however, did not differ significantly between breast CT and tomosynthesis when detecting an experimental model of 5 mm tumors [45]. Breast CT has an advantage over tomosynthesis when patient comfort is in question because with tomosynthesis breast compression is needed, while breast CT does not require breast compression.

Breast CT and PET/CT

Current studies demonstrate that positron emission tomography (PET) scans are capable of identifying some lesions not visible on standard mammograms [46]. A study by Raylman et al. showed that some tumors were better defined with a positron emission mammography (PEM) system [46]. PET scans are also useful in determining the spread of breast cancer to the axillary lymph nodes and other sites. Bowen et al. evaluated the performance of PET/CT in detecting breast lesions experimentally using a phantom, and clinically on a total of seven breasts in four patients [47]. The authors reported a registration error between PET and CT of 0.18 mm, and an accurate visualization of suspected lesions in three dimensions. They used both iodinated contrast and fluorodeoxiglucose (18-FDG), and this provided information about two types of kinetics related to the tumor: angiogenesis and glucose metabolism. In this small series, the investigators demonstrated 100% accuracy for cancer detection, including one case of DCIS. There is still need for further clinical studies in PET/CT of the breast [47]. PET scans are not currently recommended for breast cancer screening because of the prohibitive costs, the radiation doses, and the specialized nuclear medicine facilities that are required.

The use of contrast in breast CT

Use of iodinated contrast media has shown remarkable promise in the diagnosis of small breast lesions. According to Boone et al., on the basis of the combined contrast and noise data, the contrast-to-noise ratio (CNR), and the corresponding signal-to-noise ratio (SNR), lesions as small as 2 or 3 mm in diameter may be detected on breast CT [8]. For comparison, the median lesion diameter detected by using film-screen mammography has been reported to be between 11 and 16 mm [8,48,49].

Lindfors et al. performed contrast-enhanced breast CT on four patients with BI-RADS category 5 mass lesions (Figure 12.14). In the study, Lindfors and colleagues injected 100 mL of iodixanol (320 mg of iodine per mL (Visipaque 320; GE Healthcare, Princeton, NJ) intravenously by using a power injector (Mark V Plus; Medrad, Pittsburgh, PA) over 25 seconds. Breast CT was then performed after a 90–140-second delay. Three of four patients who underwent contrast-enhanced breast CT had invasive ductal carcinoma on pathology. In one patient, two enhancing spiculated masses were noted near the chest wall on breast CT. Film-screen mammography identified only the posterior mass. Both masses were shown to represent invasive ductal carcinoma on pathologic examination [12].

Prionas et al. used breast CT with contrast to analyze 54 breast lesions in 46 subjects. With the use of contrast, malignant lesions were significantly better seen as compared

(a)

(b)

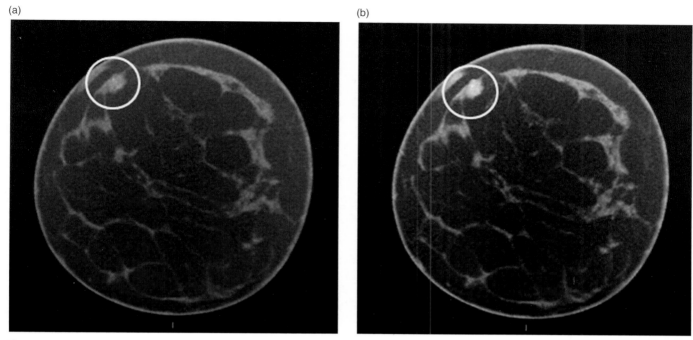

Figure 12.14 (a) Non-enhanced CT shows a poorly visualized small mass (circle) with faint microcalcifications. (b) Contrast-enhanced CT improves visualization of this mass (circle). Pathology revealed DCIS. Courtesy of Dr. Karen Lindfors, University of California, Davis, Sacramento, CA.

to non-enhanced breast CT and mammography. Moreover, on contrast-enhanced breast CT, microcalcifications were better visualized relative to non-enhanced breast CT, and visualized as well as with mammography. The amount of enhancement with malignant lesions was significantly higher than with benign lesions (55.9 HU versus 17.6 HU, respectively, $p < 0.001$). On average, DCIS enhanced even more than other malignant lesions. Further studies are needed to evaluate contrast dynamics with breast CT and the ability to classify lesions based on their enhancement curves similar to the current classification with washout curves on MRI [23].

Contrast use has also been introduced in digital mammography, and has further improved the detection of breast lesions as well. Studies by Jong *et al.* have suggested that contrast-enhanced digital mammography may be useful in identifying lesions in dense breasts [50]. These authors found that out of 10 patients with diagnosed malignant breast lesions, enhancement was observed in eight of the patients with contrast-enhanced mammography. Enhancement was observed in 89% of the invasive cancers, and no enhancement was observed in 58% of the benign lesions [50].

Breast CT in radiation therapy planning

An additional use of breast CT is for radiation therapy guidance. Investigators have used breast CT to verify appropriate positioning for prone accelerated breast partial irradiation (ABPI) [51]. Cai *et al.* concluded that although pretreatment breast CT guidance reduced initial setup errors for APBI, verification of patient position during treatment was

also needed [51]. Topolnjak *et al.* reported that breast CT significantly reduced setup uncertainties as compared to electronic portal images [52]. Hasan *et al.* recommended considering online image guidance using breast CT for ABPI [53]. Breast CT was also used to document the motion of surgical clips relative to the surgical cavity after breast excision. The clips may be used to monitor radiotherapy delivery [54].

Future improvements

With the majority of work on breast CT being fairly recent, there is room for improvement and technical development, including new algorithms and new methods of image analysis in order to limit the radiation dose and/or obtain a higher-resolution image. In addition, there is also need for better characterization of dynamic contrast enhancement curves. There is also need for more clinical studies, with more emphasis on imaging/pathology correlation. Breast CT is faster than MRI, and a breast CT unit takes less space than a MRI unit. In addition, breast CT could be used in the future for procedure guidance, including core biopsies and needle localizations [10]. In addition, it is thought that breast CT may play an important role in specimen imaging following surgery.

Dose reduction

There are several papers describing new algorithms and techniques to reduce radiation dose with breast CT. Lai *et al.* described a technique using volume-of-interest (VOI) breast CT, and this led to greatly decreased radiation dose at the periphery of the phantom, and also, to a lesser extent, in the center of the phantom. This technique also significantly decreased the scatter to primary ratio, and improved the contrast signals more than the noise levels, leading to an overall increase in the contrast-to-noise ratio (CNR) [22].

Based on their experimental work, He *et al.* suggested that the use of x-ray tube current modulation could produce substantial reduction in organ and effective dose for cone-bream CT [55]. Winey *et al.* concluded that it is possible to reduce the radiation dose to other structures by proper selection of the beam angle and the imaging field size [56]. Cai *et al.* described algorithms for scatter correction in clinical breast CT breast imaging [57]. Decreased scatter will lead to a better signal-to-noise ratio (SNR).

Improved resolution

In general, CT has limited resolution when compared to plain radiography. Its resolution is even more limited when comparing breast CT to mammography, because mammography is the highest-resolution modality in radiography. Detecting small breast lesions and microcalcifications is critical for early diagnosis and treatment. Using a small field of view in breast CT has given breast CT better resolution than in body CT imaging, but breast CT's resolution still needs improvement. A study from Finland demonstrated excellent visibility of in-vitro breast cancer with the use of high-resolution analyzer-based x-ray imaging CT, but this technique required a high mean glandular dose of 12–13 mGy, compared to < 1 mGy for mammography. The authors suggested a valuable role for this technique in the future after further reductions in dose and when compact synchrotron radiation sources become available [58].

In conclusion, breast CT has promise as a means of detection and analysis of breast cancers manifesting primarily as soft tissue density masses, but without probably unacceptable increases in radiation dose, its ability to identify microcalcifications is thought to be limited.

References

1. Chang CH, Sibala JL, Gallagher JH, *et al.* Computed tomography of the breast: a preliminary report. *Radiology* 1977; **124**: 827–9.

2. Gisvold JJ, Karsell PR, Reese EC. Clinical evaluation of computerized tomographic mammography. *Mayo Clin Proc* 1977; **52**: 181–5.

3. Chang CH, Sibala JL, Fritz SL, *et al.* Computed tomographic evaluation of the breast. *AJR Am J Roentgenol* 1978; **131**: 459–64.

4. Gisvold JJ, Reese DF, Karsell PR. Computed tomographic mammography (CTM). *AJR Am J Roentgenol* 1979; **133**: 1143–9.

5. Chang CH, Sibala JL, Fritz SL, *et al.* Computed tomography in detection and diagnosis of breast cancer. *Cancer* 1980; **46**(4 Suppl): 939–46.

6. Chang CH, Nesbit DE, Fisher DR, *et al.* Computed tomographic mammography using a conventional body scanner. *AJR Am J Roentgenol* 1982; **138**: 553–8.

7. Muller JW, van Waes PF, Koehler PR. Computed tomography of breast lesions: comparison with x-ray mammography. *J Comput Assist Tomogr* 1983; **7**: 650–4.

8. Boone JM, Nelson TR, Lindfors KK, Seibert JA. Dedicated breast CT: radiation dose and image quality evaluation. *Radiology* 2001; **221**: 657–67.

9. Chen B, Ning R. Cone-beam volume CT breast imaging: feasibility study. *Med Phys* 2002; **29**: 755–70.

10. Boone JM, Kwan AL, Yang K, *et al.* Computed tomography for imaging the breast. *J Mammary Gland Biol Neoplasia* 2006; **11**: 103–11.

11. Ning R, Conover D, Yu Y, *et al.* A novel cone beam breast CT scanner: system evaluation. *Proc SPIE* 2007; **6510**: 651030. DOI: 10.1117/12.710340.

12. Lindfors KK, Boone JM, Nelson TR, *et al.* Dedicated breast CT: initial clinical experience. *Radiology* 2008; **246**: 725–33.

13. O'Connell A, Conover DL, Zhang Y, *et al.* Cone-beam CT for breast imaging: radiation dose, breast coverage, and image quality. *AJR Am J Roentgenol* 2010; **195**: 496–509.

14. McKinley RL, Tornai MP, Samei E, Bradshaw ML. Initial study of quasi-monochromatic x-ray beam performance for x-ray computed mammotomography. *IEEE Trans Nucl Sci* 2005; **52**: 1243–50.

15. Tornai MP, McKinley RL, Brzymialkiewicz CN, *et al.*, eds. Design and development of a fully-3D dedicated x-ray computed mammotomography system. *Proc SPIE* 2005; **5745**: 189–97. DOI: 10.1117/12.595636.

16. Lai CJ, Shaw CC, Chen L, *et al.* Visibility of microcalcification in cone beam breast CT: effects of x-ray tube voltage and radiation dose. *Med Phys* 2007; **34**: 2995–3004.

17. O'Connor JM, Glick SJ, Gong X, Didier C, Mah'd M. Characterization of a prototype, tabletop x-ray CT breast imaging system. *Proc SPIE* 2007; **6510**: 65102T. DOI: 10.1117/12.713751.

18. Yang WT, Carkaci S, Chen L, *et al.* Dedicated cone-beam breast CT: feasibility study with surgical mastectomy specimens. *AJR Am J Roentgenol* 2007; **189**: 1312–15.

19. O'Connor JM, Das M, Didier C, Mah'D M, Glick SJ. Using mastectomy specimens to develop breast models for breast tomosynthesis and CT breast imaging. *Proc SPIE* 2008; **6913**: 691315. DOI: 10.1117/12.772666.

20. Chen L, Shaw CC, Altunbas MC, *et al.* Feasibility of volume-of-interest (VOI) scanning technique in cone beam breast CT: a preliminary study. *Med Phys* 2008; **35**: 3482–90.

21. Chen L, Shen Y, Lai CJ, *et al.* Dual resolution cone beam breast CT: a feasibility study. *Med Phys* 2009; **36**: 4007–14.

22. Lai CJ, Chen L, Zhang H, *et al.* Reduction in x-ray scatter and radiation dose for volume-of-interest (VOI) cone-beam breast CT: a phantom study. *Phys Med Biol* 2009; **54**: 6691–709.

23. Prionas ND, Lindfors KK, Ray S, *et al.* Contrast-enhanced dedicated breast CT: initial clinical experience. *Radiology* 2010; **256**: 714–23.

24. von Smekal L, Kachelriess M, Stepina E, Kalender WA. Geometric misalignment and calibration in cone-beam tomography. *Med Phys* 2004; **31**: 3242–66.

25. Kyriakou Y, Deak P, Langner O, Kalender WA. Concepts for dose determination in flat-detector CT. *Phys Med Biol* 2008; **53**: 3551–66.

26. Russo P, Lauria A, Mettivier G, Montesi MC, Villani N. Dose distribution in cone-beam breast computed tomography: an experimental phantom study. *IEEE Trans Nucl Sci* 2010; **57**: 366–74.

27. Russo P, Mettivier G, Lauria A, Montesi MC. X-ray cone-beam breast computed tomography: phantom studies. *IEEE Trans Nucl Sci* 2010; **57**: 160–72.

28. Ning R, Conover D, Yu Y, *et al.* A novel cone beam breast CT scanner: preliminary system evaluation. *Proc SPIE* 2006; **6142**: 614211. http://dx.doi.org/10.1117/12.655741.

29. Crotty DJ, McKinley RL, Tornai MP. Experimental spectral measurements of heavy K-edge filtered beams for x-ray computed mammoto-mography. *Phys Med Biol* 2007; **52**: 603–16.

30. Glick SJ, Thacker S, Gong X, Liu B. Evaluating the impact of x-ray spectral shape on image quality in flat-panel CT breast imaging. *Med Phys* 2007; **34**: 5–24.

31. Vedantham S, Karellas A, Suryanarayanan S, *et al.* Full breast digital mammography with an amorphous silicon-based flat panel detector: physical characteristics of a clinical prototype. *Med Phys* 2000; **27**: 558–67.

32. Floyd CE, Warp RJ, Dobbins JT, *et al.* Imaging characteristics of an amorphous silicon flat-panel detector for digital chest radiography. *Radiology* 2001; **218**: 683–8.

33. Lee SC, Kim HK, Chun IK, *et al.* A flat-panel detector based micro-CT system: performance evaluation for small-animal imaging. *Phys Med Biol* 2003; **48**: 4173–85.

34. Conover DL, Ning R, Yu Y, *et al.* Small animal imaging using a flat panel detector-based cone beam computed tomography (FPD-CBCT) imaging system. *Proc SPIE* 2005; **5745**: 307–18. DOI: 10.1117/12.595582.

35. Stock M, Pasler M, Birkfellner W, *et al.* Image quality and stability of image-guided radiotherapy (IGRT) devices: a comparative study. *Radiother Oncol* 2009; **93**: 1–7.

36. Boone JM, Shah N, Nelson TR. A comprehensive analysis of DgN(CT) coefficients for pendant-geometry cone-beam breast computed tomography. *Med Phys* 2004; **31**: 226–35.

37. Thacker SC, Glick SJ. Normalized glandular dose (DgN) coefficients for flat-panel CT breast imaging. *Phys Med Biol* 2004; **49**: 5433–44.

38. Pan X, Siewerdsen J, La Riviere PJ, Kalender WA. Anniversary paper. Development of x-ray computed tomography: the role of medical physics and AAPM from the 1970s to present. *Med Phys* 2008; **35**: 3728–39.

39. World Health Organization. Breast cancer: prevention and control, 2011. www.who.int/cancer/detection/breastcancer/en/index1.html (accessed April 2012).

40. International Agency for Research on Cancer. *World Cancer Report.* Lyon: IARC, 2008.

41. Jackson VP, Hendrick RE, Feig SA, Kopans DB. Imaging of the radiographically dense breast. *Radiology* 1993; **188**: 297–301.

42. Mandelson MT, Oestreicher N, Porter PL, *et al.* Breast density as a predictor of mammographic detection: comparison of interval- and screen-detected cancers. *J Natl Cancer Inst* 2000; **92**: 1081–7.

43. Bird RE, Wallace TW, Yankaskas BC. Analysis of cancers missed at screening mammography. *Radiology* 1992; **184**: 613–17.

44. Berg WA, Gutierrez L, NessAiver MS, *et al.* Diagnostic accuracy of mammography, clinical examination, US, and MR imaging in preoperative assessment of breast cancer. *Radiology* 2004; **233**: 830–49.

45. Gong X. A computer simulation study comparing lesion detection accuracy with digital mammography, breast tomosynthesis, and cone-beam CT breast imaging. *Med Phys* 2006; **33**: 1041–52.

46. Raylman RR, Abraham J, Hazard H, *et al.* Initial clinical test of a breast-PET scanner. *J Med Imaging Radiat Oncol* 2011; **55**: 58–64.

47. Bowen SL, Wu Y, Chaudhari AJ, *et al.* Initial characterization of a dedicated breast PET/CT scanner during human imaging. *J Nucl Med* 2009; **50**: 1401–8.

48. Curpen BN, Sickles EA, Sollitto RA, *et al.* The comparative value of mammographic screening for women 40–49 years old versus women 50–64 years old. *AJR Am J Roentgenol* 1995; **164**: 1099–103.

49. Arnesson LG, Vitak B, Manson JC, Fagerberg G, Smeds S. Diagnostic outcome of repeated mammography screening. *World J Surg* 1995; **19**: 372–7.

50. Jong RA, Yaffe MJ, Skarpathiotakis M, *et al.* Contrast-enhanced digital mammography: initial clinical experience. *Radiology* 2003; **228**: 842–50.

51. Cai G, Hu WG, Chen JY, *et al.* Impact of residual and intrafractional errors on strategy of correction for image-guided accelerated partial breast irradiation. *Radiat Oncol* 2010; **5**: 96.

52. Topolnjak R, Sonke JJ, Nijkamp J, *et al.* Breast patient setup error assessment: comparison of electronic portal image devices and cone-beam computed tomography matching results. *Int J Radiat Oncol Biol Phys* 2010; **78**: 1235–43.

53. Hasan Y, Kim L, Wloch J, *et al.* Comparison of planned versus actual dose delivered for external beam accelerated partial breast irradiation using cone-beam CT and deformable registration. *Int J Radiat Oncol Biol Phys* 2011; **80**: 1473–6.

54. Topolnjak R, de Ruiter P, Remeijer P, *et al.* Image-guided radiotherapy for breast cancer patients: surgical clips as surrogate for breast excision cavity. *Int J Radiat Oncol Biol Phys* 2011; **81**: e187–95.

55. He W, Huda W, Magill D, Tavrides E, Yao H. Patient doses and projection angle in cone beam CT. *Med Phys* 2010; **37**: 2359–68.

56. Winey B, Zygmanski P, Lyatskaya Y. Evaluation of radiation dose delivered by cone beam CT and tomosynthesis employed for setup of external breast irradiation. *Med Phys* 2009; **36**: 164–73.

57. Cai W, Ning R, Conover D. Scatter correction for clinical cone beam CT breast imaging based on breast phantom studies. *J Xray Sci Technol* 2011; **19**: 91–109.

58. Keyrilainen J, Fernandez M, Bravin A, *et al.* Comparison of in vitro breast cancer visibility in analyser-based computed tomography with histopathology, mammography, computed tomography and magnetic resonance imaging. *J Synchrotron Radiat* 2011; **18**: 689–96.

Cases

Michael N. Linver and Robert D. Rosenberg

Introduction

Tamara Miner Haygood

This chapter is an atlas of digital mammography intended to introduce the reader to the appearance of various benign and malignant entities as they may appear on digital imaging. Cases 1–17 were contributed by Robert D. Rosenberg, and cases 18–34 are from Michael N. Linver.

Dr. Rosenberg's practice switched from film-screen mammography to computed radiographic technique using Fuji equipment with 50 μm pixel size, and approximately two years later switched again to Hologic direct digital radiographic technique with a 70 μm pixel size. Therefore, his digital images are a combination of these two image types. When it makes a difference which type of image is being shown, the Fuji computed radiographic images are designated as CR images, and the Hologic direct digital radiographic images as DR images.

Dr. Linver's practice moved from film-screen mammography directly to Hologic direct digital mammography with a 70 μm pixel size, so all of his digital mammography images are obtained with that equipment.

Digital Mammography: A Practical Approach, ed. Gary J. Whitman and Tamara Miner Haygood. Published by Cambridge University Press.
© Cambridge University Press 2013.

Case 1: Typical infiltrating ductal cancer
BI-RADS assessment: category 5

(a)

(b)

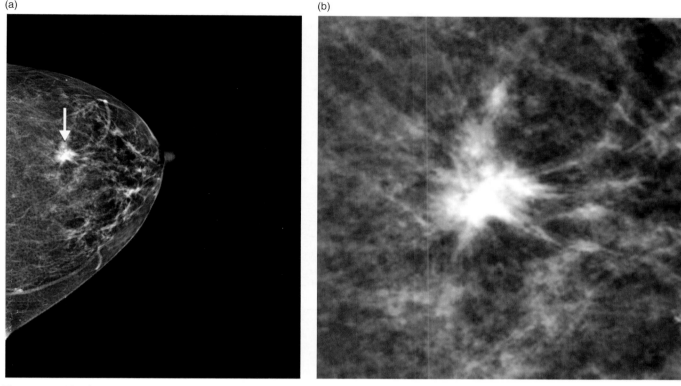

Figure 13.1 (a) Left CC view: arrow on spiculated mass. (b) Close-up of spiculated mass.

Finding

Spiculated mass.

Background

Screening mammogram, 65-year-old patient with normal 2-year-old comparisons.

Pathology

Grade II invasive ductal carcinoma, not otherwise specified.

Teaching points

There is a spiculated mass in the left breast (Figures 13.1a, 13.1b). The spicules may be better depicted on digital mammograms due to edge enhancement. While there are no calcifications in this case, ductal carcinoma in situ (DCIS) with or without calcifications may be found nearby at pathology. Typically these cancers are seen on ultrasound as hypoechoic masses with an irregular echogenic margin and are amenable to biopsy with ultrasound guidance.

This is a typical appearance of a screen-detected breast cancer. The larger the mass, the easier it is to detect, but frequently the shape of the lesion is similar; it just enlarges. Benign masses with this appearance would include post-surgical scars or other trauma. However, without a clear history of a specific trauma, biopsy is indicated. It is often useful, therefore, to get a mammogram after excisional biopsy to establish a new baseline for the next screening study, or to follow suspected abscesses closely clinically or with imaging.

Case 2: Inflammatory mass
BI-RADS assessment: category 4B

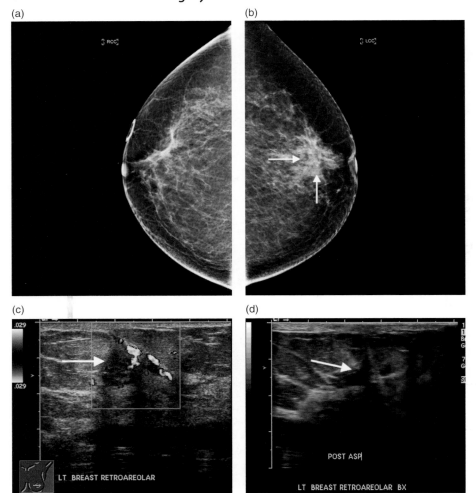

(a)

(b)

(c)

(d)

Figure 13.2 (a) Right CC view: the normal breast. (b) Left CC view: arrows point to spiculated mass. (c) Left breast ultrasound: arrow points to hypoechoic lesion with hyperemic rim. (d) Left breast ultrasound after aspiration: arrow shows a much smaller hypoechoic lesion.

Finding

Irregular mass and asymmetry on mammography. Ultrasound demonstrates a complex cystic lesion.

Background

This patient was sent for a diagnostic mammogram because of a palpable breast mass. She had also been recently treated for infection, so the breast was mildly tender at the time of the mammogram. The patient did not relay her history of infection to the radiologist until immediately before the biopsy. The "mass" was aspirated to confirm pus. If the mass did not aspirate, a biopsy or early follow-up would be necessary, as cancer is the next most likely etiology in this setting. Aspiration was done with a 13 G introducer, often used for coaxial biopsy for a 14 G needle. The ability to aspirate thick fluids is greatly enhanced with a larger needle, and if no pus was aspirated, biopsy through the introducer could have been quickly accomplished.

Pathology

White cells on Gram stain; no organisms on culture.

Teaching points

Asymmetry in the retroareolar area (Figure 13.2b, arrows) may be harder to recognize because of the complexity of the area, although this case shows a relatively large mass on the left. Minor changes in positioning will also complicate findings, as the nipple commonly appears as a "mass" in this area. The ultrasound demonstrates an obvious mass with at least low-level echoes, and increased flow at Doppler only at its borders (Figure 13.2c). The post-biopsy images show a markedly smaller mass, with the abscess wall remaining (Figure 13.2d).

Although this is a common area for breast abscesses, infections may mimic cancer. Aspiration with antibiotics may be curative, although some patients require open surgical drainage. Inflammatory breast cancer, an uncommon presentation of cancer, may mimic infection.

Case 3: Oil cyst
BI-RADS assessment: category 2

(a)

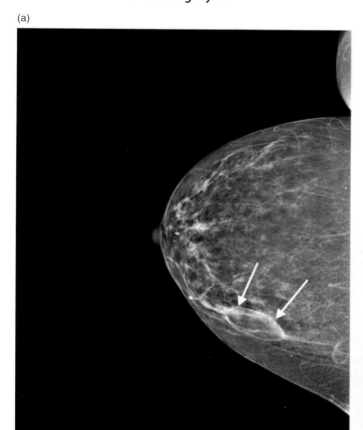

(b)

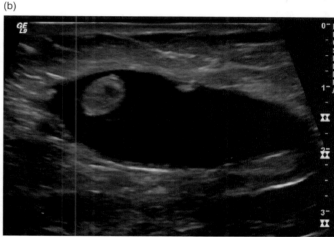

Figure 13.3 (a) Right CC view: arrows point to a fat-density mass in the medial breast. (b) Ultrasound: oil cyst.

Finding

A large fat-containing mass on mammogram (Figure 13.3a, arrows) corresponds to the ultrasound finding. The ultrasound images demonstrate a complex cyst with a mural nodule and subtle low-level echoes (Figure 13.3b). Evidence of blood flow at Doppler was absent.

Background

This patient had a recently diagnosed breast cancer in the opposite breast, and the oil cyst was noted as a palpable abnormality. Her history of previous benign surgery resulting in the oil cyst was not known at the time of ultrasound.

The ultrasound images are of a complex cyst, one with cystic and seemingly solid elements. The mammogram study was benign, with a fat-containing mass only. MRI study (not shown) was entirely benign in this area.

Pathology

No biopsy was performed on this case.

Teaching points

Digital mammography clearly demonstrated an entirely fatty mass, and further history confirmed surgery as the cause. This case illustrates the frequently complementary information of mammography and ultrasound.

Ultrasound of a fat-containing palpable mass may be misleading. A mammogram may be helpful with location correlation using a BB or other skin marker. The upper inner quadrants of the breasts are a common area for oil cysts, probably from the shoulder harness of seat belts. The traumatic incident is frequently forgotten and the breast mass develops later. Occasionally in younger patients an oil cyst or fat necrosis with a palpable mass on ultrasound may trigger biopsy. Fat necrosis may mimic cancer on MRI if seen at a stage prior to complete evolution to a fully formed oil cyst.

Case 4: New calcifications
BI-RADS assessment: category 4B

(a)

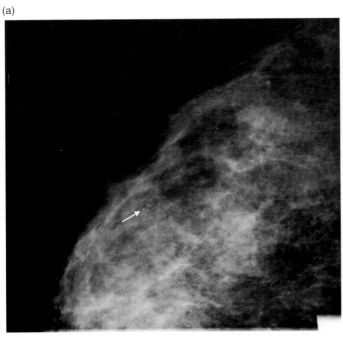

(b)

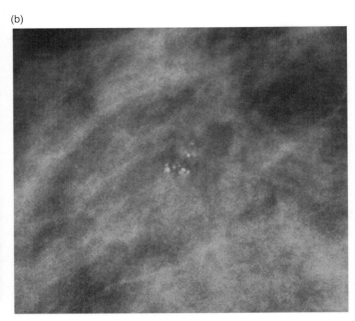

Figure 13.4 (a) Coned right CC view: arrow points to clustered microcalcifications in the lateral breast. (b) Magnification view of the same microcalcifications.

Finding

A new cluster of microcalcifications (Figure 13.4a, arrow). They are minimally pleomorphic, and are not round.

Background

Screening mammogram, with comparisons.

Pathology

Multifocal DCIS.

Teaching points

New or growing non-fatty masses are usually subject to biopsy if they are not shown to be cysts. New calcifications also generate additional concern, but their morphology is particularly important, as many benign findings such as fibrocystic calcifications and involuting fibroadenomas may cause new calcifications and may not necessitate biopsy.

As this case illustrates, calcifications are less specific for histology. While this case was proven to be DCIS, fibroadenomas or proliferative breast processes such as sclerosing adenosis or ductal hyperplasia with or without atypia might appear similar and are more likely causes of calcifications with the features seen here. Calcification analysis is complex: the number of calcifications seen is not a useful feature for distinguishing benign from malignant. Morphology is much more important, with distribution (clustered or segmental, common malignant features, versus diffuse or scattered, common benign features) also a useful criterion. There are many specific types of calcification that can be recognized by experienced mammographers as demonstrating unequivocal benign features and can be followed routinely. The positive predictive value of calcifications is generally lower than for masses. As this case and experience with MRI illustrate, the extent of calcifications on the mammogram may not accurately depict the full extent of DCIS present.

Finally, pathologists struggle with the separation of low-grade DCIS from atypical ductal hyperplasia (ADH) and other proliferative conditions. Since the criteria are not exact, and because pathologists vary in expertise and judgment, the difference in a diagnosis of ADH versus DCIS may be the pathologist interpreting the biopsy. It should come as no surprise, therefore, that the radiologic diagnosis of DCIS is difficult.

Case 5: Benign calcification cluster: comparison of digital and computed mammography
BI-RADS assessment: category 2

(a)

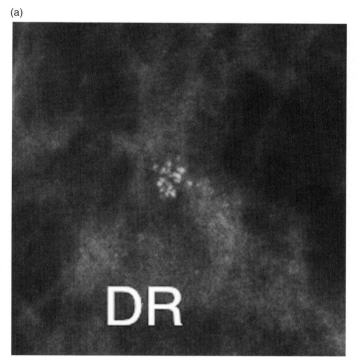

(b)

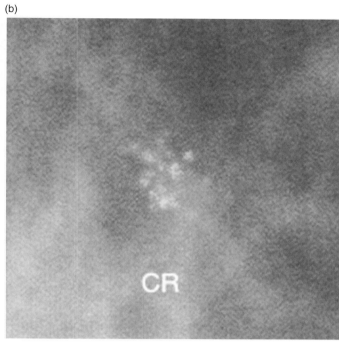

Figure 13.5 (a) DR image of microcalcifications. (b) CR image of the same microcalcifications.

Finding
Clustered calcifications. Round and stable for several years. No associated mass.

Background
Screening mammograms with comparisons.

Pathology
No biopsy performed.

Teaching points
These calcifications may be classified by some as nonspecific, as they lack layering and vary somewhat in size. However, they are all very dense and round without any malignant features and are typical of calcifications located in the lobule. These highly magnified images demonstrate the pixelated nature of digital images (Figure 13.5a). At this magnification level, no calcification looks round and well marginated. The lower resolution and processing of any type of digital mammograms, whether DR or CR, compared to film-screen requires some adjustment in the radiologist's mammography interpretation criteria.

Round calcifications, those that arise from the breast lobules, are benign. Calcifications are ideal candidates for improved detection with image processing of digital mammograms. It seems that many were present in the past but not appreciated/recognized. Careful comparison of the current DR images against prior CR studies (Figure 13.5b) seems to reveal them as previously more subtle, but not necessarily changed in appearance.

A primary value of comparing to prior images is improved specificity of mammography. Finer, smaller calcifications may be more difficult to classify. Unfortunately, the smaller the calcification, the less information is available for analysis. BI-RADS assessment 3 for calcifications should rarely be used, as changes over short periods are unusual, and the likelihood of cancer with these calcifications seems very low in the few published series.

Finally, digital mammography and computer-aided detection (CADe) have made calcifications more apparent and easier to find. One important caution is that as the digital images are edge-enhanced, making a comparison with film-screen images or even differently processed images may be difficult. One approach is to try to discern if the now obvious calcifications are actually changed in number and extent, rather than just having been made to look more obvious by the digital processing.

Case 6: Discordant biopsy and radial scar
BI-RADS assessment: category 4B

(a)

(b)

(c)

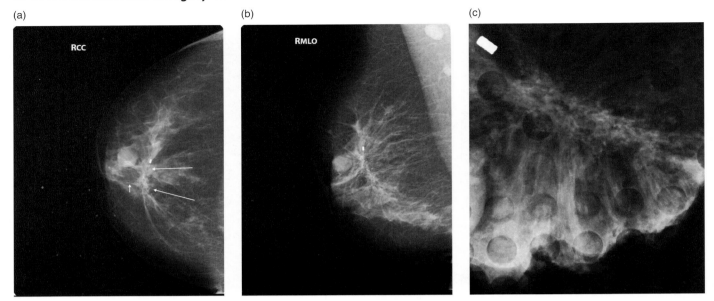

Figure 13.6 (a) Right CC view: long arrows show architectural distortion. Small arrow shows one of the many radiating lines; marker clip is visible. (b) Right MLO view of the same architectural distortion. (c) Specimen radiograph after excisional biopsy: the marker clip is visible, which confirms that the area in question was removed.

Finding

This is a classic if unusually large architectural distortion (Figure 13.6a, long arrows). It has little if any central mass, with fat within the center and many radiating lines (Figure 13.6a, short arrow).

Background

This area of architectural distortion was visible on both CC and MLO (Figure 13.6b) views. The lesion was initially subjected to a large-core biopsy, with the marker left on one end of the lesion and visible in all accompanying figures. The core biopsy was benign without atypia, but no specific histopathologic diagnosis was made. The pathology results were deemed discordant, and an excisional biopsy was performed (Figure 13.6c). In addition to the architectural distortion, there was a round, smooth mass located between the architectural distortion and the nipple. This incidental mass had been present for several years and was stable.

Pathology

Radial scar, no atypia. The incidental mass was confirmed to be benign as well.

Teaching points

Radiologic–pathologic correlation is critical for image-guided core biopsy. In this case, the initial core biopsy results were benign and nonspecific and thus discordant with the imaging findings.

Core biopsy has been shown in expert hands to be as accurate as needle localization, but it also requires recognition of occasional discordant lesions that may have been incompletely sampled. In this case, the mammographic finding is likely benign, but approximately 15% of lesions showing typical features of a radial scar may be tubular cancers. Radial scars with associated calcifications may have a higher incidence of DCIS. The radial scars are often considered high-risk lesions, and are usually subject to excisional biopsy. Some experts will initially use needle localization for this type of finding, although there is variability in approach. Also, smaller radial scars may not be as classic as in this case, and undergo core biopsy as the initial interventional diagnostic procedure. Excisional biopsy is often done in those cases, but often depends on clinician, pathologist, and radiologist preferences as well as the presence or absence of other risk factors.

Case 7: Palpable masses

BI-RADS assessment: category 4A

(a)

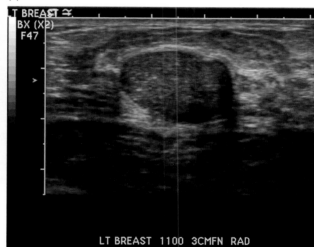

(b)

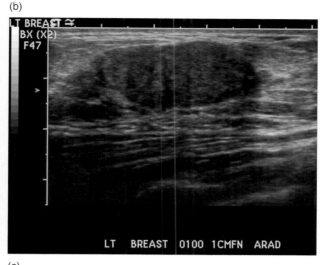

(c)

Figure 13.7 (a) Left CC view, with BBs indicating palpable masses. (b) Breast ultrasound with hypoechoic mass at 1 o'clock. (c) Breast ultrasound with hypoechoic mass at 11 o'clock.

Finding

Extremely dense mammograms, mass medially with partially obscured border, and laterally a vague asymmetry only in the area of symptoms for the lesion. Ultrasound demonstrated the two lesions as large, solid, well-marginated oval masses without malignant features.

Background

A young, symptomatic patient with two palpable breast masses in the left breast on physical examination.

Pathology

There were two masses identified on ultrasound. One was a pseudoangiomatous stromal hyperplasia (PASH) at 1 o'clock (Figure 13.7b); the other was a fibroadenoma (11 o'clock lesion) (Figure 13.7c).

Teaching points

Digital mammograms were not very helpful in identifying the pathology in this case. The ultrasound easily demonstrated two masses, with probably benign features for both the 11 o'clock mass and the 1 o'clock mass (thin echogenic capsule, not as complete as for the 11 o'clock lesion).

Even though digital mammography had improved sensitivity in dense tissues in the DMIST trial, palpable masses in patients with dense breast tissue on mammography require ultrasound imaging. By history the masses in this case were enlarging, and, given their size, biopsy was performed. Many patients, especially young ones, express a preference for biopsy of palpable masses, even small ones with features of a benign fibroadenoma, for reassurance. There is evidence that for experienced breast imagers, palpability does not significantly alter the likelihood of a lesion being malignant.

Case 8: Low-grade DCIS
BI-RADS assessment: category 4B

(a)

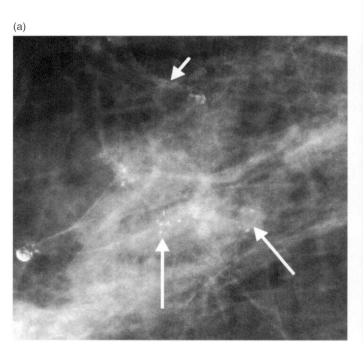

(b)

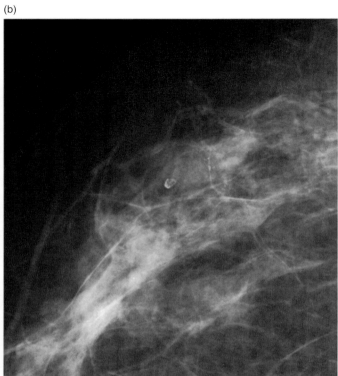

(c)

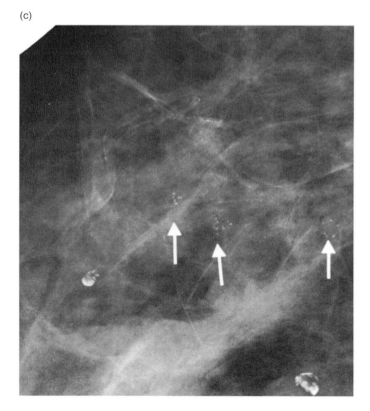

Figure 13.8 (a) Coned right CC view, with longer arrows pointing out microcalcifications. Short arrow demonstrates typically benign calcifications. (b) Right CC view obtained the previous year in the same area. (c) Magnification view.

Finding

There are minimally pleomorphic clustered calcifications (Figure 13.8a, long arrows), new from 2009 (Figure 13.8b). Several typical benign calcifications are also present nearby (Figure 13.8a, arrow head and short arrow). The magnification view defines all of the calcifications better, including the distinct multiple clusters (Figure 13.8c, arrows).

Background

Screening mammogram with comparisons, followed by magnification images.

Pathology

Low-grade DCIS.

Teaching points

These new calcifications are indeterminant but relatively problematic, as they are clustered and appear to be changing over time. No associated mass is present. There is a benign, coarse group of calcifications nearby, typical for a degenerating fibroadenoma, and there are vascular calcifications as well.

Digital images are best for detection of the calcifications, but not necessarily better for analysis. The magnification views are of help in confirming the calcifications, but the calcification size is near the limits of resolution of the DR system, with each calcification requiring a handful of pixels on the imaging detector device. The screening images demonstrate some bright individual pixels of noise simulating calcifications. Most biopsies of this type of calcification would be benign.

Case 9: Fibrocystic calcifications
BI-RADS assessment: category 2

(a)

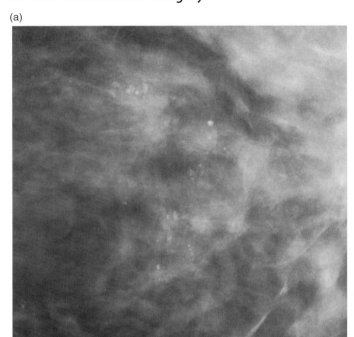

(b)

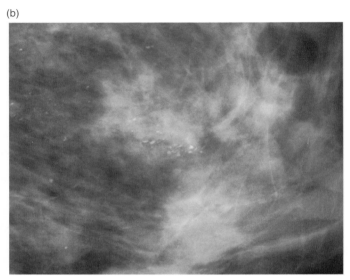

Figure 13.9 (a) Magnification image of calcifications in CC projection. (b) Magnification image of calcifications in LM projection showing layering of the calcifications.

Finding

Round calcifications on CC view (Figure 13.9a), and layering calcifications on lateral view (Figure 13.9b). This combination of features is known as "teacups and saucers," or "teacups and pearls." Many of the calcification shapes change dramatically between the two views.

Background

Screening mammogram with additional magnification images.

Pathology

Milk of calcium, no biopsy performed.

Teaching points

Layering is a benign finding diagnostic of fibrocystic calcifications known as milk of calcium. The CC views may not show calcifications as well as the MLO view as there is less density through the thin layer. On the MLO view they often look pleomorphic as some are more linear, some rounder with varying density. On 90-degree lateral views, where the x-ray beam passes through the maximum amount of calcification, and where the calcium will layer parallel to the path of the x-ray beam, the layering property is manifest and easily seen. Biopsy is not indicated in these cases. Another problem in evaluating calcifications is that there are often multiple clusters, and one can find it confusing when attempting to determine which cluster on one view is the same as which cluster on the other view. Clusters also may overlap on one view, further complicating the assessment. Occasionally, step oblique images are required to clarify which cluster is which.

Case 10: Architectural distortion
BI-RADS assessment: category 4B

(a)   (b)

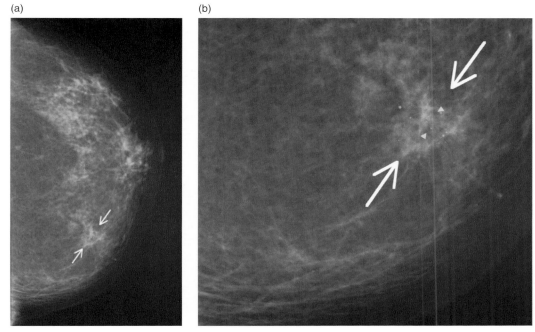

Figure 13.10 (a) Left CC view: arrows show small area of architectural distortion. (b) Coned left CC view.

Finding

Architectural distortion with several small calcifications (Figures 13.10a, 13.10b, arrows). The lesion is spiculated, with the spicules best seen on the anterior border, and the lesion clearly contains fat centrally.

Background

Screening mammogram.

Pathology

Radial scar. No DCIS.

Teaching points

Radial scars are subtle lesions to detect. In this case, cancer was not found, but tubular cancers or infiltrating lobular cancer may present similarly. Lesions with these features may be thought of as non-mass-like lesions, a term borrowed from breast MRI. The tissue pattern in these lesions is not a completely normal one, and they are of low density, similar to normal breast tissue, and without typical mass features. These may also be described as asymmetries.

Case 11: Secretory calcifications: comparison between DR and film-screen images
BI-RADS assessment: category 2

(a)

(b)

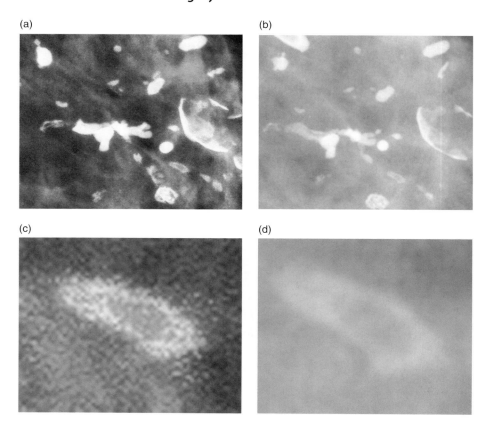

(c)

(d)

Figure 13.11 (a) Digital image of secretory calcifications. (b) Film-screen image of secretory calcifications. (c) Closely coned digital image of one of these calcifications. (d) Closely coned film-screen image of one of these calcifications.

Finding

This demonstrates many periductal and intraductal benign secretory calcifications.

Background

DR screening mammogram with film-screen comparison images.

Pathology

The lesion is benign and was not biopsied.

Teaching points

The calcifications are typical benign secretory calcifications. These may be periductal, which surround a duct and therefore have lucent centers or ductal, which usually are solid. While some ductal calcifications are considered worrisome, these dense linear calcifications are benign. Occasionally in their early development secretory calcifications might be confused with comedo-type malignant calcifications; however, such a situation would be unusual.

The DR and film-screen images are different, reflecting primarily the processing of digital images (Figures 13.11a, 13.11b). The highly magnified views demonstrate the pixels that make up digital images, clearly larger than the grain size of film-screen images (Figures 13.11c, 13.11d). A scanning artifact is present on the larger film-screen image as a white line.

Case 12: Low exposure
BI-RADS assessment: NA – technical issue

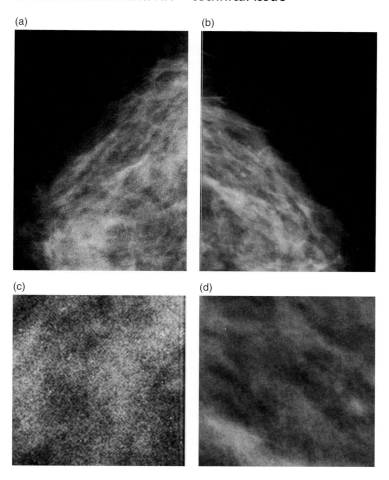

(a) (b) (c) (d)

Figure 13.12 (a) Coned right CC view, 9 mAs. (b) Coned left CC view, 90 mAs. (c) Close-up: zoomed view of a portion of the right CC. (d) Close-up: zoomed view of a portion of the left CC.

Finding
In this case, the two CC views had a 10-fold difference in exposures, with approximately 9 mAs for one (Figures 13.12a, 13.12c) versus 90 mAs for the other (Figures 13.12b, 13.12d). This difference was most obvious when the images were zoomed larger, with the right CC being distinctly more noisy than the left CC.

Background
With film-screen images, the degree of exposure is clearly demonstrated by the brightness of the images: overexposure is dark, and underexposure light. With digital imaging, the software automatically sets the window width and level for each image, and adjusts for the actual exposure, "fixing" the image. It was not clear what caused the photo-timer to cut off too early for one image.

Pathology
None.

Teaching points
Underexposure is more difficult to see on digital imaging than on film-screen imaging, as software "fixes" the differences in brightness and contrast. A decrease in contrast-to-noise ratio is the result.

Digital images generally contain all of the exposure parameters in the DICOM headers, but may not display them on the images unless prompted. Each digital system has a digital exposure value, often the "S" number also displayed on the images. Unfortunately, the digital systems do not flag an improperly exposed image.

Increasing the exposure will not result in darker images but does result in less noise on the images. Calcifications seem most sensitive to this phenomenon. Thus, increasing the exposure indices of magnification images through the use of higher kVp or mAs may improve the appearance of calcifications in borderline cases. This technique may also be useful with the spot digital systems employed in stereotactic biopsy.

For the same reason, a diffusely denser breast from edema or diffuse tumor involvement will look similar to the normal side: the digital system applies the "correct" contrast and density setting to the abnormal side. Skin thickening may be the only imaging sign to indicate the underlying pathology present. A review of the technical factors, especially kVp and mAs, at the time of interpretation will confirm this problem and avoid serious interpretation errors. An experienced technologist may also bring this situation to the physician's attention.

Case 13: Silicone "mass"

BI-RADS assessment: category 2

(a)

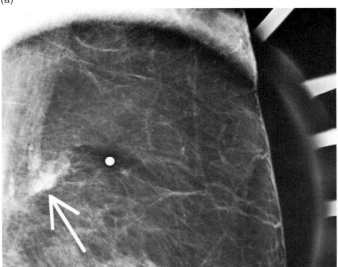

(b)

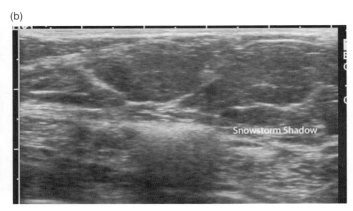

Figure 13.13 (a) Spot compression view in the MLO projection. (b) Ultrasound of the palpable abnormality.

Finding

There is a small, dense, irregular mass corresponding to a palpable abnormality.

Background

The patient had prior surgery for implant removal and noticed a new mass recently.

Pathology

Not biopsied, but typical for silicone in the soft tissues.

Teaching points

A small, irregular mass is seen on mammogram (Figure 13.13a, arrow) and corresponds to the palpable abnormality indicated by the BB on this spot compression oblique DR image. The ultrasound finding of a "snowstorm" appearance is indicative of free silicone. The snowstorm finding is quite sensitive for detecting free silicone near ruptured implants or after implant removal, or for detecting silicone trapped within regional lymph nodes. Air within the soft tissues may sometimes give a similar appearance.

Case 14: Fibroadenoma calcifications

BI-RADS assessment: category 2

(a)

(b)

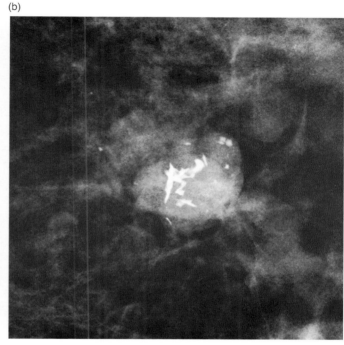

Figure 13.14 (a) CR coned image of a typical fibroadenoma. (b) DR coned image of the same typical fibroadenoma.

Finding

Popcorn calcifications.

Background

Screening mammogram with comparison images.

Pathology

Not biopsied, but a typical benign fibroadenoma.

Teaching points

This case illustrates both CR and DR images of a typical benign involuting fibroadenoma (Figures 13.14a, 13.14b). The DR images are more processed, giving more contrast and edge enhancement than the CR images, which are closer in appearance to conventional film-screen images. The calcifications in this case are classic for this benign entity, but often in the early stages of development the calcifications within fibroadenomas are pleomorphic or crushed-stone in appearance, indistinguishable from DCIS. Cancer arising from a fibroadenoma is rare.

Case 15: Developing density
BI-RADS assessment: category 4B

(a)

(b)

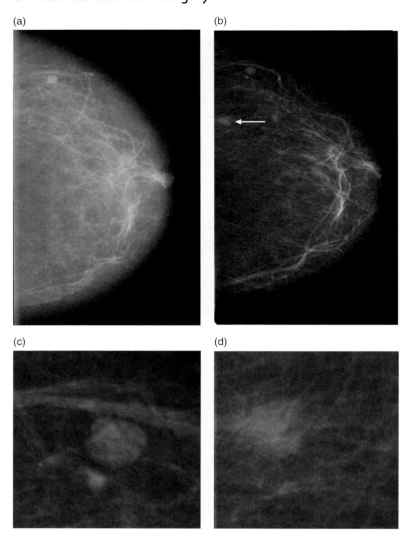

Figure 13.15 (a) Comparison left CC view, 2009. (b) Left CC view, 2010. (c) Close-up of the benign lymph node. (d) Close-up of the new, small mass.

(c)

(d)

Finding
Developing mass and benign lymph node.

Background
Screening mammography from 2010, with comparison images from 2009.

Pathology
Mucinous or colloid cancer.

Teaching points
The comparison image (Figure 13.15a) shows a benign lymph node. The new mammogram has a new mass that was readily apparent on the CC view (Figure 13.15b, arrow) but was seen as only a vague developing area on the MLO image (not shown). Additional imaging documented the mass on spot MLO mammogram but failed to demonstrate it on targeted ultrasound. Biopsy was therefore done with stereotactic guidance.

This case is a good example of the juxtaposition of a benign well-marginated lymph node with a small cancer. The cancer (Figure 13.15d) lacks the definitive sharp margins of the lymph node (Figure 13.15c), emphasizing the sometimes subtle differences between a benign mass and a well-marginated cancer. Because this mass was new, it should not qualify as a BI-RADS 3 (probably benign finding). Colloid cancer is one of the benign-appearing masses found in the 1–2% of masses assigned to BI-RADS category 3 that ultimately prove to be malignant. Some of the more common benign entities presenting as developing masses include cysts, fibroadenomas (usually in premenopausal patients), and pseudoangiomatous stromal hyperplasia (PASH).

Case 16: Calcifications captured three ways
BI-RADS assessment: NA – technical issue

(a) (b) (c)

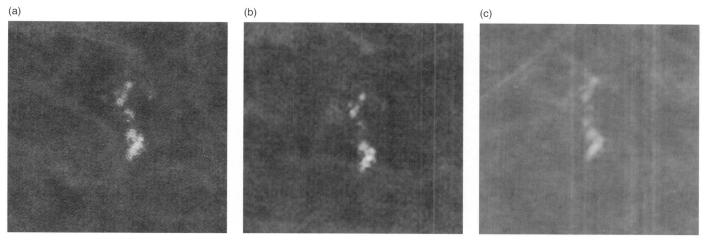

Figure 13.16 (a) CR image of microcalcifications obtained with system operating with 50 µm pixel size. (b) CR image of microcalcifications obtained with system operating with 100 µm pixel size. (c) Scanned film-screen image of the same microcalcifications.

Finding
Stable calcifications for several years in a screening mammography patient.

Background
This same group of calcifications was captured three ways: on CR at both 50 and 100 µm pixel size (Figures 13.16a, 13.16b), and on a film-screen mammogram image subsequently scanned at higher resolution (Figure 13.16c).

Pathology
None.

Teaching points
The pixilation of the images varies significantly. Although they are of lower resolution, the digital images make detection of the calcifications easier. However, analysis of fine detail is somewhat better on film-screen mammography.

Case 17: Pseudo calcifications
BI-RADS assessment: NA – technical issue

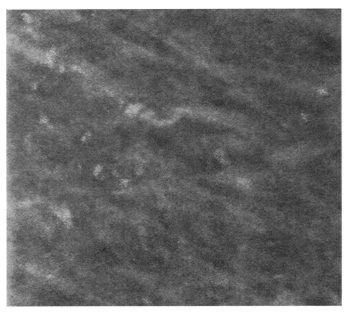

Figure 13.17 Coned digital image showing microcalcifications that disappeared on subsequent diagnostic evaluation.

Finding

Numerous pleomorphic calcifications noted near the inframammary fold. These disappeared on subsequent imaging.

Background

Screening mammogram and immediate workup study.

Pathology

None.

Teaching points

These "calcifications" were not present on immediate callback imaging. Given their appearance and location, a foreign substance on the patient's skin is the likely culprit. The enhanced detection of subtle edges and density differences with digital mammography make it more sensitive in demonstrating external artifacts.

The axillary region is the typical location for talc or other deodorant artifacts. Other skin findings including moles may contain calcifications which can sometimes be confused with DCIS within the breast. In this case, the inframammary fold contained a foreign substance, which appeared on the images in a form suggesting worrisome calcifications.

Case 18: Cyst aspirations with pneumocystograms
BI-RADS assessment: category 2

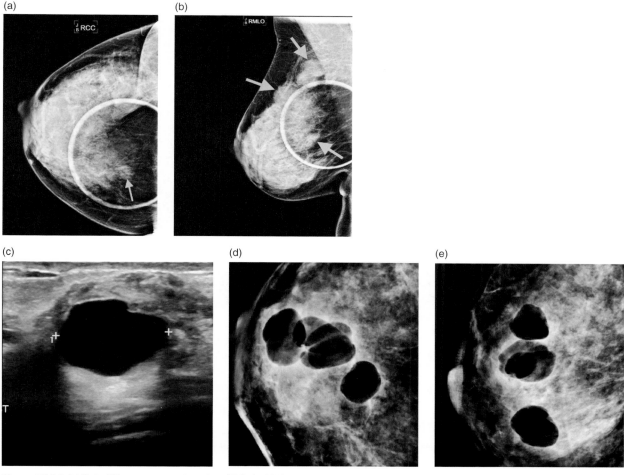

(a) (b)

(c) (d) (e)

Figure 13.18 (a) Right CC spot compression view. (b) Right MLO spot-compression view. (c) Ultrasound: right breast. (d) Pneumocystogram: right CC view. (e) Pneumocystogram: right ML view.

Finding
Multiple circumscribed masses on mammography.

Background
A 55-year-old woman presents with multiple painful palpable masses in the right breast. Diagnostic mammogram with spot compression views showed mass densities with smooth margins around only a portion of some of these masses (Figures 13.18a, 13.18b). Ultrasound showed all of the palpable masses to have features of benign cysts (Figure 13.18c). Because of constant pain, the patient desired cyst aspirations under ultrasound guidance. These were performed, as well as pneumocystography (Figures 13.18d, 13.18e). Aspirated fluid was not sent for pathology, as it was not bloody or purulent. The patient's breast pain subsided completely over the next few weeks.

Pathology
None required.

Teaching points
Pneumocystography is easy to perform and is useful for several reasons. About three-quarters as much air is injected in each cyst as there was fluid removed, and CC and 90-degree mammograms are performed after the procedure for pneumocystography. These images provide a good look at the internal margins of the cysts to ensure their smooth benign nature. Pneumocystography also offers a therapeutic advantage in that cysts very rarely recur after this procedure. Another potential advantage is that if the fluid requires cytologic evaluation and shows abnormal cells, the air will remain as a "marker" for the location of the cyst for approximately one week. Thus, the area of the abnormal cells can be located without use of a marker clip. Pneumocystography is easy to do, and the injected air costs the radiologist and the patient nothing!

Case 19: Skin mole
BI-RADS assessment: NA – technical issue

(a)

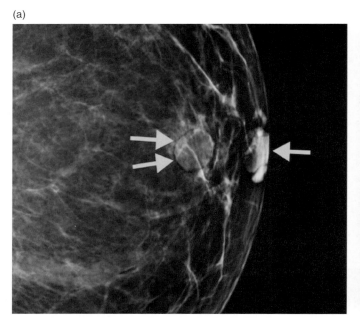

(b)

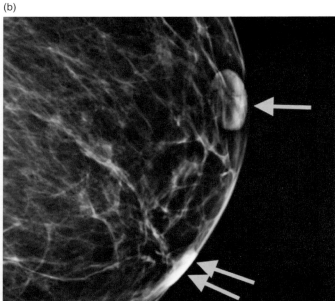

Figure 13.19 (a) Left CC view: zoomed image. (b) Left MLO view: zoomed image.

Finding
Circumscribed superficial mass

Background
A 50-year-old woman presents for screening mammogram. On the left CC view (Figure 13.19a), an ovoid, well-circumscribed, bilobed, superficial mass is seen, marked by an arrow. The nipple (marked by two arrows) is not in profile, and also appears as a round, well-circumscribed mass, well outlined by a thin rim of air. On the left MLO view (Figure 13.19b), the breast is properly positioned, with the mass marked again by an arrow, and the nipple (marked by two arrows) in profile. No "mass" is now appreciated at the nipple site. The true superficial mass proved to be a large skin mole.

Pathology
Not relevant.

Teaching points
This case illustrates the clarity in visualizing skin lesions that digital mammography provides. The case also shows the importance of positioning the nipple in profile, so as not to mistake it for a true breast mass.

Case 20: Granulomatous mastitis

BI-RADS assessment: category 4C

(a)

(b)

(c)

(d)

(e)

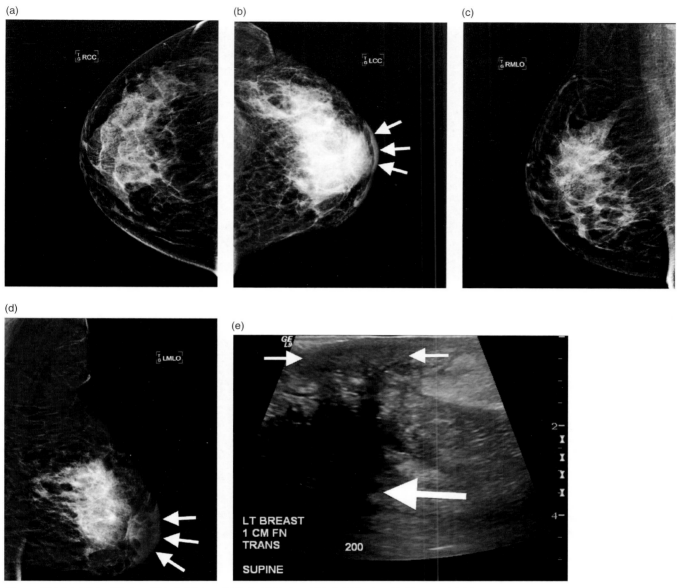

Figure 13.20 (a) Right CC view. (b) Left CC view. (c) Right MLO view. (d) Left MLO view. (e) Ultrasound: left breast.

Finding

Irregular mammographic mass.

Background

This 35-year-old patient presented with a large palpable mass in her left breast. The mammogram shows an irregular dense mass in the left breast with marked skin thickening, marked by arrows (Figures 13.20b, 13.20d). On ultrasound, there is a large, irregular, hypoechoic mass with shadowing (single large arrow) and considerable edema (two smaller arrows) throughout the surrounding tissues (Figure 13.20e).

Pathology

Granulomatous mastitis.

Teaching points

This appearance is worrisome for inflammatory breast cancer, among other possibilities (infection, other invasive cancers). At surgery, this proved to be granulomatous mastitis, a benign condition. However, any lesion with this clinical and imaging presentation must be considered malignant until proven otherwise.

Case 21: Tubular carcinoma
BI-RADS assessment: category 4B

(a)

(b)

(c)

(d)

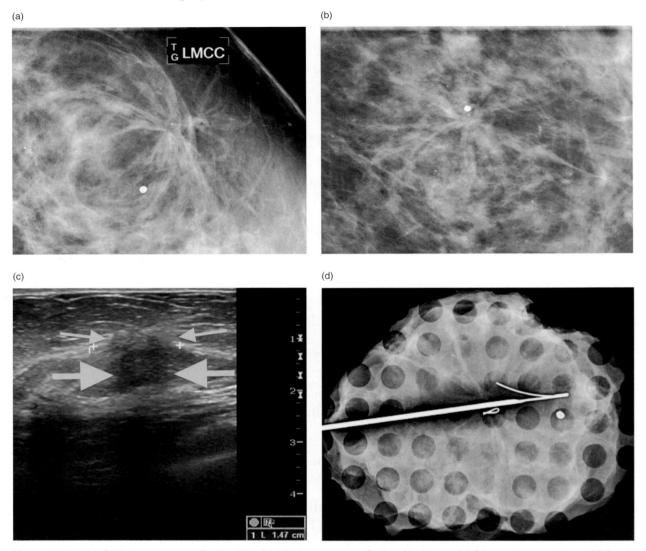

Figure 13.21 (a) Left CC view: spot magnification. (b) Left MLO view: spot magnification. (c) Ultrasound: left breast, transverse image. (d) Specimen radiograph: left breast, surgical specimen.

Finding
Architectural distortion.

Background
A 60-year-old female was recalled from screening for architectural distortion on the left. On spot magnification views, marked distortion is seen, with a few calcifications centrally (Figures 13.21a, 13.21b). On ultrasound, a spiculated, hypoechoic mass (smaller arrows) with posterior shadowing (bigger arrows) is seen (Figure 13.21c). Surgical specimen radiograph confirms the extensive spiculation and calcifications (Figure 13.21d).

Pathology
Tubular carcinoma.

Teaching points
The differential diagnosis in the absence of previous surgery or trauma lies primarily between radial scar and tubular carcinoma. This lesion proved to be a tubular carcinoma.

Note should be made of the large black "bloom" artifact around the needle on the specimen radiograph (Figure 13.21d). This artifact is created by excessive edge enhancement around very dense objects with digital imaging, and can potentially hide significant pathology within the "bloom" created around these objects.

Case 22: Invasive ductal carcinoma with high-grade DCIS

BI-RADS assessment: category 5

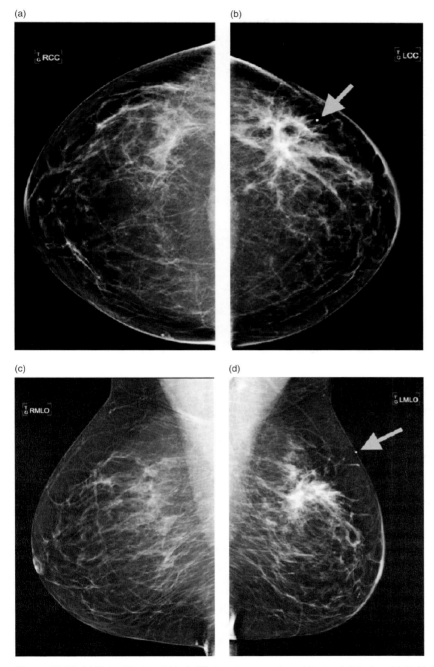

(a)

(b)

(c)

(d)

Figure 13.22 (a) Right CC view. (b) Left CC view. Arrow marks architectural distortion. (c) Right MLO view. (d) Left MLO view. Arrow points towards architectural distortion. (e) Left CC view: spot magnification. Arrows denote area of microcalcifications. (f) Ultrasound: left breast, with calipers on the outer edges of the mass. (g) Ultrasound: left axilla. (h) Bilateral MRI: axial MIP image.

(e)

(f)

(g)

(h)

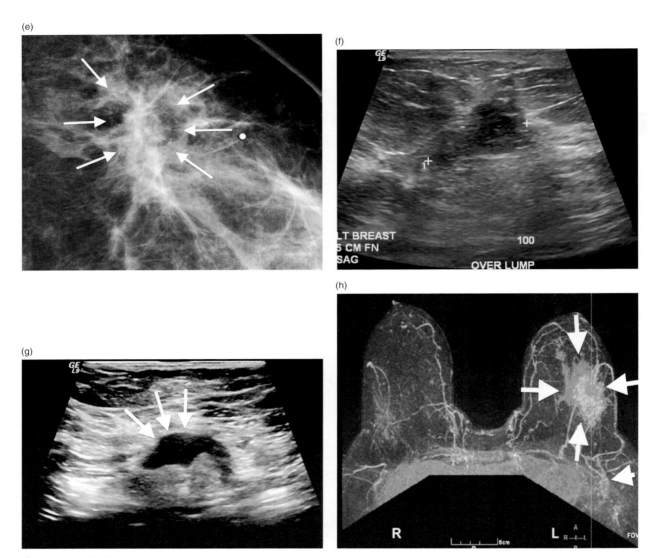

Figure 13.22 (*cont.*)

Finding

Architectural distortion and calcifications.

Background

A 47-year-old woman presented with a palpable lump in the left breast, and a large area of architectural distortion on mammography (Figures 13.22a–13.22d). On spot magnification CC view (Figure 13.22e), the distortion is more obvious, and underlying malignant-appearing calcifications are noted centrally within the tumor, as marked by the arrows. Ultrasound shows a hypoechoic mass here (Figure 13.22f). Ultrasound evaluation of the left axilla shows bulbous expansion of a portion of the cortex of a lymph node, as marked by the arrows, suggesting metastatic involvement (Figure 13.22g).

On MRI (Figure 13.22h), the primary tumor on the left is much larger than on either mammography or ultrasound, measuring at least 6 cm, as marked by the four arrows. The abnormal node in the left axilla is also seen, marked by the single short arrow.

Pathology

Invasive ductal carcinoma with high-grade DCIS, with metastasis to left axillary lymph nodes.

Teaching points

Even large cancers can be difficult to perceive, in the absence of significant mass effect. Digital technique accentuates the architectural distortion and subtle calcifications associated with many cancers, as in this case.

Case 23: Invasive ductal carcinoma, missed on previous digital mammogram due to "gray" images

BI-RADS assessment: category 4C

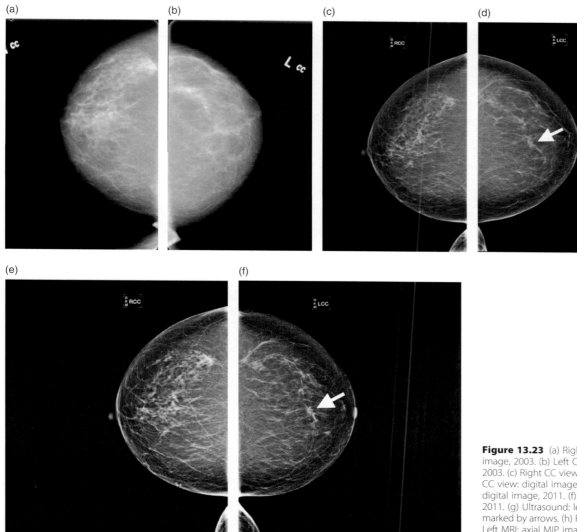

Figure 13.23 (a) Right CC view: film-screen image, 2003. (b) Left CC view: film-screen image, 2003. (c) Right CC view: digital image, 2010. (d) Left CC view: digital image, 2010. (e) Right CC view: digital image, 2011. (f) Left CC view: digital image, 2011. (g) Ultrasound: left breast, 2011. Small mass marked by arrows. (h) Right MRI: axial MIP image. (i) Left MRI: axial MIP image. Satellite lesions marked by arrows with the larger mass between them.

Finding

Spiculated mass.

Background

A 63-year-old female underwent a baseline screening mammogram with film-screen technique in 2003 (Figures 13.23a, 13.23b), interpreted as normal. She returned seven years later, in 2010, at which time a screening digital mammogram was performed, also interpreted as normal (Figures 13.23c, Figures 13.23d). However, in retrospect, there was a subtle new spiculated mass on the left on this study (Figure 13.23d, arrow), made more difficult to perceive because of relatively low contrast on the digital images. When she returned for her screening mammogram the next year, in 2011, the digital image algorithms had been modified for much higher contrast (Figures 13.23e, 13.23f). The spiculated mass on the left (Figure 13.23f, arrow) had changed very little since the previous digital mammogram, but this year was much easier to perceive. This was detected at screening at this time, with diagnostic workup including ultrasound, which showed a hypoechoic irregular mass (Figure 13.23g, arrows). Breast MRI showed the spiculated

Figure 13.23 (cont.)

(g)

(h)

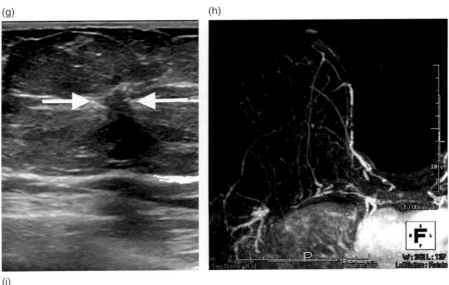

(i)

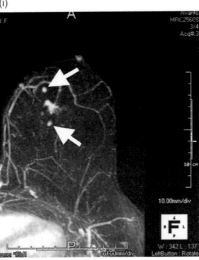

mammographic mass as expected, but also demonstrated two tiny satellite lesions (Figures 13.23h, 13.23i, arrows), not seen on either mammography or ultrasound.

Pathology

Invasive ductal carcinoma, multifocal.

Teaching points

Differences in display parameters on digital images can create difficulties in perceiving pathology. In this case, it appears that a subtle new cancer on the 2010 digital mammogram was missed in part because of relatively low contrast on the digital images.

Case 24: Invasive lobular carcinoma

BI-RADS assessment: category 5

(a)

(b)

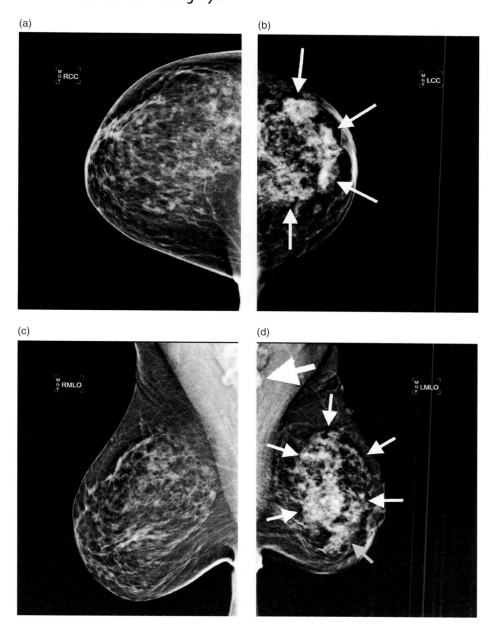

(c)

(d)

Figure 13.24 (a) Right CC view. (b) Left CC view. (c) Right MLO view. (d) Left MLO view. (e) Repeat left MLO view. (f) Ultrasound: left breast. (g) Ultrasound: left axilla. (h) Right MRI: axial MIP image. (i) Left MRI: axial MIP image.

Finding

Shrinking breast and multiple masses.

Background

A 49-year-old woman presents with a firm left breast. On the initial mammograms (Figures 13.24a–13.24d), there is marked increased density with architectural distortion and suspected masses throughout the left breast (small arrows). The breast also appears markedly smaller than the right, with some skin thickening as well. Note that on the left MLO view, the axilla shows an incompletely imaged lymph node medially (Figure 13.24d, larger arrow). A repeat MLO view demonstrates the lymph node completely (Figure 13.24e, arrow), with an absent fatty hilum now appreciated, a worrisome sign for metastatic tumor in the node. On ultrasound, the irregular mass/masses throughout the left breast are seen (Figure 13.24f), with extensive

(e)   (f)   (g)

(h)   (i)

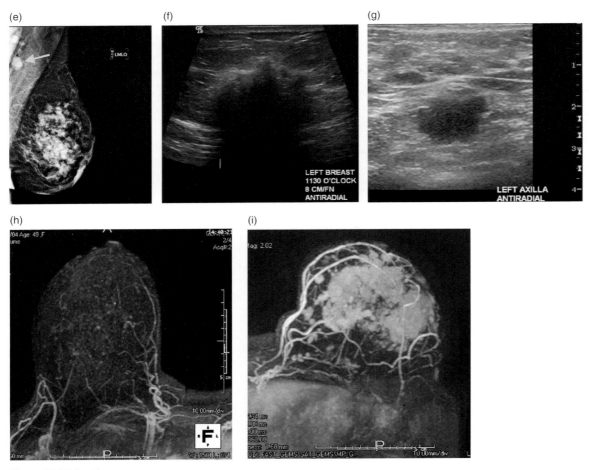

Figure 13.24 (cont.)

posterior shadowing, consistent with the mammographic and clinical findings. Left axilla ultrasound shows a markedly abnormal lymph node, with irregular margins, and no fatty hilum (Figure 13.24g), consistent with the findings on mammogram. Breast MRI shows the shrunken left breast filled with a large vascular enhancing mass (Figure 13.24i).

Pathology

Invasive lobular carcinoma, with metastatic involvement of left axillary lymph nodes.

Teaching points

The "shrinking breast" is a finding associated most frequently with invasive lobular carcinoma, although invasive ductal carcinoma can present this way as well. Often, the breast will not appear shrunken clinically, and only appears so on mammography because of its lack of compressibility compared to the normal side.

Even in digital mammography, positioning remains vitally important in displaying potential pathology. Here, the abnormal lymph node in the left axilla was initially almost completely cut off by suboptimal positioning.

Case 25: Large hamartoma
BI-RADS assessment: category 2

(a)

(b)

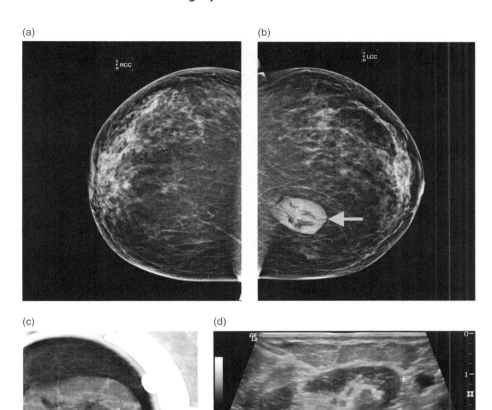

Figure 13.25 (a) Right CC view. (b) Left CC view. (c) Left CC: spot compression view. (d) Ultrasound: left breast.

(c)

(d)

Finding

Circumscribed fat-containing mass.

Background

This screening digital mammogram on a 42-year-old female shows a large, well-circumscribed mass on the left (Figure 13.25b, arrow). The mass persists on spot compression view, with a central lucency (Figure 13.25c, arrows). On ultrasound, there is a mixed echotexture to the mass (Figure 13.25d).

Pathology

Presumed hamartoma (adenofibrolipoma).

Teaching points

Most large benign lesions are equally well displayed in both film-screen and digital mammography, although the well-circumscribed margins are more clearly delineated on digital images.

This particular case does demonstrate the danger of performing an ultrasound on a fat-containing circumscribed mass such as a hamartoma. The ultrasound shows a potentially confusing mixed echogenic pattern, with hyperechoic appearance to the fatty elements. The mammographic features alone are pathognomonic of virtually all well-circumscribed fat-containing masses, obviating the need for ultrasound altogether.

Case 26: Calcified residual capsule from removed implant
BI-RADS assessment: category 2

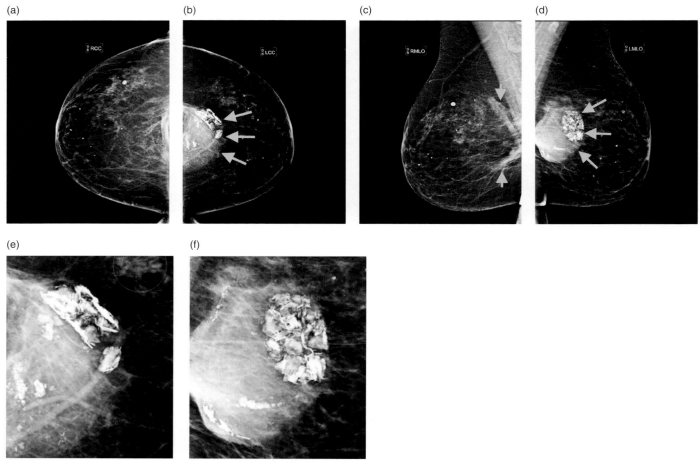

(a) (b) (c) (d)

(e) (f)

Figure 13.26 (a) Right CC view. (b) Left CC view. (c) Right MLO view. (d) Left MLO view. (e) Zoomed left CC view. (f) Zoomed left MLO view.

Finding
Circumscribed mass with calcifications

Background
A 45-year-old female presents for a screening mammogram, which shows some architectural distortion posteriorly on the right on the MLO view (Figure 13.26c, two arrows). On the left, there is a large circumscribed mass with sheet-like calcifications peripherally on both the CC and MLO views (Figures 13.26b, 13.26d, three arrows), better seen with zooming (Figures 13.26e, 13.26f). Pertinent history is recent explantation of silicone implants.

Pathology
None required here.

Teaching points
When implants are removed, there is often a potential space remaining, which in turn fills with fluid, much like the seroma that forms in a lumpectomy cavity. This creates a "pseudo-mass," which can be confusing, especially without appropriate history. In this case, there is extensive dystrophic calcification of the fibrous capsule, which apparently was not removed with the implant on the left, outlining the "seroma" that filled the implant cavity. The appearance of the sheet-like calcification is virtually pathognomonic for this entity. Thus, the diagnosis of a benign mass is made easily in this situation. The architectural distortion on the right is also a finding often associated with implant explantation.

Case 27: Benign stable linear calcifications
BI-RADS assessment: category 2

(a)

(b)

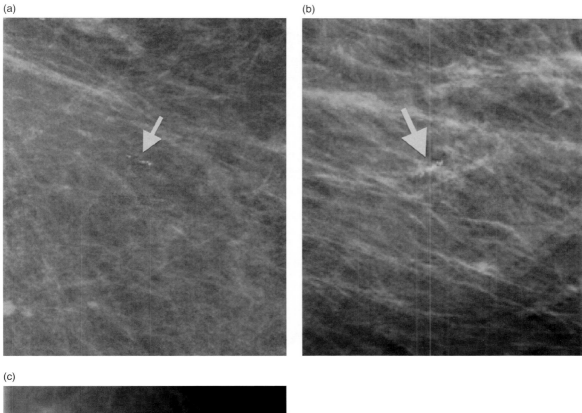

(c)

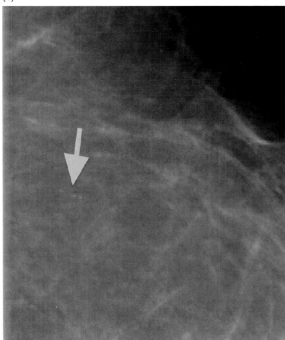

Figure 13.27 (a) Left CC view, current digital study: spot magnification. (b) Left MLO view, current digital study: spot magnification. (c) CC view of calcifications on left: previous film-screen image, magnified at photography.

Finding

Linear calcifications, seen better on digital than on film-screen mammography.

Background

A 52-year-old female presents for first digital mammogram. She had previously undergone film-screen mammogram three years earlier, available for comparison. A tiny cluster of somewhat worrisome linearly oriented calcifications was seen on the left, best seen on spot magnification views (Figures 13.27a, 13.27b). However, a careful search of the previous film-screen images from three years earlier (Figure 13.27c) led to the discovery of these same calcifications, faintly seen but unchanged in the current digital images (Figures 13.27d) and therefore felt to be benign.

Pathology

Benign process (presumed).

Teaching points

Due to better contrast and edge enhancement on digital images, subtle calcifications which were present but not appreciated on previous film-screen images become readily apparent on subsequent digital studies. These are often then labeled as "new," sometimes leading to unnecessary biopsies. Therefore, it is imperative that a very careful search of the previous film images be performed in an effort to find the calcifications for comparison to the digital images. It is often useful to digitize the film images with a high-resolution digitizer. Once digitized, these images can then be manipulated to change the contrast and brightness, just like the true digitally acquired images, allowing for better visualization of tiny calcifications. One can also apply edge enhancement, further enhancing one's ability to see any subtle calcifications on the digitized previous film images.

Case 28: Massive skin calcifications
BI-RADS assessment: category 2

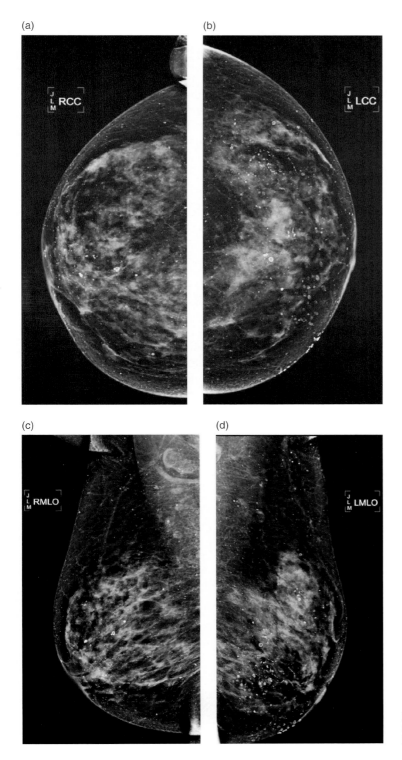

(a)

(b)

(c)

(d)

Figure 13.28 (a) Right CC view. (b) Left CC view. (c) Right MLO view. (d) Left MLO view. (e) Zoomed left CC view. (f) Zoomed left MLO view.

(e) (f)

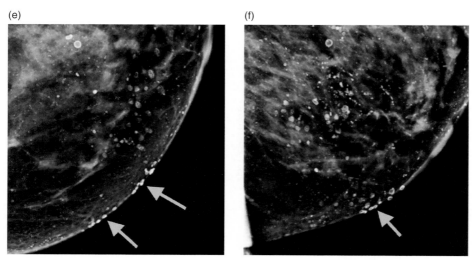

Figure 13.28 (*cont.*)

Finding

Multiple bilateral skin calcifications.

Background

A 48-year-old woman undergoing screening mammography, which shows multiple bilateral calcifications (Figures 13.28a–13.28d). Zoomed views show most of the calcifications to have benign morphologic features, with many of these contained within the skin (Figures 13.28e, 13.28f, arrows).

Pathology

Benign skin calcifications (presumed).

Teaching points

Skin calcifications are extremely well seen in digital format. In film-screen technology, such calcifications are often completely "burned out" and therefore not visible when in tangent at the skin surface. In this case, although myriads of skin calcifications are seen bilaterally, no further evaluation is needed, as the easily visualized skin line shows many of these calcifications to be in the skin itself, a finding which is pathognomonic of benignity. Most of the calcifications that do not project in the skin on these images have smooth, oval borders and lucent centers, an appearance that is also typical of skin calcifications.

Case 29: Invasive ductal carcinoma presenting as palpable lump on the left, with DCIS found on additional workup on the right

BI-RADS assessment: category 4B

(a)

(b)

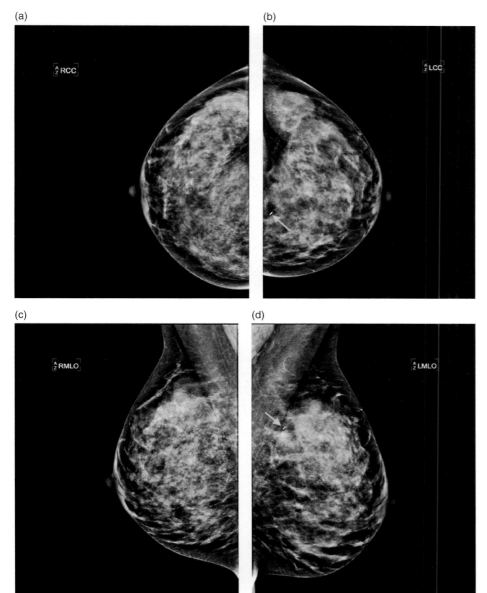

(c)

(d)

Figure 13.29 (a) Right CC view. (b) Left CC view. (c) Right MLO view. (d) Left MLO view. (e) Left ultrasound over palpable lump. (f) Spot magnification view of calcifications on right: CC view. (g) Spot magnification view of calcifications on right: LM view. (h) Ultrasound of right breast, in area of calcifications. (i) Bilateral MRI: axial MIP image. (j) Right MRI: sagittal MIP image. (k) Left MRI: sagittal MIP image.

Finding

Palpable lump due to invasive ductal carcinoma on left, with additional workup of incidental calcification on right showing DCIS.

Background

Patient presented with a palpable mass on the left at 11 o'clock, at the site of a clip placed during previous benign biopsy (Figures 13.29b, 13.29d, arrow). Mammography showed no definite mass,

but ultrasound disclosed a small irregular hypoechoic mass here (Figure 13.29e). Ultrasound biopsy yielded invasive ductal carcinoma. However, note was then made of several clusters of subtle powdery calcifications in the opposite (right) breast (Figures 13.29f, 13.29g, arrows), most of which appeared suspicious and new since a previous study five years earlier, performed with film-screen technique. A vague mass was seen in the same area on the right on ultrasound (Figure 13.29h). Biopsy on the

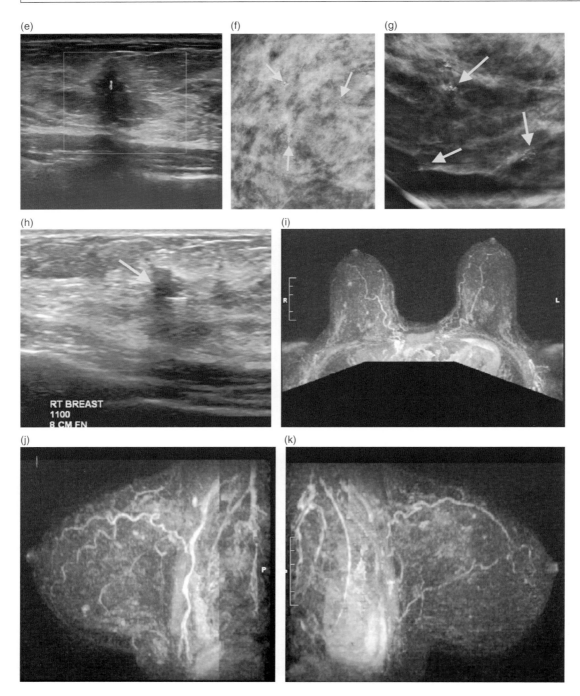

Figure 13.29 *(cont.)*

right with ultrasound showed intermediate grade DCIS. Pre-operative MRI interestingly showed almost no findings on either side (Figures 13.29i–13.29k).

Pathology

Left: Intermediate-grade invasive ductal carcinoma. Right: Intermediate-grade DCIS.

Teaching points

Careful evaluation with digital mammography and ultrasound of both breasts, once a cancer is found on either side, is a valuable part of the preoperative workup with digital as with film-screen mammography. In this case, the cancer on the right would not have been detected, even on the preoperative MRI, if a careful mammographic evaluation of the subtle calcifications on the right had not been undertaken.

Case 30: High-grade DCIS, not initially found in mastectomy specimen
BI-RADS assessment: category 4C

(a)

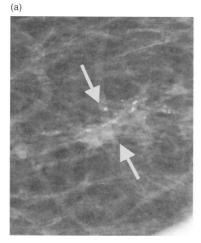

(b)

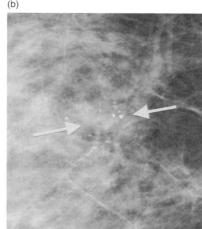

(c)

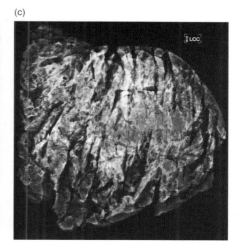

(d)

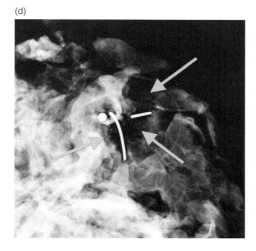

Figure 13.30 (a) Spot magnification: right CC view. (b) Spot magnification: right ML view. (c) Specimen radiograph: left mastectomy specimen. (d) Specimen radiograph, left mastectomy specimen: spot magnification view, with two pins and a localizing wire placed through the known malignant calcifications by the radiologist.

Finding

Malignant calcifications in mastectomy specimen (missed by the pathologist).

Background

A 50-year-old woman underwent screening mammography, showing a focus of calcifications on the right. Spot magnification views showed suspicious linear and branching features (Figures 13.30a, 13.30b, arrows). Stereotactic biopsy yielded high-grade DCIS. The clip placed at the time of stereotactic biopsy was found to have migrated approximately 5 cm from the biopsy site. The patient opted for mastectomy, but the pathologist was unable to find any cancer in the mastectomy specimen. The radiologist evaluated the mastectomy specimen with a digital specimen radiograph (Figure 13.30c), and was able to find the tiny focus of residual malignant calcifications (indicated by arrows) in the specimen (Figure 13.30d), assuring that the cancer had indeed been removed. Once the radiologist pointed out the

location, the pathologist was able to confirm the cancer and also confirm that it had been removed with clean margins.

Pathology

High-grade DCIS, with good margins eventually found on mastectomy specimen.

Teaching points

The radiologist can find digital mammography very useful when the pathologist cannot find any malignant calcifications on needle biopsy specimens or mastectomy specimens which contain calcifications. The ability of digital mammography to display even the tiniest calcifications can prove valuable in leading the pathologist to the correct area of tissue to be examined microscopically, especially in a large mastectomy specimen such as this, where the location of the clip placed at the time of stereotactic biopsy was of no value in identifying the area of concern.

Case 31: Widespread DCIS, missed on film-screen study three years earlier
BI-RADS assessment: category 4C

(a)

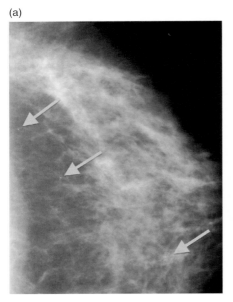

(b)

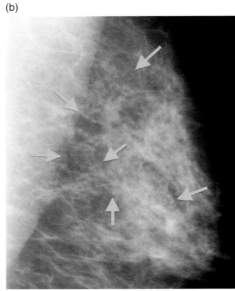

(c)

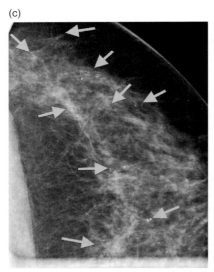

(d)

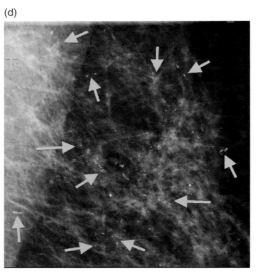

Figure 13.31 (a) Left CC view, lateral half: film-screen image, 2006. (b) Left MLO view, upper half: film-screen image, 2006. (c) Left CC view, spot magnification: digital image, 2009. (d) Left ML view, spot magnification: digital image, 2009. (e) Left ultrasound-guided vacuum biopsy: pre-biopsy image, 2009. (f) Left ultrasound-guided vacuum biopsy: specimen radiograph, 2009. (g) Bilateral MRI: axial MIP image.

Finding

Malignant-appearing calcifications.

Background

A 49-year-old patient had her first film-screen mammogram in 2002, interpreted as normal. The patient did not return for follow-up screening mammogram until 2006. The film images obtained at that time were also interpreted as normal. On closer retrospective evaluation, there were several calcifications in the upper outer quadrant of the left breast in 2006 (Figures 13.31a, 13.31b, arrows),

new since the 2002 study. They were missed in part because of poor visualization in these dense breasts with film technique. This patient did not return again for mammographic screening until 2009. Digital images showed widespread clearly malignant-appearing calcifications with linear and branching forms in the left upper outer quadrant, better seen on spot magnification views (Figures 13.31c, 13.31d, arrows), in the same area as the new calcifications overlooked on 2006 film images. On ultrasound, a vague mass was seen in the region (Figure 13.31e, arrow), and ultrasound-guided vacuum-assisted core biopsy of these yielded

(e)

(f)

Figure 13.31 (*cont.*)

(g)

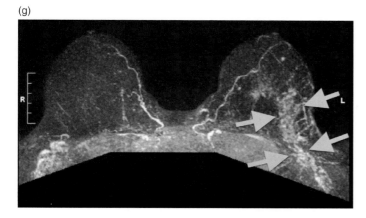

calcifications in the specimens (Figure 13.31f, arrows), and high-grade DCIS on pathology. Preoperative MRI shows non-mass-like enhancement in the same region over a 6 × 8cm area (Figure 13.31g, arrows), all found to be DCIS at surgery.

Pathology

Widespread high-grade DCIS.

Teaching points

The first calcifications seen with some forms of high-grade DCIS are often difficult to discern at screening. Certainly, the improved visualization of small calcifications with digital mammography, especially in dense breasts, provides a great benefit as compared to film-screen technique.

Case 32: High-grade DCIS
BI-RADS assessment: category 4C

(a)

(b)

(c)

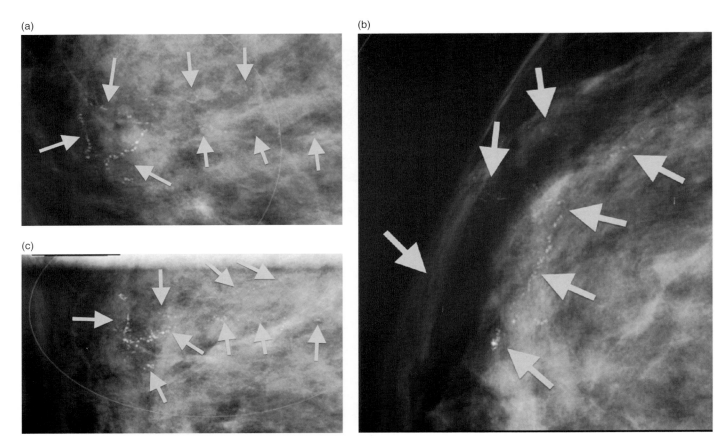

Figure 13.32 (a) Right MLO zoomed view. (b) Right CC view: spot magnification. (c) Right ML view: spot magnification.

Finding
"Snake skin" calcifications of high-grade DCIS.

Background
Screening mammogram in a 38-year-old showed an area of suspicious calcifications buried in dense tissue in the retro-areolar region of the right breast (Figure 13.32a, arrows). Spot magnification views showed the linear branching "snake

skin" appearance of these, so typical of high-grade DCIS (Figures 13.32b, 13.32c, arrows).

Pathology
High-grade DCIS.

Teaching points
Classic high-grade DCIS shows up nicely on digital images, even in very dense breast tissue, as was the case here.

Case 33: Calcified fibroadenomas
BI-RADS assessment: category 2

(a)

(b)

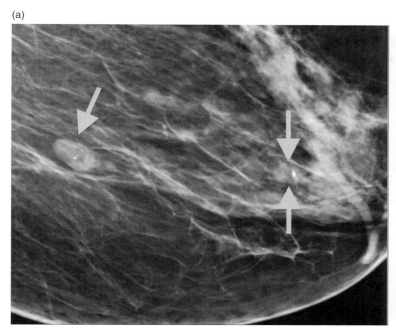
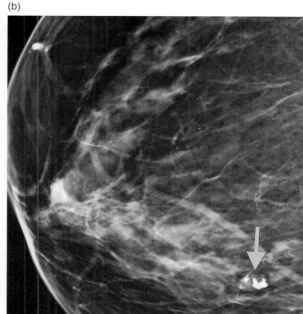

Figure 13.33 (a) Left MLO zoomed view. (b) Right CC zoomed view.

Finding
Benign calcified fibroadenomas.

Background
A 64-year-old woman underwent screening mammography, showing two calcified nodules on the left and one calcified nodule on the right. The more posterior nodule on the left (Figure 13.33a, one arrow) and the nodule on the right (Figure 13.33b, arrow) were well circumscribed, whereas the more anterior nodule on the left (Figure 13.33a, two arrows) had partially obscured margins. All three contained calcifications indicating these to be benign fibroadenomas.

Pathology
Benign fibroadenomas (presumed).

Teaching points
This patient demonstrates the various stages of calcification which benign fibroadenomas often undergo. In the left breast are two fibroadenomas with tiny, soft calcifications seen when they first begin to calcify (Figure 13.33a). In the right breast is a fibroadenoma, which shows dense, irregular, larger calcifications, often called "staghorn" or "popcorn" calcifications, for obvious reasons (Figure 13.33b). The calcifications indicate a more extensive and mature degenerative process within these lesions. More importantly, they are pathognomonic for the benign nature of these lesions, obviating the need for further evaluation or biopsy.

Case 34: Bloom artifact around calcifications
BI-RADS assessment: NA – technical issue

(a)

(b)

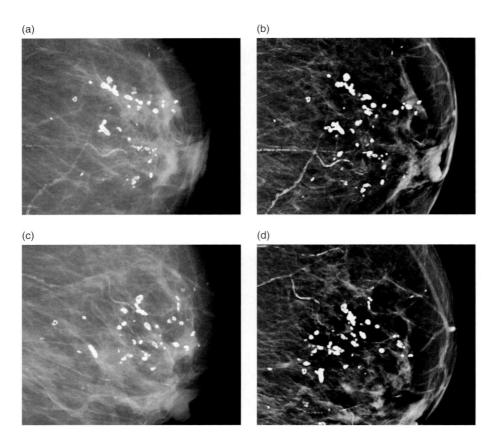

Figure 13.34 (a) Left CC view: previous film-screen image. (b) Left CC view: current digital image. (c) Left MLO view: previous film-screen image. (d) Left MLO view: current digital image.

(c)

(d)

Finding
Bloom artifact around dense benign calcifications.

Background
71-year-old woman with screening mammograms over two years, the first a film-screen exam, and the second a digital exam (Figures 13.34a–13.34d). There are very dense dystrophic calcifications seen in the retroareolar area of the left breast, with very little change in their appearance between the previous film images and the current digital ones. The morphology of the calcifications is clearly benign, consistent with old trauma and/or plasma cell mastitis. However, there is a black halo around many of the most dense calcifications on the digital study, with a resultant loss of information.

Pathology
Old trauma and/or plasma cell mastitis (presumed).

Teaching points
Sometimes the edge enhancement seen with digital mammography can work as a disadvantage. In this case, the dense dystrophic calcifications are nicely demonstrated on both the previous film-screen images and the current digital ones. However, note the large black areas around many of the calcifications on the digital images. These are created by a huge bloom artifact of edge enhancement, thereby masking any real lesions seen in the area of "bloom." Thus, subtle soft lesions in this "dead zone" can be missed. This artifact is especially troublesome on specimen radiographs, with the artifact hiding potentially important calcifications in the zone of bloom artifact around the localizing wire.

Comparison of commercially available systems

Karla A. Sepulveda, Lindsay Hwang, and William R. Geiser

Digital mammography units

See table 14.1.

Computer-aided detection (CADe)

See table 14.2.

Breast tomosynthesis

At the time of writing, Hologic has gained US Food and Drug Administration (FDA) approval in the United States for a breast tomosynthesis platform, the Selenia Dimensions machine, which can perform both ordinary two-dimensional digital mammography and tomosynthesis.

Suggested parameters for digital breast tomosynthesis include [1–3]:

- 4–15-second scan over a range of 15–60 degrees

- detector and acquisition geometry to maximize the field of view
- rapid reconstruction of thin slices separated by 1 mm
- total radiation dose similar to or less than conventional mammography
- high detective quantum efficiency (DQE) detector to minimize noise
- large-field-of-view detector to accommodate all breast sizes
- breast compression no greater than conventional mammography

Breast computed tomography

At the time of writing, there are no commercially available breast computed tomography units in the United States. Breast computed tomography is considered to be in the experimental phase.

References

1. Machida H, Yukara T, Mori T, *et al.* Optimizing parameters for flat-panel detector digital tomosynthesis. *Radiographics* 2010; **30**: 549–62.

2. Helvie MA. Digital mammography imaging: breast tomosynthesis and advanced applications. *Radiol Clin North Am* 2010; **48**: 917–29.

3. Diekmann F, Bick U. Breast tomosynthesis. *Semin Ultrasound CT MRI* 2011; **32**: 281–7.

Digital Mammography: A Practical Approach, ed. Gary J. Whitman and Tamara Miner Haygood. Published by Cambridge University Press. © Cambridge University Press 2013.

Table 14.1 Digital mammography units.

	Hologic Selenia	Hologic Selenia Dimensions 2D/3D	GE Senographe DS	GE Senographe Essential	Siemens Novation 2D	Siemens Inspiration 2D/3D	Philips Sectra MicroDose L30	Planmed Nuance	Planmed Nuance Excel	Fuji Aspire	Giotto Image 3D
Conversion method	Direct	Direct	Indirect	Indirect	Direct	Direct		Direct	Direct	Direct	Direct
Conversion material	a-Se	a-Se	Cesium iodide	Cesium iodide	a-Se	a-Se	Chrystalline Si	a-Se	a-Se	a-Se	a-Se
Detector temperature control	Integrated	Integrated	Separate component	Separate component	Integrated	Integrated	Integrated	Integrated	Integrated	Integrated	Integrated
DEL resolution	70 μm	70 μm	100 μm	100 μm	85 μm	85 μm	50 μm	85 μm	85 μm	50 μm	85 μm
X-ray tube anode	Molybdenum or tungsten	Tungsten	Molybdenum/rhodium	Molybdenum/rhodium	Tungsten	Tungsten	Tungsten	Tungsten	Tungsten	Tungsten	Tungsten
Filtration	Molybdenum/rhodium	Rhodium/silver	Molybdenum/rhodium	Molybdenum/rhodium	Molybdenum/rhodium	Molybdenum/rhodium	Beryllium	Rhodium/silver	Rhodium/silver	Rhodium	Rhodium
Grid type	HTC	HTC	Reciprocating linear	Reciprocating linear	Reciprocating linear	Reciprocating linear	None	Reciprocating linear	Reciprocating linear	Reciprocating linear	Reciprocating linear
Grid retraction	Automatic	Automatic	Motorized with manual removal	Motorized with manual removal	Automatic	Automatic	N/A	Automatic	Automatic	Automatic	Automatic
Magnification factor	1.8x	1.5x, 1.8x	1.5x, 1.8x	1.5x, 1.8x	1.5x	1.5x	2.0x	1.6x, 1.8x, 2.0x	1.6x, 1.8x	1.8x	1.5x, 1.8x
Field of view	24 x 29 cm	24 x 29 cm	19 x 23 cm	24 x 31 cm	24 x 30 cm	24 x 30 cm	24 x 26 cm	17 x 24 cm	24 x 31 cm	24 x 30 cm	24 x 30 cm
Average glandular dose	1.2 mGy	1.2 mGy	1.3 mGy	1.3 mGy	1.2 mGy	1.2 mGy	0.8–1.0 mGy	0.8–0.9 mGy	0.8–0.9 mGy	1.27 mGy	0.8 mGy
MTF@ 2 lp/mm	≥90%	≥90%	≤60%	≤60%	≤85%	≥85%	85%	>80%	>80%	71.5%	≥90%
MTF@ 4 lp/mm	70%	70%	≤25%	≤25%	≤65%	≤65%	58%	>60%	>60%	51.6%	63%
FDA approved	Yes	Yes	Yes	Yes	Yes	Yes	Yes	Yes	Yes	Yes	Yes
Tomosynthesis ready?	No	Yes	No	Yes	No	Yes	No	No	No	No	Yes
Tomosynthesis FDA approved	No	Yes	No	No	No	No	No	No	No	No	No

a-Se, amorphous selenium; Si, silica; DEL, detector element; μm, micron; mA, milliampere; HTC, High Transmission Cellular; N/A, not applicable; cm, centimeter; mGy, milliGray; MTF, modulation transfer function; lp, line pairs; FDA, US Food and Drug Administration.

Table 14.2 CADe Systems.

	Hologic (R2 Cenova)	iCAD (Second Look)
Platform	Intel server Windows XP	Intel server Windows XP
Additional software application	Yes Volumetric assessment (R2 Quantra) Digitized film image processing (R2 DigitalNow HD)	No
Remote access	Hologic Connect	Via VPN
Centroid marking	Yes	No
Anatomic marking	Anatomic outline	Region outline
Calcification	Individual outlines	Rectangle
Mass	Central density outline	Ellipse
Architectural distortion	Yes	Ellipse
Mass + calcifications	Yes	No
Variable-sized marks (based on prominence of features)	Yes (EmphaSize)	No
Ancillary data (lesion distances, size, CADe feature information)	Yes	No
Operating points	9 (3 calcifications × 3 masses)	3 (combined)
Sensitivity	Calcifications (95–97%) Mass (83–90%) Overall (88–93%)	Overall (90–96%)
Case throughput (4-view study)	30–60/hour	30/hour
PACS workstation compatability	All	Some

PACS, picture archiving and communication system; VPN, virtual private network.

Index